Praise for
SUPER GUT

"*Super Gut* reveals how virtually every aspect of our health is fundamentally influenced by the vast array of microscopic organisms living upon and within us. Dr. Davis makes it clear that so many issues related to living in our modern world challenge this relationship and set the stage for illness. But the good news, as *Super Gut* so eloquently portrays, centers on our newfound ability to improve the health and functionality of the vast array of microbes upon which we depend. It's clear that we can manipulate this relationship to our advantage. And Dr. Davis shows us how."
—David Perlmutter, MD, author of #1 *New York Times* bestseller *Grain Brain* and *Drop Acid*

"Reading *Super Gut* is reading an incredibly important manual on building the super 'hard drive' for a long, healthy, and productive life....With easy-to-implement, inexpensive recommendations, it won't be long before you're forever grateful you took the time to read and implement....All disease begins in the gut. So build a Super Gut!"
—Dr. Tom O'Bryan, author of *The Autoimmune Fix* and *You Can Fix Your Brain*

"*Super Gut* brings the conversation into new territory. Bacteria are not the bad guys! Dr. Davis's plan helps you replenish the microbiome and eliminate those culprits that are depleting us of essential natural probiotics that maintain a healthy gut. Microbiome medicine is an essential part of good health, disease prevention, vitality, and longevity. Bravo to Dr. Davis on this newest addition to the literature."
—Dr. Raphael Kellman, founder of Microbiome Medicine, author of *The Microbiome Diet*, *The Microbiome Breakthrough*, and *Microbiome Thyroid*

"An intriguing look into the science of the gut microbiome, and its implications for human health. Dr. Davis brings his usual light to this area of science and follows that up with some practical advice."

—Dr. Jason Fung, *New York Times*
bestselling author of *The Obesity Code*

"Unlike other books on the microbiome, Dr. Davis has taken the conversation several steps further by showing how lost microbes can be restored and how an epidemic of overgrowth of undesirable species can be pushed back with often spectacular results. He packs the book with specific strategies and recipes so that the reader is well equipped to regain health, vigor, even youthfulness."

—Mark Hyman, MD, *New York Times*
bestselling author of *The Pegan Diet*

SUPER
GUT

Also by William Davis, MD

Wheat Belly: Lose the Wheat, Lose the Weight,
and Find Your Way Back to Health

Wheat Belly 10-Day Grain Detox: Reprogram
Your Body for Rapid Weight Loss and Amazing Health

Wheat Belly Slim Guide: The Fast and Easy Reference
for Living and Succeeding on the Wheat Belly Lifestyle

Undoctored: Why Health Care Has Failed You and
How You Can Become Smarter Than Your Doctor

Wheat Belly Total Health: The Ultimate Grain-Free
Health Guide and Weight-Loss Life Plan

Wheat Belly 10-Day Detox

Wheat Belly 30 Minutes (or Less!) Cookbook

Wheat Belly Journal: Track Your Path Back to Health

Wheat Belly Cookbook

Lose the Wheat, Lose the Weight! Cookbook

SUPER GUT

A Four-Week Plan to Reprogram Your Microbiome,
Restore Health, and Lose Weight

WILLIAM DAVIS, MD

hachette
BOOKS
NEW YORK

Copyright © 2022 by William Davis, MD

Cover design by Sara Wood
Cover copyright © 2022 by Hachette Book Group, Inc.

Hachette Go, an imprint of Hachette Books
Hachette Book Group
1290 Avenue of the Americas
New York, NY 10104
HachetteGo.com
Facebook.com/HachetteGo
Instagram.com/HachetteGo

First Trade Paperback Edition: February 2023
Hachette Books is a division of Hachette Book Group, Inc.

The Hachette Go and Hachette Books name and logos are trademarks of Hachette Book Group, Inc.

The publisher is not responsible for websites (or their content) that are not owned by the publisher.

Print book interior design by Linda Mark.

Library of Congress Cataloging-in-Publication Data
Names: Davis, William, 1957– author.
Title: Super gut : a four-week plan to reprogram your microbiome, restore health, and lose weight / William Davis, MD.
Description: First edition. | New York : Hachette Go, 2022. | Includes bibliographical references and index.
Identifiers: LCCN 2021035884 | ISBN 9780306846977 (hardcover) | ISBN 9780306846953 (ebook)
Subjects: LCSH: Gastrointestinal system—Microbiology. | Health.
Classification: LCC QR171.G29 D38 2022 | DDC 612.3/2—dc23
LC record available at https://lccn.loc.gov/2021035884

ISBNs: 978-0-306-84696-0 (paperback), 978-0-306-84697-7 (hardcover), 978-0-306-84695-3 (ebook)

Printed in the United States of America

LSC-C

Printing 1, 2022

Dedicated to the memory of Professor Ilya Ilyich (Élie) Mechnikov, biologist and keen observer, who, more than a century ago, was the first to recognize the power of the microbiome in health and aging, and who also was a lover of yogurt

CONTENTS

INTRODUCTION   ix

PART I
BOWEL BLUES

  1 GUT-WRENCHING   3

  2 A MICROBIOME ONLY A MOTHER COULD LOVE   13

  3 GHOSTS OF MICROBES PAST   21

  4 THE FECALIZATION OF AMERICA   35

  5 MIND YOUR MUCUS   47

PART II
FRANKENBELLY AND FRIENDS

  6 SIBO: FRANKENBELLY   61

  7 SIFO: FUNGAL JUNGLE   93

  8 CONQUERING YOUR FRANKENBELLY:
      MANAGING SIBO AND SIFO   109

PART III
GUT REACTION

  9 TAKE A WALK ON THE WILD SIDE   135

 10 BOWEL POWER   159

PART IV
BUILD YOUR OWN SUPER GUT: A FOUR-WEEK PROGRAM

WEEK 1: PREPARE THE SOIL 175

WEEK 2: RESEED YOUR GARDEN 195

WEEK 3: ADD WATER AND FERTILIZER 205

WEEK 4: GROW YOUR SUPER GUT
MICROBE GARDEN 215

SUPER GUT RECIPES 227

SUPER GUT SAMPLE THREE-DAY MENU PLAN
AND SHOPPING LISTS 275

AFTERWORD: SWEAT THE SMALL STUFF 281

ACKNOWLEDGMENTS 287

APPENDIX A: RESOURCES 291

*APPENDIX B: ERADICATING YOUR FRANKENBELLY:
SUPER GUT SIBO AND SIFO PROTOCOLS* 307

APPENDIX C: ERADICATING H. PYLORI 313

REFERENCES 317

INDEX 339

INTRODUCTION

> DR. FRANKENSTEIN: "You know, I don't mean to embarrass you, but I'm a rather brilliant surgeon. Perhaps I can help you with that hump."
>
> IGOR: "What hump?"
>
> *Young Frankenstein*, 1974

IN MARY SHELLEY'S TALE OF *FRANKENSTEIN*, THROUGH BUMBLING experiments and a crude stitching together of body parts electrified to life, Dr. Victor Frankenstein creates a monster, unnatural and not entirely human, a creature terrible to behold who escapes to terrorize the countryside.

Nobody here is stitching loose heads and arms to torsos or passing 220 volts through organs to bring them back to life. Instead, a peculiar alchemy of human health has been occurring these last fifty years or so, creating modern health horrors all during a time—most of us have believed—of unprecedented medical advancement. So it's all the more surprising that a universe of primitive creatures dwelling directly below our diaphragm, behind our belly button, but beneath our conscious awareness—and that of our doctors—is only now coming to light as a hugely important phenomenon in human health.

Eleven years ago, in the first of my series of Wheat Belly books, I described how agricultural scientists and farmers had changed this plant called "wheat," transforming a traditional five-foot-tall plant into an eighteen-inch-tall, thick-stalked, large-seeded crop, a change that required thousands of genetic experiments. The final genetically altered result did indeed produce a high-yield crop, enabling farmers to harvest several-fold more bushels per acre than of traditional strains, a boom in yield that helped feed the hungry in starvation-plagued underdeveloped countries. But this new crop also inflicted a collection of unexpected effects on the humans who consumed it, effects ranging from appetite stimulation to temporal lobe seizures, seborrhea to a 400 percent increase in celiac disease. Formerly rare type 1 and type 2 diabetes became mainstream conditions, and humans who used to eat to live were transformed into a population with insatiable all-you-can-eat appetites. The health consequences of consuming modern wheat are so destructive, so unnatural, that I labeled it "Frankengrain."

I found that removing Frankengrains from the diet yielded substantial, often life-changing, health benefits. Thousands of people experienced effortless weight loss and transformations in their health, restoring them to 1950s-like flat tummies and freeing them of numerous modern health conditions. And yet, a substantial proportion also reported something like this: "I lost forty-seven pounds without even trying, and I'm no longer hungry all the time. I am no longer prediabetic and I'm off two blood pressure pills. My rheumatoid arthritis is about 70 percent better and I was able to stop the several-thousand-dollar-per-month injectable drug. But I still have some flare-ups and had to resume the steroids and naproxen." In other words, removing Frankengrains from the diet and adding in the handful of nutritional supplements I recommended, which reversed health phenomena such as insulin resistance, did not fully address all of people's health issues. Some people reported losing, say, seventy pounds, with only another thirty pounds to go—but their weight loss stalled despite doing everything right. The Wheat Belly lifestyle includes basic efforts to recultivate healthy microbial species dwelling in the gastrointestinal tract, that is, the intestinal microbiome, but something was still missing.

The Wheat Belly community, large, international, and enthusiastically engaged, was also (and remains) a *collaborative* community, all of us sharing experiences and looking for better answers on how to achieve 100 percent success and finally conquer residual health issues. This community, in effect, is an enormous crowdsourcing of wisdom, with hundreds of thousands of people all seeking answers to similar questions. (Don't worry: if you are unfamiliar with the strategies of the Wheat Belly lifestyle, which, despite its shortfalls, is still quite powerful, I articulate its tenets later in the book in addition to introducing new and powerful strategies you can use to build a Super Gut.)

Over the last few decades, outside the Wheat Belly experience, an explosion of research made it clear that common mental and emotional struggles such as depression, social isolation, hatred, anxiety, and attention deficit hyperactivity disorder (ADHD) could be blamed on disruptions to the intestinal microbiome. It also became clear that health conditions as unrelated as obesity, autoimmune conditions, and neurodegenerative diseases likewise could be blamed on changes inflicted on the microbes dwelling beneath our diaphragms. Because I am personally interested in both improving human health and performance and decreasing people's reliance on the health-care system, I wondered whether such microbiome disruptions could explain the persistence of health issues in the individuals who were following my programs. It was this chain of logic that sent me searching for evidence of lost microbes, bacterial species that might have vanished from the modern human microbiome. And, indeed, I did find several candidates that, when restored to the human gut, yielded impressive improvements in people's health, and even in their appearance.

But I also found that the disappearance of several key microbes could not explain all persistent health problems. Hints of a more comprehensive answer kept trickling in from the worldwide Wheat Belly community as some people continued to complain about their sleep struggles, persistent joint pain even after partial relief with wheat and grain elimination, and stubborn food intolerances from before the Wheat Belly program that would not resolve. Why would so many people have intolerances to everyday foods such as tomatoes, kidney beans, and peanuts? Digging into the idea that disrupted microbiomes could also account for these health phenomena made it clearer and clearer that I'd find the answers in the microbial universe. Then additional developments, such as the availability of a smartphone-enabled consumer device that can detect microbial gas production in the breath, clinched it: the answers would come from the microbiome.

I wanted to discover ways to put the power of a healthy microbiome to work beyond the usual "take a probiotic and get plenty of fiber." I wanted to address not just people's residual health problems but also ways they could supercharge their health to reach new heights of day-to-day functioning.

I am certain beyond any doubt that modern lifestyles have disrupted the composition of microbes in the human gastrointestinal (GI) tract, and these microbial imbalances are to blame for the residual health issues the Wheat Belly community and others were encountering. Modern lifestyle factors that disturb our inner ecosystem are also responsible for a long list of other health problems—no body system is immune to the effects of this monster we have created called the modern human microbiome. The microbiome of our hunter-gatherer ancestors and that of our predecessors just fifty years ago were very different from the one we have today. A combination of factors associated with modern life—from modern processed foods to stomach acid–blocking drugs—has created a gut that is almost no longer human; it's something I call a "Frankenbelly," and it's as destructive to our health or perhaps more so than Frankengrain. Real health horrors result from a Frankenbelly: from irritable bowel syndrome and constipation to ulcerative colitis and Crohn's disease, from polycystic ovary syndrome and colon cancer to depression and despair, from social isolation to thoughts of suicide. These are all effects of this thing we, as a society and as individuals, have created: a Frankenbelly of disruptions in the microbiome.

Now we have to figure out how to kill off this thing and resurrect something closer to the natural human condition. Unfortunately, the medical community is poorly equipped to handle the ailments resulting from a disturbed microbiome, never mind understand their source. Rather than address the proliferation of unhealthy bacterial and fungal species responsible for generating dark emotions, anxiety, and suicidal impulses, doctors prescribe antidepressant and antianxiety medications to block their effects. Rather than chart the location of errant microbes that underlies conditions like hypertension and atrial fibrillation, they prescribe medications that push blood pressure down and suppress abnormal heart rhythms. Rather than decipher the microbial disruptions that cause weight gain and type 2 diabetes, they resort to gastric bypass and medications that forcibly regulate blood sugar. All these conventional but misguided efforts also come, of course, with a considerable price tag and long lists of side effects. I'm sure you can appreciate the fact that coming to an understanding of all the microbial havoc that's been inflicted on modern humans will turn our entire idea of health and disease topsy-turvy. Solutions will be different too—we will certainly need tools beyond those you can obtain through your doctor's prescription pad.

We need to rebuild the very microbial core of our health to achieve freedom from disease and to regain youthfulness and overall quality of life. And you know what? The sorts of benefits we can reap from restoring the healthy human microbiome will go farther than just relief from, say, being overweight or having acid reflux. The strategies that I shall share with you can also yield smoother skin, accelerated healing, and increased feelings of empathy for other people—benefits that you likely had no idea originated with the microbial universe within. First, we must reestablish order in this monstrous microbial mess we have created, then I will show you how to cultivate a Super Gut.

QUIT YOUR BELLYACHING

If you could ask an organism like *Escherichia coli* (*E. coli*), "What is the purpose of human life?" *E. coli* would answer, of course, "Your purpose is to support me and my fellow microbes." You may see a higher purpose to life, but from the vantage point inside your colon or duodenum, you are little more than a microbe factory.

All living creatures on this planet have a unique and individual microbiome: spiders and mosquitos, squirrels and chipmunks, trout and turtles. Humans likewise have a microbiome unique to our species but that differs for each individual. But the practices of modern life—shopping in a grocery store and eating food served from a drive-through window rather than killing or foraging your next meal; bathing in a hot shower in place of a dip in a lake or river; taking a course of antibiotics for a sinus infection instead of toughing it out—add up to wreak cataclysmic alterations in the composition and location of the microbes we harbor in and on our bodies.

Even though the microorganisms inhabiting your GI tract don't have names or addresses and can't like your Facebook page, they play a crucial role in such diverse phenomena as your level of optimism, your skin's appearance, your energy level, your empathy for other people, and your romantic life. They even influence how fast you age and how long you live.

The trillions of bacterial and fungal creatures inhabiting your GI tract have been playing a major role in the movie that is your life. Even if you follow healthy habits and are free of modern conditions like diabetes and obesity, the creatures comprising your microbiome can still determine whether you succumb to the helplessness of Alzheimer's dementia or will be blowing out 105 candles on your birthday cake, surrounded by great-great-grandchildren, with your mental capacity and memories of last Tuesday's social gathering intact. Few things in this world play a role so critical yet remain so anonymous.

It wasn't that long ago that the microbes inhabiting the human body were thought to be important only for their role in causing infections. But the administration of antibiotics, which has wreaked havoc on people's microbial balance over the last century, reveals that a multitude of microorganisms are actually necessary for health. Bacterial species dwelling in the GI tract, for instance, produce B vitamins such as folate and vitamin B_{12}, or increase feelings of love for family and friends, or stimulate vivid, colorful dreams during the restorative rapid-eye-movement (REM) phase of sleep, which are essential components for normal mental health.

Like it or not, all of us today are under the profound influence of trillions of anonymous microscopic creatures. Who would have realized even ten years ago that this collection of microorganisms can determine whether you develop Parkinson's disease, how rapidly you heal from an injury, and whether you can tolerate the foibles and quirks of your spouse? It's unsettling to think that microscopic creatures might make the difference between writing a book that earns the Nobel Prize for Literature and gunning down people in a church. But that is the impressive power of this population of microbes we carry, a universe of life that can serve or work against us.

Thankfully, many of the health struggles that can be blamed on a disrupted microbiome can be reversed simply by shifting toward a healthier diet, addressing common nutrient deficiencies, and restoring healthier bacterial species to the GI tract after we've beaten back undesirable microbes.

But what about someone who, having accumulated all the microbial disruptions of prior years, now has a disastrous case of bacterial and fungal overgrowth that has careened out of control? All the microbe-disruptive factors of modern life enable the proliferation of unhealthy bacterial and fungal species in our bodies, most concentrated in the gastrointestinal tract, a situation labeled "dysbiosis." Dysbiosis confined to the colon, that is, the last five feet of the GI tract, poses risks for health conditions such as ulcerative colitis and colon cancer. But it is not uncommon for unhealthy bacterial species to ascend from the colon where they belong into the ileum, jejunum, duodenum (parts of the small intestine), and stomach, a situation labeled "small intestinal bacterial overgrowth," or SIBO. The disruptions of bacterial populations that cause SIBO often also enable fungal species to similarly proliferate and climb up the length of the GI tract to inhabit places they do not belong, and this condition is called "small intestinal fungal overgrowth" (SIFO). Sadly, it is the rule, rather than the exception, that doctors fail to recognize these situations but "treat" the varied diseases they cause that show on the surface. You can see how someone with unrecognized SIBO, for instance, who suffers from conditions that are not readily reversible such as diverticulitis, Hashimoto's thyroiditis, or colon cancer, can end up taking a long list of prescription drugs and even undergoing serious medical procedures such as gallbladder or weight loss surgery. However, if the SIBO or SIFO is caught early enough and reversed—and a healthy microbiome is restored—many of the accompanying chronic conditions will fade away in the face of good health in symbiosis with a balanced internal microbial universe.

The key, therefore, is to be keenly aware of dysbiosis, SIBO, and SIFO and all their signs and consequences, then take action to correct these common situations. I shall show you how to recognize the telltale signs of these conditions, how to confirm their presence, and how to deal with them. It's not all doom and gloom. I go several steps further to show you how to take your healing program to new heights so that you can look in the mirror and be proud of what you see and visit your doctor, who will be speechless at the superior level of your health, and answer all the questions coming at you from people wanting to know why and how you look so darned good: slender, firm, muscular, with thick, moist skin, adept mental capacity, libido fully intact. Understanding and reestablishing order in your microbial universe—shifting their population composition, limiting where they are allowed to reside, and reducing the flood of their toxic by-products—bring on a tsunami of positive health, weight loss, and age-reversing effects.

We are embarking on a journey that, I believe, will allow you to find answers to questions that may have stumped doctors, who usually ignore the fact that you have lost crucial microbes and acquired a host of unhealthy species in their place. While they continue to prescribe drug after drug to treat the symptoms of a disturbed microbiome, offer ineffective advice such as "move more, eat less," and blame you for moral weakness, gluttony, or bad genes, you will learn to recognize and address this microbial switch, and then you are on your way to magnificent health.

Dust off your yogurt maker, cancel the Botox appointment, and pull up a chair, as you are about to go on a bacterial journey that can change the course of your life. Let's begin by detailing exactly how and why so much has gone wrong in the human microbiome.

PART I

BOWEL BLUES

1

GUT-WRENCHING

You may, in many ways, be a lot like your parents and grandparents. Perhaps you inherited your mom's curly hair or your grandfather's aversion to cilantro. But, unlike genes, which determine traits such as hair texture and taste preferences, the microbiome you carry in your gut is not the microbiome of your ancestors, the generations of humans who preceded you. It's different even compared to your parents' and grandparents'. The collection of microbes you carry inside has almost unrecognizably changed.

As inhabitants of the twenty-first-century world, we are witness to troubling changes in the global climate: ocean acidification, shrinking coral reefs, receding polar ice caps, extreme droughts, wildfires, flooding—it's all part, of course, of Earth's changing environment under human influence.

If humans are capable of affecting oceans and polar ice caps, could we also be introducing disastrous change into the thirty-foot ecosystem of our gastrointestinal (GI) tract? Absolutely. A parallel environmental catastrophe has occurred from our mouths on down. There are no hurricanes, of course, but human efforts have dramatically altered the internal microbial environment, influencing where they take up residence and whether their toxic by-products are allowed to pollute our system. There's no need to run for higher ground, but the gastrointestinal equivalent can be every bit as catastrophic.

The modern human microbiome bears little resemblance to the microbiome of isolated pockets of people living the hunter-gatherer lifestyle in Africa and South America. These are the few remaining peoples whose way of life reflects the way humans lived for the preceding several million years, unexposed to antibiotics and other modern microbiome-disruptive factors. Indigenous people who live a traditional lifestyle harbor microbial species that we lack, while we have acquired species that traditional people do not have. Revealingly, the health of hunter-gatherers with these microbiomes includes virtually no stomach ulcers, acid reflux, hemorrhoids, constipation, irritable bowel syndrome, diverticular disease, colon cancer, or other health conditions—what anthropologists label "diseases of civilization"—that commonly afflict modern people.[1]

Over thousands of human generations, microorganisms have evolved to coexist with us, their hosts, in a relationship so close and intimate that there are bacterial species that exist *only* in the human gastrointestinal tract and no other place on Earth—not in swamps, not under rocks, not in garbage dumps, but only in the thirty feet of the human GI tract. These creatures struck a balance with human life and took up residence inside us.

But over the last several decades, this quiet coexistence has experienced a major disruption. Species have been lost—what microbiologists call "the disappearing microbiome"—old species have been replaced with new, and microbes we ordinarily associate with infection now dominate the microbiome in many people. And, in a shocking number of us, microbes have taken up residence along the entire length of the gastrointestinal tract, bottom to top, creating, in effect, a thirty-foot-long infection, hot with inflammation. You might experience this shift in residence as a persistent and annoying eczematous rash or as depression that responds poorly to every antidepressant your doctor prescribes; the root cause is living and reproducing along the length of your GI tract.

Modern conveniences have distanced us from the raw, desperate scramble that defined human life over the preceding several million years. We don't wear the skins of animals we've killed on our backs and feet but buy clothes and shoes manufactured in some faraway factory. Meat is prekilled for us; vegetables are purchased in plastic bags or are served in a salad bar, not picked off plants, trees, and bushes or dug from the ground. The distance we've created from butchering and digging has created a squeaky-clean, sanitized, and antibiotic- and industrial chemical–filled present.

Convenience, mass food commercialization, and the lack of blood and dirt under our fingernails have contributed to a silent but massive health epidemic. Many of us were delivered by C-section and fed synthetic baby formula that led to food allergies, obesity, and diverticular disease later in life. We survive a urinary tract infection or pneumonia by taking antibiotics, only to develop ulcerative colitis or compulsive behaviors months or years later. We refrigerate food to prolong its shelf life but deprive ourselves of the fertile growth of microorganisms that appear naturally in fermenting foods, and thereby set ourselves up for autoimmune thyroid disease and rosacea.

The Centers for Disease Control and Prevention (CDC) tracks conditions of the gastrointestinal tract and has reported an alarming increase in cases of ulcerative colitis over the last few years, with a 50 percent increase in cases just from 1999 to 2015.[2] Colon cancer, once a disease of the elderly, is now increasingly a disease of people in their thirties, forties, and fifties, one of the many canary-in-the-coal-mine phenomena that signal a dramatic shift in human health, likely due to changes in the microbiome.[3]

Because medical doctors are largely unaware of this epidemic health situation, they continue to treat the outward symptoms of dysbiosis with conventional remedies—pain medication, anti-inflammatory drugs, antidepressants, statin cholesterol drugs, food-avoidance strategies—or they look for late manifestations using tests like colonoscopies, but the underlying condition remains unrecognized and uncorrected. Failure to recognize and manage this dysbiotic situation not only allows conditions such as ulcerative colitis and colon cancer to run rampant but also allows many other long-term health consequences to emerge.

SHINING A LIGHT INTO THE SMALL INTESTINE

The microbiome disruptions most modern humans have experienced often are confined to the colon, the last way station before you and I wave good-bye to the indigestible remnants of food and microbes that we flush away. But, in a good number of people, the problem has gotten much worse. When unhealthy bacterial species dominate in the colon, they then head northward to colonize the small intestine and end up occupying some or all twenty-four feet of the small intestine, from the ileum up through the jejunum and duodenum, plus the stomach. When the entire length of small bowel is involved, there can be thirty feet of GI tract occupied by unfriendly microbes. As you can imagine, this much larger infestation holds greater health implications: more intestinal inflammation, greater numbers of pathogenic microbes—trillions—that live and die and create a greater burden of toxic by-products from the remnants of dying microbes.

The small intestine has been something of a blind spot in health care, largely because of its inaccessibility. During an upper endoscopy, a gastro-enterologist can visualize the esophagus, stomach, and duodenum but rarely any farther down the GI tract, given the multiple turns and the length of the device, which is typically limited to four feet, which leaves the small bowel unseen. Likewise, during colonoscopy, a six-foot-long colonoscope can visualize the five feet of colon all the way to the cecum, a short blind sac that marks the beginning of the colon, but no farther. This means that twenty-some feet—greater than the length of your car—of small bowel between the duodenum and cecum cannot be visualized. This has proven to be a perennial problem in pinpointing, for instance, a source of bleeding from the small bowel, which could be a leaking two-millimeter blood vessel twelve feet down from the duodenum, twelve feet up from the cecum, and completely inaccessible to a scope.

Likewise, for many years dysbiosis was thought to be a phenomenon confined to the colon. Bowel flora composition is usually assessed from a sample of stool, a waste product whose makeup is largely influenced by the colonic microbiome. But the small intestine is proving to be a microbial hotspot, a major player in the microbiome. When dysbiotic microbes from the colon travel up the small intestine, they create the nasty situations that define small intestinal bacterial overgrowth (SIBO) and small intestinal fungal overgrowth (SIFO): undesirable bacterial and fungal species that have proliferated and ascended into the small intestine.

SIBO was identified eighty years ago but only through examinations of surgically removed small bowel or at autopsy, and so it was thought to be an uncommon situation, found only in people with serious and life-threatening intestinal disease. The availability of breath testing (which I discuss in detail later, including do-it-yourself at-home breath testing), a technique validated by researchers such as SIBO expert Dr. Mark Pimentel of Cedars-Sinai Medical Center in Los Angeles that essentially maps out the location of microbes in the GI tract, has simplified the ability to identify SIBO, thereby circumventing the limitations of stool testing and scopes. Over the last ten to fifteen years, breath testing has changed our perceptions of SIBO: it is now clear that SIBO is far more common than previously thought.

In fact, I argue later in this book that SIBO is so widespread and common that the number of people affected exceeds the size of the type 2 diabetes and prediabetes epidemics, and it's all occurring in plain view of doctors, yet not gaining mention in headlines, hospitals, or workplace wellness programs. I believe that SIBO is so ubiquitous that it now reaches across all societal levels regardless of geography, sex, income, or age. If you wear shoes or brush your teeth, there is a very good chance that this issue applies to you and is impairing your health, restraining your day-to-day functioning, and limiting your hopes of feeling good.

SIBO manifests in a breathtaking variety of ways. SIBO and, to a lesser degree, SIFO can appear as the aches and pains of fibromyalgia, the bowel urgency of irritable bowel syndrome, sleep-disrupting restless leg syndrome, gallstones, food intolerances and allergies, skin rashes, social isolation and feelings of hatred, anxiety, or depression, and hundreds of other health conditions and social situations. These microbial disturbances can complicate type 2 diabetes, obesity, seizure disorders, and heart and autoimmune diseases. They can also manifest as everyday health phenomena such as anxiety, eczema, insomnia, constipation, and painful menstrual cycles. Evidence increasingly points toward autism and premature menstrual cycles in young girls as being part of these microbial imbalances. Once you learn to recognize the signs, you will begin to understand that *everyone's* health issues need to be viewed through the lens of these ubiquitous conditions.

Examination of surgically removed sections of small bowel with SIBO shows that the presence of excessive numbers of unhealthy bacterial species inflames the intestinal wall, occasionally causing ulceration (a break in the mucous membrane), blunts the ability of the hair-like villi to absorb nutrients, and disrupts the digestive process, leading to diarrhea and failed absorption. Impaired digestion of fat and protein is especially common, resulting in some of the telltale signs that I shall discuss, such as seeing fat droplets in the toilet after a bowel movement, which signifies that unhealthy microbes have blocked the process of fat digestion in the small intestine.

Like humans, bacteria and fungi live and die. Although their relations don't conduct funerals for them or erect headstones over their graves, their life cycles, unlike our many decades, are measured in hours to days, reflecting a lightning-fast rate of turnover. With that much life and death cycling in your GI tract, involving trillions of creatures, where do the by-products go upon their death? Without wills or estates to settle, the remains of trillions of microbes are recycled by other microbes, some are metabolized by you, and others are passed out into the toilet. But in dysbiosis, some remnants also invade our bloodstream and thereby are "exported" to other parts of the body. In 2007, a French research group reported on this critical phenomenon. They labeled this flood of toxic bacterial breakdown products "metabolic endotoxemia," and it has been found to underlie numerous modern health conditions, especially those driven by inflammation, such as type 2 diabetes, heart disease, and neuro-degenerative diseases.[4] The main driver of endotoxemia is something called lipopolysaccharide, or LPS, which originates in the cell walls of or-ganisms such as *Escherichia coli* (*E. coli*) and *Klebsiella*, common inhabitants of the colon and stool. When those microbes die, their cell wall contents are liberated, and if the integrity of the intestinal wall has been compro-mised by pathogenic species, the LPS can pass through this broken barrier into the blood. The consequences of endotoxemia are especially powerful when all thirty feet of the GI tract are filled with unhealthy microbes.

Because the blood vessels that feed the GI tract drain into the portal circulation that leads to the liver, it's the liver that first receives this flood of microbial toxins. Blood circulating out of a GI tract with SIBO contains as much as tenfold greater LPS levels than blood from a healthy GI tract. After passing through the liver, microbial toxins then enter the systemic circulation, which flows through all other body organs. The trillions of bacteria and fungi inhabiting the length of the GI tract therefore have an impact on all the other organs of the body. This explains how, for instance, microbial proliferation in the GI tract can be experienced as an inflamed fatty liver, or rosacea of the skin, or the progressive cognitive decline of dementia, or the ceaseless leg movement of restless leg syndrome—health phenomena that occur far away from their microbial origin. Modern medicine is useful for mechanically ablating the source of abnormal heart rhythms and reducing the aching muscles and joints of fibromyalgia, but it fails to address the microbial proliferation and endotoxemia that cause, or at least worsen, these conditions.

Labeling these situations "SIBO" and "SIFO," however, underestimates the health disruptions they introduce. Rather than "small intestinal bacterial overgrowth," we should simply call it "bacterial overgrowth," because the effects range far and wide outside the small intestine. Although it's not as ubiquitous as bacterial overgrowth, fungal overgrowth similarly involves a proliferation and expansion of fungal species that, like bacterial overgrowth, extend their effects outside the small intestine (we explore fungal overgrowth in Chapter 7).

BACTERIAL "BLUES"?

It's been known for years that about a third of people who experience depression, a potentially debilitating condition that is often poorly responsive to prescription antidepressant medication, show increased measures of inflammation such as C-reactive protein and other markers. But what could this source of inflammation be that drives depression in the absence of, say, a red, swollen knee or pneumonia? The same people who show increased markers of inflammation with depression are also those most likely to prove resistant to prescription antidepressant medication.

In a number of clinical studies, brave volunteers without depression have willingly received injections of the LPS endotoxin derived from the cell walls of bacteria. Within hours of receiving this artificial increase in LPS, they developed the signature emotions of depression: dark moods, anxiety, loss of motivation, disinterest in everyday activities, impaired cognitive function. Imaging of brain function in these people revealed all the brain hallmarks of depression.[5] The unavoidable conclusion: the products of bacterial breakdown that enter the bloodstream play a role in causing depression, especially depression unresponsive to conventional treatments. Not surprisingly, this has prompted the pharmaceutical industry to explore adding various anti-inflammatory drugs to conventional antidepressants in order to block some of these inflammatory mediators—once again, disregarding the cause of the inflammation, namely, factors associated with bacterial overgrowth, and only treating the symptoms.

Lost from these observations, however, is the fact that, outside of these artificial situations in which LPS is directly injected, the high levels of LPS circulating in the bloodstreams of many people in everyday life originate with bacterial overpopulation that leads to endotoxemia. I believe that addressing disruptions to healthy, balanced bacterial populations and the endotoxemia/excess LPS that results makes a lot more sense than focusing on a downstream symptom.

SIBO and SIFO are situations that many of us—including me—formerly dismissed as uncommon, even rare, but they are proving to be—given the scientific evidence, widespread availability of stool testing, and direct-to-consumer devices that detect the various forms of microbial overgrowth—as common as ordering paper towels or baking mixes through Amazon. Although few Americans have heard of SIBO and SIFO, tens of millions of us are affected by them. We now know that 35–84 percent of the thirty-five million Americans diagnosed with irritable bowel syndrome, as well as the equal number who remain undiagnosed but grin and bear bowel urgency and bloating, have SIBO.[6] We also know that of the twelve million Americans with the pain and disability of fibromyalgia, up to 100 percent have the bacterial overgrowth of SIBO, as do the majority of people with restless leg syndrome, fatty liver, diverticular disease, various food intolerances, gallstones, autoimmune and neurodegenerative conditions, and type 2 diabetes.[6-12] The bacterial overgrowth of SIBO is also present in about 50 percent of the 150 million American adults who are overweight or obese.[13] We also know that about a third of people with SIBO also have SIFO.[14] It may not pillage the countryside or terrorize people in their cottages, but it is a monster that modern life has created, and it dwells in the thirty feet of your GI tract.

Tally up the numbers and you will recognize that, although the type 2 diabetes and prediabetes epidemics now encompass over a hundred million Americans, the number of those with SIBO handily matches or exceeds this number. Critics will inevitably challenge these estimates, but the evidence confirms that bacterial and fungal overgrowth and related conditions are common—the exception is to have normal, healthy bowel flora.

This presents a health challenge of unprecedented scale. Look to your left, look to your right, and you will see at least one person, if not many, with this condition. It's hard to overstate the power of this tidal wave of change in human physiology and microbial collaboration.

But even if you do not have SIBO or SIFO, it is likely—virtually guaranteed—that you have, at the very least, dysbiosis. Substantial disruptions of the bacterial and perhaps fungal species inhabiting your colon still pose implications for health, whether or not you are regular or require a stack of magazines for bowel habit success.

Beyond toxic microbial breakdown products, even microbes themselves can, in the worst situations, trespass into internal organs, places where they do not belong. Pick an organ, any organ, and you can find bacteria living there and exerting peculiar health effects. We now recognize that bacteria that have taken up residence in places like the bile duct and gallbladder, for instance, play a role in creating gallstones. The bacterial species occupying these unexpected locations tend to be species like *E. coli* and others from the *Pseudomonas* and *Enterococcus* groups, species that are usually found in the colon and stool.

Unhealthy bacteria and fungi have been recovered from arteries, breasts, prostate glands, even the human brain, representing an invasion of microbes whose health effects are only beginning to be appreciated.[15–17]

Like bacteria, fungi such as *Candida albicans*, *Candida glabrata*, and *Malassezia* can ascend the entire length of the GI tract and release their toxic breakdown products, which are distributed to the rest of the body. In some people, fungi manage to escape the GI tract and take up residence in other places.[14] This explains why people with intestinal fungal overgrowth commonly also experience fungal infections of the underarms, throat, esophagus, vagina, groin, and brain. Although less well studied than bacterial overgrowth, the health implications of fungal overgrowth are now likewise proving to be far greater than originally thought. The recent discovery that people who die of Alzheimer's dementia have brain tissue riddled with fungi, an observation that we shall discuss further, is especially concerning.

This is not infection in the conventional sense in which a single bacterial or fungal species proliferates unchecked, creates a pus-filled abscess, and damages the organ it is trying to dominate. SIBO is more properly labeled "infestation," that is, occupation without full takeover, much like ants in your cupboards—they don't run you and your family out of the house, but they are still a nuisance and ruin your stash of Oreos.

It's therefore not just a matter of microbial overpopulation. Microbes in the GI tract impact other organs of the body via the spread of their toxic products and they can even trespass into those organs. Over the span of just two human generations, since bell-bottom jeans were in fashion and Grandma lamented the loss of gentlemanly manners, the species of bacteria and fungi in the human GI tract have changed, production of their by-products has expanded exponentially, and the consequences on us human beings as their hosts have become more serious. Accordingly, the rules of engagement with them must also change.

Dysbiosis, and certainly SIBO and SIFO, may not be diagnosed by doctors, be discussed on the TV morning news, or be the topic of panicked talk on social media, but these conditions present enormous implications for your health. They are situations so dramatically unnatural that taking a costly probiotic or eating kimchi alone will not remedy them. To gain an understanding of how this disaster of an internal environment emerged, let's start at the beginning of every individual's life: Mom.

2

A MICROBIOME ONLY
A MOTHER COULD LOVE

OUR MOTHERS GET US STARTED ON THE GREAT MICROBIAL adventure of our lives. First by passing through the birth canal, and then by breastfeeding and physical contact with Mom, newborns receive their mother's microbiome. Birth and early life therefore begin the process of populating an infant's body with microbes, part of the intimate and wonderful bond that mothers and their children share.

But in modern times this bond has been corrupted. One major disruptive factor in a healthy balance of intestinal microbes in children is the unfortunate commercialization of motherhood. By "commercialization" I mean that financial interests have entered into this natural phenomenon called bearing children. Obstetricians fearful of malpractice lawsuits and motivated by greater fees for performing Cesarean sections, followed by aggressive marketing of synthetic infant formulas in place of breast milk, sever the normal passage of the maternal microbiome to the infant. No question: there is a time and place for practices like C-section, but commercial interests have tipped the scales, putting children at a disadvantage from the very start.

The 32 percent of children delivered by C-section and/or the 17 percent of children who are not breastfed begin life without the advantages of sharing in their mother's microbial bounty.[1,2] The one in three children born by C-section begins life with a different microbiome than a vaginally delivered child's. They acquire bacterial species that reflect the populations of microbes that inhabit hospitals, and their microbiome is dominated by undesirable species from the Enterobacteriaceae family of bacteria, the same species that originate in fecal material from the colon and characterize bacterial overgrowth. These differences persist for years after delivery.[3,4] But even vaginal delivery is no guarantee that healthy flora will be transferred to a newborn because most childbearing women have suffered the same microbiome-disruptive factors that the rest of us have experienced, so they don't have a balanced microbiome to pass along to their children. To make matters worse, new mothers are often given antibiotics around the time of delivery for episiotomies and prevention of neonatal streptococcal infection. Likewise, infants who are not breastfed obtain microbes only from their mother's skin and from food and the environment, yielding a different landscape of microbes, one that is missing the bacterial species, antibodies, and nutrients found in breast milk. Premature infants experience the most extreme microbiome disruption of all because they are administered aggressive courses of antibiotics, often for extended periods during their stay in the intensive care unit apart from their mothers.

What if, like so many other modern people, a woman of childbearing age drinks sugary or diet soft drinks, takes nonsteroidal anti-inflammatory drugs to relieve menstrual cramps, previously relied on birth control pills or intrauterine devices for contraception, is exposed to the herbicide glyphosate in grains—in short, she carries a microbiome monstrously changed? The potential consequences include delayed *in utero* development of her baby and premature delivery. (Think about it: disturbances in a pregnant mother's microbiome can trigger premature delivery, an astounding association.[5]) Mothers who have ulcerative colitis or Crohn's disease and other health conditions pass on a different microbiome than moms without these conditions. And the situation of an altered microbiome persists in the infant long after birth.[6] Reflecting the powerful influence of a mother's microbiome on her infant, even mothers with gingivitis—yes: gum disease in the mouth, many inches and a bodily system away from the uterus and baby—may be at increased risk for premature birth and delivering a low-birth-weight newborn.[5]

But then, imagine a baby born from a healthy mom via vaginal delivery who is breastfed for the first two years of life (exclusively breastfed for the first six months, and then consuming a combination of breast milk and formula until two years of age, as well as some solid foods, as recommended by the World Health Organization). This child is not given antibiotics or other prescription drugs, lives on healthy foods free of glyphosate and herbicide and pesticide residues, and is allowed to interact with the environment, meaning they touch soil, pets, and other children—in other words, this child is allowed to develop a healthy and supportive microbiome because the factors that disrupt a healthy balance of microbes are minimized and the factors that promote a healthy biome are encouraged. If we were to analyze the composition of bowel flora in this child, it would reveal a healthy mix of microbial species in the colon, with sharply declining bacterial and fungal numbers as we ascend into the ileum and jejunum. This microbiome would be rich in health-supportive species such as *Lactobacillus*, *Bifidobacterium*, and *Akkermansia* species; hospital-acquired and pathogenic stool species would be in the minority. This child has regular bowel movements, is free of skin rashes and allergies, does not suffer from food intolerances, and enjoys normal mental, emotional, and physical development. This child would be at the extreme end of positive human health, with favorable bowel flora that support a long and healthy life. Unfortunately, such a theoretical healthy child is becoming the exception in our modern world.

At the other extreme is a child born via C-section, who is hastily transitioned to bottle-fed formula within a few weeks of birth, administered antibiotics at delivery and several times during childhood, fed commercial foods such as fruit juices, animal crackers, and fast-food french fries. Over time, this child develops intolerances to common foods along with asthma, skin rashes, intermittent diarrhea, and behavioral and learning issues. Examination of the bowel flora of this child would reveal species like *Staphylococcus aureus*, *Citrobacter*, *Klebsiella*, and *Salmonella* present not just in the colon but also all the way up the GI tract. The pediatrician prescribes inhalers, steroid creams, drugs to firm up bowel movements, and drugs for attention deficit hyperactivity disorder. This child's health struggles continue through their teenage years and into young adulthood, when they are diagnosed with irritable bowel syndrome (IBS), migraine headaches, acne, and eczema, all followed by struggles with weight, prediabetes, and fatty liver.

Sadly, I bet this last situation rings familiar to you.

Formal explorations of the connection between a disrupted microbiome and various childhood diseases have unearthed a complex tangle of changes in bowel flora. Disrupted microbiomes have been documented in both the airways and the bowels of children with asthma, for example, and in the bowels of those at risk for developing type 1 diabetes and children experiencing slowed growth. Children who experience diarrhea during the first two years of life show cognitive delay and slowed growth as older children.[7–9]

This is not about some theoretical change in intestinal bacteria of interest only to microbiologists. This represents dramatic change in the composition of the microbial partners we have in this coexistence, changes that hold potential for profoundly influencing health from birth onward.

FORMULA FOR FAILURE

There is no synthetic infant formula, no matter how well conceived, that matches the health benefits of a mother's breast milk. The composition of breast milk is the result of millions of years of human evolution. It is a natural source of factors such as antibodies, prebiotic fibers and oligosaccharides, probiotic microbes, phospholipids, bacteriocins (natural microbe-produced antibiotics) that suppress growth of unhealthy bacteria, and other components crucial to the infant's health and growth. No synthetic formula on the market even comes close to re-creating the composition of human breast milk. No synthetic formula was administered to infants fifty thousand, one hundred thousand, or one million years ago upon their emergence from the birth canal—only mother's breast milk.

No question: Formula manufacturers have worked to improve their products, even introducing innovations such as organic ingredients and prebiotic fibers and converting to A2 casein dairy (which mirrors the human form of casein protein) to reduce potential for autoimmune disease. But the catch-up process continues to include blunders in formulation such as the use of nonfat milk (human breast milk is 4–5 percent fat, a similar fat content to whole cow's milk) and inclusion of genetically modified ingredients with all their associated problems, including disruption of the infant's microbiome.

Before such improvements were introduced, the infant formula industry was marked by scandal. Nestlé, for instance, heavily marketed its products to women in Africa, suggesting to these women that formula was superior to breast milk. These poor women, eager to join the modern world, were thereby encouraged to purchase a product that came to be associated with the deaths of millions of children from malnutrition (largely because mothers would dilute the formula to reduce costs). In the United States, the *New York Times* reported on how formula manufacturers provided financial perks to doctors and hospitals to encourage them to hand out packages for new mothers at discharge that included formula samples, a practice that resulted in as much as a sixteen-fold increase in the rate of infections in infants during the first two months after birth.[10]

There are real consequences to failing to feed an infant human breast milk. Breastfed infants have greater populations of probiotic *Lactobacillus* and *Bifidobacterium* species, whereas *Enterococcus* and *Enterobacter* species—species that typically inhabit the colon and characterize bacterial overgrowth—dominate in formula-fed children.[11] In an analysis commissioned by the Department of Health and Human Services Office on Women's Health, children who were breastfed for at least the first three months of life experienced 42 percent less atopic dermatitis, 27–40 percent lower risk of developing asthma, and 50 percent fewer ear infections.[12] Later in life, they were also less likely to become obese or develop type 2 diabetes, and they ranked higher in intelligence quotient (IQ). There is power in providing a child with a healthier microbiome that begins with a mother's priceless contributions.

The microbe *Bifidobacterium infantis* plays an especially critical role in the early health of an infant, as it is meant to dominate an infant's intestinal microbiome. This species is uniquely able to metabolize oligosaccharides present in breast milk (not present in synthetic formula). But 90 percent of modern infants lack this species altogether. Evidence tells us that supplying this microbe as a probiotic allows the child to metabolize milk oligosaccharides while it also reduces the numbers of unhealthy stool organisms.[13] (Later in the book, I will show parents how to make a B. infantis yogurt that moms can consume and thereby provide this microbe to the newborn the way it was supposed to be passed on: by the baby's passage through the birth canal and via breast milk.)

Antibiotics are the most frequent class of drugs prescribed for children. It is estimated that up to 50 percent of antibiotic prescriptions are unnecessary, prescribed for viral, not bacterial, upper respiratory and middle ear infections that antibiotics are ineffective against. Pediatricians often choose broad-spectrum antibiotics that eradicate a wide range of bacterial species and that encourage fungal proliferation (due to reduced competition from bacteria) rather than narrow-spectrum antibiotics with fewer consequences. Children who have received antibiotics are more prone to becoming overweight, developing allergy and autoimmune diseases, and experiencing increased susceptibility to infections.[14] Only an occasional child grows into adulthood who hasn't taken at least one, if not many, courses of antibiotics with wide and enduring consequences.

Many of us are off to a rough microbial start as infants and children, and the unfortunate situation continues into adulthood. The adult microbiome is the cumulative result of microbiome disruptions that occurred through infancy, childhood, and teenage years, as well as deficiencies passed on from generation to generation. One out of every two or three adults will be prescribed an antibiotic this year alone.[15] But adults do far more than take antibiotics that disrupt the microbial communities of their bodies. They take prescription drugs that reduce stomach acid, the natural barrier to microbes that descend the esophagus as well as those that ascend from the colon, setting the stage for bacterial colonization of the full length of the GI tract.[16] Millions take nonsteroidal anti-inflammatory drugs (NSAIDs) such as ibuprofen or naproxen for arthritis pain, menstrual cramps, migraine headaches, and other reasons. Not only do many people develop asymptomatic damage to the small intestine with NSAID use, but these drugs also invite bacterial species from the colon to take up residence in the upper bowel.[17] Engaging in a diet that includes sugary soft drinks and snacks, that is, dietary habits followed by millions of Americans, also cultivates bacterial colonization in the small intestine, where these species don't belong.[18] Abundant evidence shows that exposure to herbicide and pesticide residues in food alters the microbiome, as does the herbicide used on genetically modified corn and soy, glyphosate, which is also a potent antibiotic.[19–21] And, in a disturbing intersection between global climate change and the human microbiome, increasing levels of ground-level ozone, the product of automobile exhaust exposed to sunlight, has been found to alter bowel flora composition.[22]

As we've discussed, toxic by-products of microbial life and death transported outside the GI tract, called endotoxemia, trigger inflammation and disease in distant parts of the body, from big toe to brain. This is how, for instance, bacteria in the GI tract cause the facial skin rash called rosacea, the musculoskeletal pain of fibromyalgia, and the premature delivery of an infant. You can also begin to appreciate how a topical anti-inflammatory drug for rosacea, an oral anti-inflammatory drug for fibromyalgia that blocks pain pathways, and a drug for depression that raises serotonin levels do nothing to address the underlying cause—unhealthy expansion of bacterial populations and the flood of toxic metabolic by-products they produce—and may even make the situation worse. A prescription drug may provide temporary relief from the aches and pains of fibromyalgia, or a low-FODMAPs diet can reduce the bloating and diarrhea of IBS (FODMAPs, fibers and sugars metabolized by microbes, are an issue I shall discuss further later in the book), but you remain exposed to all the other consequences of uncorrected bacterial overgrowth, intestinal and otherwise.

HAS IT GONE TOO FAR?

Modern lifestyle habits have therefore primed your body for unhealthy microbial expansion. If there is no benefit to curtailing your carbon footprint or erecting levees against the equivalent to rising oceans in your body, what can you do to turn the tide against microbial expansion and invasion? Thankfully, you can do plenty.

Later, I discuss the consequences of bacterial and fungal overgrowth and endotoxemia. We shall then go over what you can do to subdue these processes and even evict microbial squatters from places where they are not welcome. I shall also show you the tricks for cultivating genuinely beneficial bacterial species in your microbiome so that you can obtain specific, often spectacular, health effects. Yes, you can achieve some pretty magnificent changes by attending to your inner ecosystem.

But first, let's next discuss in more detail how bacterial overgrowth shows up so that you don't mistake the consequences of eating an *E. coli*–contaminated fast-food burger for the chronic and devastating effects of bacterial and fungal proliferation.

3

GHOSTS OF MICROBES PAST

B OWEL FLORA AIN'T WHAT IT USED TO BE.
     Over and over again, life teaches us lessons that make us rethink
our daily habits: living life through the screen of a cell phone is a bad idea,
cutting short on sleep to squeeze in more work and play yields health consequences, food served from a drive-through window is not how the human diet should be conducted. Relearning the lessons of life and health is
every bit as worthwhile and necessary, perhaps more so, in the world of the
microbiome.

Let's now consider how modern life has caused the loss of a number
of bacterial species that have important functions for human health. It's
the equivalent of an inner extinction event, but one that we can thankfully
reverse.

LOST IN THE SHUFFLE

Methods to identify microbes inhabiting the human GI tract were not
available a century ago, nor even as recently as when Ronald Reagan was
president. Instead, earlier methods were crude and incomplete, relying on
the ability of sampled microbes to grow in a petri dish or similar preparation, which amounted to viewing the thirty-foot-long world of the human

GI tract through a keyhole that revealed only a fraction of the microscopic creatures in there. Up until recently, these crude methods did not allow so-called anaerobic species to grow in samples because they die upon exposure to air or oxygen, yet the human microbiome is filled with such anaerobes (organisms that live without oxygen).

Newer methods that rely on DNA markers have revealed a universe of creatures, including anaerobes, that were previously unidentified. These methods identify microbes by the code written in an organism's DNA, which is unique to that species (and strain, an issue we shall discuss later), and DNA identification methods are unaffected by the presence or lack of oxygen. New methods also allow us to make detailed comparisons between the modern microbiome and that of earlier humans who were not exposed to modern disruptive factors. Such assessments reveal that the modern microbiome is very different from the microbiomes of the past. No surprise: just think how our great-grandparents' generation, not that long ago, had less obesity, type 2 diabetes, autoimmune diseases, social isolation, and exposure to glyphosate, diet sodas, or ubiquitous industrial chemicals.

Examinations of ancient microbiomes such as those contained in bones, fossilized fecal material, and ancient dental plaque tell us that, thousands of years ago, a human's microbial inhabitants were comprised of very different species from what we harbor today. What is striking about these analyses is that they have uncovered the fact that there was considerable overlap of the microbiomes of ancient cultures across continents. Specimens discovered in tropical caves and fecal material recovered from permafrost mummies of northern latitudes show similar microbiomes. The greatest differences are seen in comparisons of *any* ancient microbiome to the microbiome of modern people.[1-3] As humans evolved from exclusively hunter-gatherer lifestyles to agricultural communities, microbiome composition shifted to accommodate the resulting changes in diet: less diversity of plants consumed, greater reliance on starchy crops like maize and wheat. The next big leap in changes of microbiome composition occurred as people became more urbanized, exposed to antibiotics, and reliant on grains, sugar, and processed foods.

In recent times, as I mentioned in Chapter 2, numerous factors, from antibiotics to ice cream, have altered the collection of microorganisms inhabiting the human body. Compare bacterial species present as recently as 1960 to the modern microbiome and it becomes clear that, compared to all our predecessors, modern humans of the twenty-first century have fewer bacterial species inhabiting our GI tracts. Factors that disrupt the microbiome have resulted in a shrinking and less-varied population of bacterial species. Many species have been lost, hit-and-runs eliminated on the great microbiome highway. When we analyze microbes in modern stool specimens, we see that many people now have few beneficial *Lactobacillus*, *Bifidobacterium*, and other species, while showing plenty of *Escherichia coli*, *Shigella*, *Pseudomonas*, and other fecal microbes, which are increasingly dominant in the modern GI tract. But something we do not see are the species that have *vanished* from the modern microbiome. Because there are no birth records or ghosts to tell us precisely which have disappeared, we resort to comparing modern microbiomes to microbiomes of the past.

Identifying the microbes we are missing is a tougher task than identifying microbes that are present and whose necessity is questioned. DNA analyses are shedding light on these differences. An international research group recently conducted a monumental effort, for example, that uncovered thousands of previously unidentified species in both Western and non-Western populations.[4] As researchers study these newly discovered species, we will learn many exciting lessons on how to take advantage of this treasure trove of microbes. Similar research methods are being applied to the microbiomes of the remaining hunter-gatherers on the planet and to the remains of ancient microbiomes, so we may soon have vast catalogs of the many species we've lost.

The communities of humans in the world who still live as hunter-gatherers provide insight into intestinal microbiomes that have not been exposed to antibiotics, prescription drugs, or the modern Western diet. These people dig in the soil for roots and tubers, use a spear to kill their next meal, drink water from rivers or streams, and don't travel by car or communicate with cell phones. When we compare modern bowel flora to that of indigenous people such as the Hadza of Tanzania, the Matsés of Peru, or the Yanomami of the Brazilian rain forest, we discover, as similarly revealed by fossilized fecal material or bone, that the composition of their microbiomes is different.[5-7] The indigenous populations have numerous species that are absent from the modern human microbiome. Interestingly, comparison among the microbiomes of indigenous peoples demonstrates that, even though these populations are separated by vast distances and live on different continents, their bowel floras are oddly similar. Bowel flora species of the Hadza in East Africa, for instance, are similar to those of the Matsés in the Peruvian rain forest; these are indigenous peoples on two different continents with no opportunity to interact. The extraordinary cross-cultural, cross-continental similarities have prompted speculation that the microbiome indigenous peoples carry is therefore representative of our ancestral Stone Age microbiome, that is, the microbiome of our ancestors, the microbiome before modern disruptions entered the picture, the microbiome that was part of human evolution. It appears certain that, as inhabitants of the twenty-first century, *our* strange microbiome *is* the exception.

The idea that modern people lack bacterial species that show up as one or another health condition has led to the concept of replacing lost or deficient species. In one recent study, for instance, researchers at Boston Children's Hospital replaced several strains of Clostridia missing from the bowels of infants who were experiencing food allergies and found that this practice showed potential to reverse them.[8] This evidence is preliminary but holds promise to help undo the numerous and sometimes dangerous food allergies to peanuts, eggs, or fish a growing number of children experience.

Another bacterial genus largely lost from most modern people is *Oxalobacter*, bacterial species that can dwell in the colon and that enthusiastically consume oxalate, a common naturally occurring compound in foods such as nuts, spinach, beets, and chocolate. In contrast, the majority of indigenous people such as the Hadza and Yanomami carry plenty of *Oxalobacter* species. As more modern people lose these species, they develop painful calcium oxalate kidney stones, especially following exposure to antibiotics. Most concerning, there has been a major increase in calcium oxalate kidney stones in children, especially after taking a course of antibiotics.[9,10] Other changes in bowel flora composition are also likely at work in people with oxalate kidney stones, such as proliferation of some species (*Methanobrevibacter smithii*) and loss or reduction of others (*Lactobacillus plantarum*). But the process appears to revolve around the loss of the *Oxalobacter* species of bacteria.

Bifidobacterium infantis is another microbial casualty, absent in 90 percent of all newborns. This species provides substantial health and growth advantages to newborn infants, but either it is not passed on from mother to baby or it is lost by exposure to antibiotics. Without *B. infantis*, infants are more likely to become overcolonized by Enterobacteriaceae stool species, a situation that has been associated with a dramatic increase in stool pH over the years (an increase in stool pH reflects a child's inability to metabolize nutrients such as breast milk oligosaccharides into acidic fatty acid by-products that nourish intestinal cells and provide other benefits). Infants in the early twentieth century, for instance, had stool pH of around 5.0, whereas modern infants without a healthy population of *B. infantis* have less-acidic stool, with a pH of 6.5 (a more than tenfold decrease in acidity on the pH scale).[11] Restoration of *B. infantis* protects premature infants from a devastating and often fatal condition called necrotizing enterocolitis in which unhealthy bacterial species invade and destroy the intestinal wall.[12] *B. infantis* is one of several "keystone" species in infants that, because it is capable of metabolizing nutrients in breast milk, supports the growth of other beneficial bacterial species as the baby grows. But even vaginal delivery and breastfeeding are no guarantee that an infant will become colonized by this crucial species because mothers themselves can lack this microbe and are thereby unable to pass it on. Beyond protection from necrotizing enterocolitis, restoration of this species provides considerable advantage to infants. Infants in whom *B. infantis* is restored are more likely to sleep through the night and nap longer, they are less likely to have diaper rash, they have less colic, and they have 50 percent fewer bowel movements per day (and thereby need 50 percent fewer diaper changes). And the benefits of this species continue beyond infancy in the form of reductions in allergic rhinitis (nasal allergy), asthma, potential for autoimmune diseases, and abdominal pain from irritable bowel syndrome, as they become older children.[13-15] But what is even better than providing an infant with *B. infantis* as a probiotic after birth? Restoring this microbe to the mom before birth, which allows the mother to pass it on to her baby, just as should occur naturally, while it also provides health benefits to the mother.

L. REUTERI: THE LOVE BUG

The bacterial species *Lactobacillus reuteri* is a star in the world of intestinal microbes, one that yields spectacular effects for its human host. Up until the mid-twentieth century, most people in the Western world enjoyed the benefits of this bacterial species dwelling in their GI tracts, which they had acquired from their mothers as infants by passage through the birth canal and breastfeeding. Indigenous people living in jungles and mountains, as well as chickens, pigs, and other creatures, carry this microorganism, suggesting that it plays an essential role in survival.

But modern life has eradicated this species from 96 percent of people in the Western world. Today, only 4 percent—fewer than one in twenty people—continue to enjoy the presence of this marvelous species.[16,17] Among the many benefits of *L. reuteri* is its unique capacity to trigger the release of the hormone oxytocin from the human brain, which has been demonstrated through an elegant series of experiments conducted at the Massachusetts Institute of Technology (MIT). Think about that: a microbe living in your GI tract determines an important aspect of your brain's functioning.[18]

Oxytocin is the hormone of empathy and connectedness. It is the hormone that surges when you are in love or feel closely connected to another person or pet your dog. Oxytocin helps you see the other side of an argument, cultivates sympathy for the plight of other people, and reduces social anxiety.

Loss of *L. reuteri* and its oxytocin-provoking effects means that modern people have lower oxytocin levels than people of fifty years ago. We live in a time plagued by increased social isolation, record-setting rates of suicide, skyrocketing divorce. Could the loss of the oxytocin-boosting *L. reuteri* be at least one cause behind these disturbing social trends? Surely, these are complex issues with many potential causes, but could the modern devastation of the helpful organisms in the thirty feet of GI tract, including the disappearance of *L. reuteri* and the accompanying loss of empathy and desire for human connection, be at least part of the explanation? I believe it is.

OXYTOCIN: HORMONE OF LOVE . . . *AND* YOUTH?

Restoring *L. reuteri*, a microbe lost by most modern people, triggers release of oxytocin from the brain and, with it, a surge in empathy and desire for the company of other people. Oxytocin is the driver of the affection between mother and child, the attachment you feel to your partner, and it's the factor that opens your mind to the opinions of other people. The microbiome of the majority of modern people is missing *L. reuteri* in an age when the social phenomena of isolation, suicide, divorce, and social discord are at record levels. Yet, as important as the effects of oxytocin are for human social life, this hormone is so much more than that.

One of the first hints at oxytocin's power to exert impressive physiological effects came from a series of animal experiments performed at MIT by a group studying cancer. They observed the following effects in elderly animals given *L. reuteri* compared to those who did not receive *L. reuteri*:

- Thick fur, more rapid hair growth (Animals that did not receive *L. reuteri* experienced dermatitis and patchy hair loss.)
- Thicker skin, with substantial increase in dermal collagen
- Acceleration of skin healing (Skin healing can be viewed as a reflection of overall youthfulness and health.)
- Lifelong slenderness (Mice without *L. reuteri* became overweight.)
- Reduced levels of the stress hormone cortisol
- Preservation of mating behavior in older mice

In other studies, *L. reuteri* or oxytocin administration restored youthful muscle in elderly mice, reversed the impaired immunity of aging, and reversed age-related bone loss.

Add it all up: Mice without *L. reuteri* got old and fat, lost fur, lost muscle and bone density, lost interest in sex, and lost immune protection. *L. reuteri*–receiving mice stayed slender, had thick fur, maintained youthful muscle and bone density, maintained youthful immunity, and continued to be sexually active—they stayed young until death. Let me repeat that for emphasis: *mice carrying L. reuteri and enjoying youthful levels of oxytocin stayed young until death.* It doesn't mean they lived longer. It means that, at an age when they might have been collecting mouse Social Security, getting around with a walker, and reading AARP magazine, they instead appeared much younger and slender and remained socially and sexually engaged.[18-21]

A growing list of these phenomena is corroborated by human experiences.[21-24] Since I have been advocating for the restoration of *L. reuteri* in modern people's microbiomes, achieved by making *L. reuteri* yogurt with high bacterial counts (recipe provided later in the book), we have indeed been witnessing the effects seen in the experimental models reproduced in many people: thicker skin, reduction in skin wrinkles, accelerated healing, restoration of youthful muscle and strength, increased libido. And, because mice cannot tell us how they feel, people consuming this *L. reuteri*–rich yogurt are reporting additional effects such as deeper sleep with vivid dreams, reduced appetite, greater optimism, and less social anxiety, effects likely resulting from the oxytocin boost caused by the bacteria.

Restoration of *L. reuteri*, therefore, doesn't just make you a better, healthier human being but also can yield a range of effects that, I believe, turn back the clock ten, maybe twenty years. All this by restoring a bacterial species that, odds are, you probably lost or never received, let alone heard of.

I discuss how you can restore this marvelous bacterial species later in the book.

Restore this lost bacterial species, and many experience a flood of empathy and desire for human connection. People report liking their families and coworkers better, a renewed desire to converse with strangers in line for coffee at Starbucks and gather with friends, and a tendency to cry more at movies. They also report being better able to understand the views and opinions of others.

L. reuteri is unique among bacteria in that it "prefers" to colonize the upper gastrointestinal tract, the stomach, duodenum, jejunum, and ileum, rather than to take up residence only in the colon, where most other probiotic species prefer to live. Living in the upper reaches of the GI tract, *L. reuteri* is an enthusiastic producer of natural antibiotics called bacteriocins that are effective against undesirable bacterial species that ascend into the small intestine where they don't belong. Loss of *L. reuteri* in modern people is therefore a likely contributing factor to the bacterial overgrowth in the small intestine that is now widespread; restoration of *L. reuteri* is therefore also part of the solution.

This is just one bacterial species, nearly vanished from the microbiomes of modern people, that when restored yields astounding effects. *L. reuteri* illustrates the power of purposeful cultivation of the human microbiome that we shall explore further. But it also raises a troublesome question: What other unknown microbes have we lost and, with them, the health-promoting, allergy-preventing, weight-managing, emotional and social benefits they provide?

Super Gut Success: Lisa, 61, New Mexico

"I'VE BEEN EATING A HALF CUP OF *L. REUTERI* YOGURT WITH blueberries or raspberries and walnuts sweetened with monk fruit sweetener almost every day for the past year. I cofermented *L. reuteri* and *L. casei* Shirota to eat during flu season this year.

"The wrinkles around my eye area are definitely diminished. My skin has a smoother texture overall. I have incredibly sound sleep and have dreams with total recall upon arising. Bowel frequency has improved as well.

"I started making *L. reuteri* yogurt in June 2019, and during the winter months I have been eating a co-ferment of *L. reuteri* and *L. casei* Shirota. I see more clarity in my skin, less wrinkles, and many compliments from others."

H. PYLORI: BRIDE OF FRANKENBELLY?

While we have lost a number of bacterial species that are beneficial, we are also in the process of losing a unique species, *Helicobacter pylori*, that has two faces: it provides some benefits, such as protection against acid reflux and perhaps obesity, but it also causes stomach and duodenal ulcers and may promote some forms of cancer. Humans acquired this microbe around the time *Homo sapiens* migrated out of Africa some sixty thousand years ago, but it has diminished in frequency among modern humans over the past fifty years. *H. pylori* currently infects the stomachs of 50 percent or more of the earth's population. In developed countries like the United States, however, the proportion of people with *H. pylori* has dropped to around 15 percent, likely because of the same reasons that we've lost species like *L. reuteri* and *B. infantis*.

For many years, stomach and duodenal ulcers were blamed on stress and consumption of acidic foods. The stomach was long believed to be free of bacteria, given its extremely acidic, low-pH environment. Then, two Australian doctors, Robin Warren and Barry Marshall, demonstrated that eradication of *H. pylori* from the stomach allowed ulcers to heal, proving that ulcers were an infectious process and that certain bacteria could survive in the stomach. Prior to this discovery, I remember the days before antibiotics were used to eradicate *H. pylori* and before stomach acid–suppressing drugs were employed to reduce ulcer pain—it was common to see people in the emergency room vomiting red blood or passing partially digested black blood in their stools from bleeding ulcers. Recognizing that stomach and duodenal ulcers are infectious processes was an enormously powerful insight.

But *H. pylori* is proving to be much more than a cause of ulcers and hemorrhage. It has since been associated with conditions such as stomach cancer, pancreatic and biliary tract cancers, autoimmune diseases, Parkinson's disease, and increased risk for type 2 diabetes.[25–28] Eradication of *H. pylori* has proven more effective in reducing the rash of rosacea and the disability of Parkinson's disease than conventional drugs for these conditions.[29,30] Harboring *H. pylori* increases the likelihood that a person develops SIBO, especially if the infestation results in loss of the person's ability to produce stomach acid, which is common after many years of the bacteria inhabiting the stomach.[31,32]

Eradicating this microbe therefore provides protection against a number of human diseases. But is it all good to get rid of this bug entirely?

Evidence suggests that *H. pylori* has a complicated relationship with its human host. Because humans and *H. pylori* have coexisted for sixty thousand years, we have adapted to each other. *H. pylori*, for instance, tolerates stomach acid and does not stimulate much of a human immune response against it. Although it is associated with the diseases mentioned above, it may also provide advantages. Noted microbiologist Dr. Martin Blaser of New York University, a critic of overuse of antibiotics, has meticulously explored the role of *H. pylori* in human health and argues that its absence is associated with increased frequency of asthma and allergies and perhaps even contributes modestly to weight gain (resulting from distortions of the hormones leptin and ghrelin).[32]

All in all, while it is among the growing list of microbes being lost by many people, in my view there are long-term advantages in not having *H. pylori* infesting your stomach, as the health conditions associated with this microbe are greater threats than the diseases reduced by its presence. Removing *H. pylori* is part of our Super Gut effort to combat dysbiosis and SIBO. The conventional solution is to identify, then eradicate this microbe after an ulcer is diagnosed. But you can take the reins in identifying its presence and eradicating it using selected natural strategies before ulcers or other health conditions arise. Should you wish to eradicate *H. pylori* on your own, see Appendix C for a suggested regimen of natural agents to do so.

A MICROBIOME POINT OF NO RETURN?

Lock up a group of humans and deprive them of food and water—is it any mystery that these poor souls would succumb to deprivation? Sadly, throughout history we have countless instances of such tortures inflicted on humans by happenstance or by other humans.

What happens if you likewise fail to support the microbes living in your GI tract by starving them of the prebiotic fibers and other nutrients they need to survive? They cannot, of course, shop at a supermarket or raise their own livestock. Through neglect, you will thereby erase dozens, perhaps hundreds, of potentially beneficial bacterial species from the confines of your microbiome.

The situation is made worse when your microbiome is exposed to factors that further disrupt bacterial populations, which also contributes to eradicating beneficial species. Glyphosate, the active ingredient in Roundup herbicide, in particular, is a guilty suspect: it has been shown to effectively eradicate probiotic species like *Lactobacillus* while being ineffective against pathogenic *Escherichia coli*, *Shigella*, and all their coconspirators in the SIBO community, thus enriching populations of unhealthy bacterial overgrowth in the intestinal microbiome.[33]

Lost microbe species don't spontaneously come back. Just as rats do not spontaneously generate out of a pile of rags, bacterial species that have been lost or eradicated from the microbiome do not regenerate but are gone forever unless, of course, we take efforts to reimplant them.

Many people have inadvertently lost species from their microbiome. Follow a strict low-carb diet—whether you call it ketogenic, paleo, carnivorous, Atkins, or something else—and fail to include a variety of prebiotic fibers, polyphenols, and other nutrients microbes need that can only be sourced from plants, not animal products, and you do damage to your microbiome because the species you've starved out will not just reappear. Eating regimes that lack microbial nutrients diminish the diversity of bacterial species, that is, the number of unique microbial species—with higher diversity generally regarded as a sign of health—that exist in the gut. Some species are lost and other bacterial species that feed on the protective mucus lining of the GI tract, such as *Akkermansia muciniphila*, proliferate. (Later in the book, I shall discuss in greater detail the implications of *Akkermansia* overproliferation that results from dietary mishaps.) This degrades the protection the intestinal mucus offers and can lead, over time, to inflammation of the intestinal wall, colitis, and other conditions.[34–36]

There is no question: Limiting dietary carbohydrates is a superior method to limiting fat or calories for weight loss and overall health. But don't make the potentially fatal mistake of forgoing the nutrients required to nourish your bowel flora, else you will add to the list of ghosts of microbes past.

Now that we've considered the microbes lost in modern humans, let's discuss how changes in microbial populations have led to the process of fecalization of the human species. Yes, it is as bad as it sounds. Undesirable stool species are waging—and often winning—the war in your GI tract.

4

THE FECALIZATION OF AMERICA

I T'S A MYSTERY NO LONGER: MODERN PEOPLE HAVE MASSIVELY changed the composition of the human microbiome. This is reflected by changes to teeth, on the skin, in the intestinal tract, in bowel habits, in overall health. In this chapter, I discuss how fecal microbes now rule the roost in many people.

Recently, I was discussing the microbiome with two friends who are radiologists, and they told me that when they review CT scans, they have been witnessing a dramatic increase in a phenomenon called fecalization. Also called small bowel feces sign, fecalization is when fecal microbes, usually restricted to the colon, appear in the small intestine, conferring the characteristic appearance of stool seen normally in the colon up into the ileum. For a CT scan, patients ingest oral contrast agents that high-light the inner contours of the GI tract. Feces retained in the colon have a characteristic appearance on a CT scan and should appear only in the colon. But my radiologist friends are now seeing an increasing number of people with fecalization, feces appearing in the small intestine where it should not be. Small intestinal fecalization has a limited number of causes, one of which is small bowel obstruction, an exquisitely painful and life-threatening emergency situation when something blocks or prevents the normal movement of the bowels. But the majority of people with fecalization are young (twenties, thirties, and forties) and are not acutely ill but have chronic abdominal complaints such as urgency, diarrhea, and bloating. (If you have had an abdominal CT for one reason or another, get a copy of the actual report: you will be surprised at how often fecalization is mentioned by the interpreting radiologist, but never mentioned by the doctor to the patient.)

Just fifty years ago, it would have been unimaginable to think that an uncommon condition called type 2 diabetes would become so commonplace as it is today, that we would be suffering the worst epidemic of overweight and obesity seen in the history of humans on the planet, and that the rate of inflammatory bowel diseases like ulcerative colitis and Crohn's disease would be exploding among Americans. But numerous factors unique to modern life have invited fecal organisms to take the seat at the head of the table called your health, and these unwanted guests in the upper GI tract don't follow the rules of etiquette by supporting their host (i.e., you); instead, they are bent on considerable destruction.

It was only a few years ago that we viewed the microbes inhabiting the human GI tract as nothing but a nuisance, like the human appendix or the dandelions in your lawn. If they caused an infection: Take an antibiotic for an upper respiratory or urinary tract infection, endure diarrhea, run through a few extra rolls of toilet paper, case closed. Or get a prescription for a course—or five—of antibiotics for a child with an ear infection, then everything goes back to normal, right?

No, not even close. Antibiotics are like a hydrogen bomb set off in the GI tract that leaves a path of microbial devastation. It takes years to rebuild the microbiome, which often never fully recovers. Antibiotics are especially good at eradicating healthy bacterial species that keep harmful species of the Enterobacteriaceae family, as well as fungal species, in check. Many of the species of Enterobacteriaceae are resistant to antibiotics. When antibiotics eradicate beneficial species, harmful microbes take advantage of the reduced competition for nutrients, which results in a bloom of undesirable microorganisms.[1] Much like an algal bloom in a pond contaminated with agricultural fertilizers, so too do the bacterial and fungal nasties surge after a course of antibiotics.

We've discussed how antibiotics are prescribed to humans with breathtaking frequency. In 2016, for example, 260 million antibiotic prescriptions were written in doctors' offices and other outpatient settings. Antibiotics are prescribed to newborns and infants at nearly twice the rate of adults.[2] In other words, if you breathe oxygen or like pepperoni pizza, you have likely taken at least one, if not a dozen or more, courses of antibiotics in your life. This does not even factor in that 70 percent of all antibiotics are not prescribed for humans but are given to livestock to accelerate growth, and you consume these antibiotics when you eat a fast-food hamburger or farm-raised salmon.[3]

C. DIFF AND THE POWER OF NORMAL

Sometimes the course of antibiotics that slashes populations of healthy microbes enables the proliferation of the bacterial species *Clostridium difficile* (called *C. diff* for short), which causes diarrhea and colitis. Even though it is a pathogenic species, *C. diff* is normally present in many people in low numbers that are kept under control by healthy microbes. When *C. diff* proliferates, as can occur in about 1 percent of people following a course of antibiotics, it results in bloody, painful diarrhea, necessitating more antibiotics. But, in recent years, antibiotics are proving to be increasingly ineffective as *C. diff* develops resistance.

The number of *C. diff* infections has doubled since 2009. It is now the number one, most common hospital-acquired infection, and this microbe has become extremely difficult to eradicate. Most concerning of all, now *C. diff* infections are happening "spontaneously" outside of hospitals and in those who have not had a preceding course of antibiotics.[4,5]

Part of the increased incidence of *C. diff* infections can be blamed on widespread consumption of stomach acid–blocking drugs and nonsteroidal anti-inflammatory drugs such as ibuprofen and naproxen, and part can be blamed on the disruption of bowel flora that occurs in people after weight loss surgery such as gastric bypass.[6,7] But spontaneous *C. diff* infection is also occurring in otherwise apparently healthy people with none of these susceptibilities.

This situation is the one that opened the door for the initially offensive notion of "fecal transplants," which have since become a popular corrective strategy. A fecal transplant is when a quantity of stool from a presumably healthy "donor" is transferred into the intestinal tract of a person with a *C. diff* infection.

Doctors have resorted to fecal transplantation for the 15–20 percent of people with *C. diff* infection who fail to respond to antibiotics and for the 30 percent of people with one or more relapses. This maneuver is associated with as much as a 92 percent success rate.[8]

Take a step back for a moment and think about this: restoration of a presumably healthy microbiome eradicates this dreaded bacterial infection in the majority of cases, *even when potent antibiotics have failed.* It is a powerful illustration of what healthy bowel flora are capable of, picking up where antibiotics leave off. What might this tell us about the bowel flora of people who develop "spontaneous" *C. diff*?

A community hospital experience in Quebec, Canada, further illustrates the power of the microbiome against *C. diff.* In 2003, the hospital experienced an unexpectedly large number of infections with a virulent strain of *C. diff* that was poorly responsive to isolation, hygiene measures, and antibiotics. Physicians therefore added a probiotic (a brand called BioK+) to all courses of antibiotics administered in the hospital. This effort resulted in an 87 percent reduction in new *C. diff* cases in the nearly forty-five thousand hospitalizations over the ensuing ten years.[9]

It is also becoming clear that people who are susceptible to *C. diff* carry an overabundance of species in the Enterobacteriaceae family of bacteria, the species most responsible for SIBO that I shall discuss further in Chapter 6.[10] This question needs to be explored further, but it is increasingly looking like people with unrecognized SIBO are the ones who develop the unrestrained spontaneous proliferation of this dreaded microorganism.

Examine someone's fecal material after a course of antibiotics and you will witness increased numbers of Enterobacteriaceae species. Examine the contents of the upper gastrointestinal tract, such as the stomach and duodenum, and you can often identify increased numbers of unhealthy stool-sourced bacteria there too. Examine the bile duct leading to the pancreas and gallbladder, the liver and other organs, and you will likewise uncover the same species of rogue stool bacteria.

Fecalization, proliferation of Enterobacteriaceae and *C. diff*—what else besides the microbial devastation inflicted by antibiotics could lead to such drastic alterations in intestinal bacterial populations?

We swim in an ocean of factors that disrupt bowel flora. Some changes are self-imposed. Smoking cigarettes or simply indulging in too much alcohol is disruptive to microbial communities.[11,12] Consumption of refined sugar triggers rapid changes in the intestinal bacterial species present, causing loss of healthy species and yielding symptoms of irritable bowel syndrome within *days* of increased sugar intake.[13] The noncaloric artificial sweeteners aspartame, saccharine, and sucralose are no safer, having been shown to trigger changes in bacterial species that exaggerate insulin resistance and lead to type 2 diabetes and obesity.[14] In addition to stomach acid–blocking and anti-inflammatory drugs, preliminary evidence suggests that unhealthy changes in bowel flora composition develop with widely prescribed statin cholesterol-reducing drugs, which cause shifts in bowel flora species to a compositional pattern that resembles the one seen in obesity and diabetes.[15]

DIETARY FAT: FRIEND OR FOE?

Butter versus low-fat nondairy spread? Eggs versus breakfast cereal? Sausage versus granola?

The low-fat diet message offered by "official" guidelines should have died out decades ago, along with culottes and bell-bottom pants, but investigations of the microbiome have, unfortunately, prompted a partial resurrection of advice to reduce dietary fat, which is actually counterproductive to health.

The fifty-year experiment that launched when dietary guidelines were based on misinterpreted and poor-quality clinical studies on reducing fat intake illustrates just how disastrous this guidance can be. It leads to weight gain, obesity, and type 2 diabetes on an unprecedented level, each condition the body's—and microbiome's—response to increased carbohydrate intake to compensate for lost fat calories.

Much of the low-fat diet message was constructed around this house of cards called cholesterol testing, a crude and woefully outdated method to gauge cardiovascular risk that is nevertheless still the prevailing standard despite availability of superior methods of measuring cardiovascular risk that have nothing to do with cholesterol. (This goes beyond the microbiome-centered discussion we are having here, and I cover it in greater detail in my other books such as *Wheat Belly Total Health* and *Undoctored*.) But, as outdated and ineffective as the low-fat message is, some in the world of the microbiome have continued to slam dietary fats.

Before we get to the rationale, let me illustrate a basic principle. Just because one thing is associated with something else does not necessarily mean that the two things have a cause-effect relationship. Imagine you smoke cigarettes. Every time you go to the convenience store to buy Marlboros, you also buy a lottery ticket—ads for big winnings are prominently displayed right by the cash register. Likewise, fellow smokers who buy their cigarettes at the store also see the ads and buy lottery tickets. One week, one of your fellow smokers wins the lottery, prompting a survey of the characteristics of people who win the lottery. Lo and behold, someone observes that people who smoke are more likely to win the lottery. Conclusion: smoking increases your chances of winning the lottery. Ridiculous? Yes, it is, but you would be shocked at the amount of dietary and health advice that is crafted on such false associations.

The fat debate has been reignited by experiments in which laboratory animals fed greater quantities of fat develop dysbiosis, fatty liver, obesity, and type 2 diabetes. Many researchers working with lab animals have therefore declared that fat consumption corrupts the microbiome and is to blame for these common health conditions. On the basis of their results, they advise you to choose low-fat products over a rib eye steak or butter.

But hold on a minute: What exactly are these "high-fat diets" composed of?

High-fat diets in experimental settings are typically diets high in corn oil, given the widely held but erroneous assumption that omega-6-rich oils like corn oil are healthy. Different fats have different effects on such factors as bacterial species in the GI tract and levels of intestinal enzymes (e.g., alkaline phosphatase) that can disable bacterial toxins. Feed an animal omega-6-rich oils and it provokes peculiar changes in its microbiome composition, changes not seen with consumption of oils that are naturally part of that animal's diet in the wild, such as saturated fat, oleic acid, or omega-3 fatty acids.[16]

High-fat diets are also prebiotic fiber–poor diets. More recent research points to the lack of prebiotic fiber and the resultant dysbiosis, including the reduction or loss of species such as *Bifidobacterium longum* and *Akkermansia muciniphila*—not fat consumption per se—as the causes of such long-term health consequences as type 2 diabetes.[17,18] Replace unhealthy fats (excessive quantities of omega-6 fats) with healthy fats (omega-3s, omega-9s or monounsaturated oleic acid, and saturated fats, including the fats obtained from meats, organs, fish, olive oil, and other foods), supplement high fat intake with prebiotic fibers that are a part of a natural diet, and the purported deleterious effects on the microbiome of high-fat feeding are miraculously erased.[19,20]

In other words, as with lottery-winning smokers, increased dietary fat is simply a marker for other changes in diet and in the microbiome. Consuming the right fats may, in fact, actually strengthen the protective mucus barrier (more on that later), reducing its penetrability by toxic intestinal contents.[21] This idea is also consistent with findings that higher intake of the right kinds of fat leads to weight loss and reduction of visceral fat, reduction of insulin resistance and hemoglobin A1c (a measure of blood sugar fluctuations over the preceding ninety days), reduction of inflammation, and other health benefits.

TMAO AND OTHER SHINY OBJECTS

Another misleading distraction in the world of the microbiome is a bacterial metabolite called trimethylamine oxide, TMAO for short. Headlines have broadcast how foods that increase blood levels of TMAO, such as fish, chicken, pork, and beef, have been associated with greater risk for coronary heart disease and heart attacks.

TMAO is the product of Firmicutes (a large grouping of bacteria) and Enterobacteriaceae, the family of species that dominate in dysbiosis and SIBO. Finding higher levels of TMAO in those who eat meat has led to the overly simplistic conclusion that consumption of animal proteins therefore causes heart disease. You can readily identify the error in logic being made here: it's not the fish, chicken, pork, or beef causing heart disease via increased TMAO; it's disruptions of bowel flora composition, enriched populations of Firmicutes and Enterobacteriaceae that produce TMAO, that are more likely to blame. Microbial disruptions are accompanied by increased bacterial endotoxemia, which is also known to contribute to heart disease.[22] We shall also discuss how a diet rich in prebiotic fibers and polyphenols and the fat, oleic acid, such as that in extra-virgin olive oil, turns off the adverse potential of increased TMAO while also reducing endotoxemia.[23]

Go ahead: enjoy the fat, ignore cholesterol content, have some beef, pork, or fish—just as humans have for the last several million years before dietary guidelines and flashy headlines muddied the waters.

The explosion of herbicides and pesticides applied in conventional farming also has a major impact on the modern microbiome. Hundreds of millions of tons of the herbicide glyphosate, for instance, now contaminate the environment; it's detectable in waterways, livestock and other foods, and the human body, given its liberal application to the major crops of corn, soy, and wheat and the lawns in your neighborhood. Although classified as an herbicide, glyphosate is also a potent antibiotic, lethal to healthy bowel flora species such as *Lactobacillus* and *Bifidobacterium* species, while it does not affect unhealthy species—in other words, it *selects for* bacterial species that are harmful.[24,25] Proliferation of several unhealthy Clostridia species accompanied by the loss of several helpful Clostridia species (you can appreciate how efforts to untangle good from bad can be challenging) is now a prime suspect in causing autism in children, a phenomenon that has been associated with exposure to this herbicide.[26] Glyphosate is therefore at the top of the list of agricultural herbicides that contribute to bacterial overgrowth.

The pesticide chlorpyrifos, also widely used and present at high concentrations in some foods, degrades the intestinal mucus barrier and allows higher levels of toxic lipopolysaccharide (LPS) into the bloodstream, disruptions that increase the potential for insulin resistance, type 2 diabetes, and obesity.[27] Numerous other associations between herbicides and pesticides and disruptions of the microbiome and protective intestinal barrier have been documented. In short, living a modern life that includes eating mass-produced food, most of it delivered anonymously in frozen packages or from a drive-through window, makes it difficult, perhaps impossible, to dodge all the microbiome-disrupting factors coming at us.

Throw into the mix ubiquitous industrial chemicals such as bisphenol A (BPA) and polychlorinated biphenyls (PCBs) contaminating our water, soil, air, and food and heavy metals like mercury and cadmium, and you have even more bowel flora–disrupting effects. Even human breast milk and infant formula have been found to be riddled with numerous industrial compounds such as dioxin, PCBs, BPA, thiocyanate, and arsenic.[28]

At the hands of antibiotics and other pharmaceutical agents, artificial sweeteners, herbicides, pesticides, and industrial chemicals, our microbiomes are the casualties, battered survivors of a massive onslaught of disruptive chemicals. Many of us began life without the advantages of a healthy microbiome, engage in unhealthy diets that worsen the situation, then are exposed to numerous factors in modern life that further favor overgrowth of unhealthy bacterial species at the expense of protective species. Given the ubiquitous disruptions, you can appreciate that your poor, unsuspecting microbiome doesn't stand a chance, and you may, like millions of others, have become fecalized.

SINK YOUR TEETH INTO THIS

You may be getting the impression that disruption of the human microbiome is a modern phenomenon unique to the last half century. No question: the last fifty years represent an unprecedented acceleration of microbial disruption in the human body. But such changes got their start many thousands of years earlier. We know this from examinations of a number of unexpected sources: human teeth and fossilized fecal material ("coprolites"), along with insights emerging from the study of naturally mummified or frozen people from ancient cultures.

Collaborations between anthropologists and microbiologists show us that the emergence of agriculture, primarily cultivation of wheat and barley in the Middle East around twelve thousand years ago, was associated with a dramatic shift in oral bacteria to a population that favored species associated with tooth decay and periodontitis.[29] A shift in oral flora to species that ferment sugars from grains acidifies the oral cavity, leading to tooth decay. People are often surprised to learn that, prior to the adoption of agriculture, dental decay was unusual among hunter-gatherers, with only 1–3 percent of all teeth recovered showing decay.[30,31] Imagine: Cultures without toothbrushes, fluoridated toothpaste, dental floss, dentists, or dental plans, whose notion of dental hygiene was using a twig or blade of grass to pry loose a fragment of wildebeest from between their teeth, lived their lives, often to old age if they had survived early childhood, with full mouths of teeth, aligned and without decay, gingivitis, or abscesses. Many examples exist of ancient people who lived into their fifties, sixties, and seventies with mouths full of straight, intact teeth.

Then came agriculture and, with it, the consumption of wild, then cultivated wheat, barley, millet, and maize. In each and every locale where grains were consumed—wheat and barley in the Middle East, millet in sub-Saharan Africa, maize in Central America—tooth decay, gingivitis, periodontitis, abscesses, and tooth loss skyrocketed, affecting 16–49 percent of all teeth recovered.

That pattern continues today: 60–90 percent of all school-children have dental decay, 20 percent of adults have periodontal disease, and 100 percent of adults have some evidence of dental decay. The World Health Organization has reported a shocking proportion of people over the age of sixty-five who are edentulous, that is, entirely without teeth, with figures as high as 58 percent in Canada, 41 percent in Finland, and 26 percent in the United States.[32]

The human oral microbiome has clearly changed. Because the oral microbiome is a determinant of the intestinal microbiome, we can only speculate on what changes it provokes in the thirty feet of GI tract that receive swallowed oral microbes.

The modern human GI tract is therefore the site of a violent coup in which pathogenic *Escherichia coli* and *Klebsiella* species have taken over, ousting healthy probiotic species. These Enterobacteriaceae are the Vladimir Putins of the intestinal world, eager to seize more land, gain more resources. But the land in question is not Crimea or Ukraine but the human GI tract. No longer content to stay in the colon, these creatures have extended their reign into the small intestine, bringing their brand of fecalization with them.

It's this process of overproliferation of the Enterobacteriaceae species that yields some of the most troublesome health problems in modern people—bacterial proliferation in the small intestine, SIBO, which we shall discuss at greater length in Chapter 6.

Let's now go on to discuss one of nature's wonderful protective mechanisms that you share with snails and frogs and that you and your gut can put to work toward better health: intestinal mucus.

5
MIND YOUR MUCUS

ANOTHER PROTECTIVE FACTOR THAT MODERN LIFE HAS DIS-rupted is the mucus lining of the GI tract, among the first lines of defense against microbial chaos. Before you say "ewwww" as I bring up the topic of mucus, I'd like to convince you that the intestinal mucus lining is your good friend that keeps you from tangling with some nasty microbes.

Mucus is something you probably don't think about too often until it proves a nuisance. It's that gooey, messy thing coughed up, for instance, during a bout of the flu or blown out your nose with an allergy. But mucus plays a critical role in health, acting as a physical barrier, a medium for the body's immune system to work in, and a lubricant. Imagine living in a home that lacked the bricks, stucco, or aluminum siding that shields the interior. If instead you lived your life out in the open, with rain, wind, and snow pummeling you—it would be miserable. We need that shield against the elements. Likewise, a life without the protective layer of mucus would be harsh, perhaps impossible. Mucus makes it possible, for instance, for the stomach to contain hydrochloric acid—a substance powerful enough to remove paint that begins the digestive process—without digesting itself. Mucus allows the intestinal tract to tolerate regular injections of caustic bile and pancreatic enzymes that break down the proteins, fats, and carbohydrates we eat. Every region of the GI tract produces its own unique form of mucus, a wondrous and fascinating orchestration of protection and digestive function.

In addition to providing a defense against the onslaught of digestive warfare, mucus defends the cells in the gastrointestinal lining against infiltration by undigested components of the diet and forms a barrier against the trillions of microbes that inhabit the GI tract. Some factors fortify the mucus layer, other factors degrade it, and they can make the difference between magnificent intestinal health and a condition like ulcerative colitis. We are all less than one millimeter of mucus away from intestinal destruction and disease. Some have proposed that the initiating event in ulcerative colitis, for example, is a defective mucus lining of the colon that permits bacteria to invade the intestinal wall. Maintaining this crucial barrier is therefore a basic requirement for health.

Mucus is primitive, harking back to the first multicellular organisms. Its persistence all the way up to modern *Homo sapiens* reflects its indispensable nature, much like water and oxygen. Whereas creatures like snails and frogs are masters at mucus production, humans are pretty good at it too, producing the proteins that comprise mucus along every inch of the entire GI tract. Imagine swallowing chewed-up food, for instance, without lubrication—that bite of apple or hamburger might stay lodged in your esophagus for days.

The dense collections of microbes in the human GI tract are not meant to make direct contact with the intestinal lining. Mucus keeps them away. Only when the mucus lining breaks down or aggressive invasive microbes enter the picture is there direct contact. And which bacterial species inhabit the GI tract plays a major role in determining whether the mucus lining stays healthy and intact or is degraded, allowing microbes to breach it to reach the intestinal wall.

The primary food source for bacteria in the human GI tract is a specific form of fiber called "prebiotic fiber." Humans lack the digestive enzymes to break down prebiotic fibers, but bacteria can metabolize them and convert them to compounds that, in turn, nourish human intestinal cells. Bacterial "digestion" is therefore crucial to human health. But, when times are hard for bacteria and prebiotic fibers are in short supply or missing, some species turn to human mucus as an alternative source of nutrition, gobbling up and thinning the mucus lining.[1] This causes potentially serious health complications for the mucus-producing host, that is, you. We shall discuss this peculiar phenomenon a bit later.

The colon has a double layer of protective mucus, which offers better protection against the greater numbers of bacteria and fungi that are normally concentrated there and meant to live there. The small intestine has a more fragile single layer of protective mucus. What happens when microbes ascend from the colon into the small intestine, as in SIBO and SIFO, and high numbers are present in the upper GI tract, where the dual-layer protection of mucus is not present? The increased populations of microbes can compromise the small intestine's single-layer mucus lining, a breach that allows their metabolic breakdown products to enter the bloodstream. Sometimes even intact microbes themselves gain entry into the intestinal wall, then bloodstream to travel elsewhere. The entire process invites plenty of body-wide inflammation that takes many different forms and that we experience as conditions such as fibromyalgia, ulcerative colitis, or Hashimoto's thyroiditis.

Mucus may be something you'd prefer to ignore, but being aware of the crucial role this gooey compound plays in the human body can be a step toward success in regaining control over your microbiome and thereby your health.

ANY MUCUS ON THE MENU?

We know that modern people are fairly miserable at including plentiful fiber in their diet. No doubt, the transition from a diet of fibrous wild plants, roots, and tubers consumed by our hunter-gatherer ancestors to a diet of modern vegetables and fruits, bred for sweetness and low fiber content, coupled with the proliferation of processed foods, has reduced human fiber intake to a fraction of what it used to be. The "fix" recommended by various agencies providing dietary advice mostly focuses on including cellulose fiber such as that found in bran-rich breakfast cereals and whole grains. Cellulose is an indigestible form of fiber that passes through the GI tract passively, untouched by both human digestion and microbial digestion, so it provides "bulk" but accomplishes little else as it passes into the toilet, unchanged and intact.

The prebiotic variety of fiber, on the other hand, is far from passive. Prebiotic fibers are the primary food source for many species of intestinal bacteria, which convert them into metabolites crucial for human health. It's a genuine symbiotic relationship: They need us and we need them. We shall discuss later how a plentiful intake of prebiotic fibers thereby provides human benefits such as reduced blood sugar, reduced insulin resistance, lower triglycerides, less potential for fatty liver, and lower blood pressure.

Beyond missing out on the metabolic benefits of microbial consumption of prebiotic fibers, neglecting intake of prebiotic fibers leads to an odd phenomenon. When the human host fails to take in plentiful prebiotic fibers, some bacterial species proliferate because, as mentioned above, when they are deprived of prebiotic fibers, they can instead consume human mucus, a unique advantage (for them, not for us) that most bacterial species do not have. The bacterial species *Akkermansia muciniphila* (*mucin* + *phila* = mucus lover), for example, provides substantial health advantages when present at moderate numbers (e.g., 3–5 percent of the total intestinal bacterial population) by producing beneficial metabolites for the human host. But a drop in prebiotic fiber intake, as often occurs with an American-style processed food diet or excessively strict low-carb or ketogenic diets, brings out *Akkermansia*'s darker side, its ability to survive on human mucus. While other prebiotic fiber–consuming species die off or are reduced in numbers when starved, *Akkermansia* proliferates, even expanding to comprise 10 percent, 15 percent, 18 percent, or more of all bacterial species in the GI tract, and enthusiastically gobbles up human mucus. The end result is a disintegration of the gut's mucus lining.[2] This leads to intestinal inflammation, increased intestinal permeability, and endotoxemia, as well as increased potential for colon cancer.

This situation means that average Americans, deficient in total fiber intake and thereby woefully deficient in prebiotic fiber intake, live our lives on the edge of microbial despair, lacking in the beneficial microbial metabolites made by the shrinking populations of good microorganisms and intermittently causing some microbes to resort to mucus consumption. It also means that many people who follow ketogenic or other low-carb diets, lulled by near-term benefits, neglect prebiotic fiber intake, which can pave a path to long-term health deterioration.

Besides disregard of prebiotic fibers, what other factors contribute to disintegration of the protective mucus lining?

HOW ABOUT A LITTLE MORE MUCUS IN YOUR DAY?

Mucus is produced continuously by intestinal cells. You eat breakfast, you produce mucus. You sit at your desk, surf the internet, or rake leaves, you produce mucus. You go to sleep, you produce mucus. The mucus lining you had yesterday, or even this morning, is not the mucus lining you have now. It is a forgiving system that can remedy temporary disruptions within minutes, no more than hours, because of around-the-clock production of mucus proteins and other factors. Despite these extraordinary built-in safeguards, modern humans have still managed to muck it up.

Even if minding your mucus is not at the top of your list of life's priorities, being aware of the factors in everyday life that disrupt it can be important to your health and well-being because of mucus's impact on intestinal health and microbiome composition.

Probiotic bacteria such as *Lactobacillus* and *Bifidobacterium* species are on your side. They stimulate mucus production, yielding a thicker, more protective lining, and produce metabolites (e.g., butyrate, propionate) from prebiotic fibers that nourish the intestinal lining.[3] This may be one of the major reasons why commercial probiotics, despite being haphazard collections of organisms, may nonetheless be modestly beneficial. But there's more you can do to fortify your intestinal mucus barrier.

We've discussed how having a balance of *Akkermansia*—not too few, and not too many—also promotes healthy intestinal mucus because this species encourages mucus production even though it can also consume it. Have too few *Akkermansia* and you won't enjoy this microbe's stimulated mucus production or its substantial metabolic benefits, such as reduced blood sugar and reduced blood pressure. Have too many, as develops when you fail to consume plentiful prebiotic fiber, and *Akkermansia* proliferates out of control and consumes the mucus lining. We prevent this last potentially dangerous effect simply by including plenty of prebiotic fibers in our diet.

But we can go further to ensure that *Akkermansia* species are vigorously stimulated by including plenty of olive oil in our diet. A lot of scientific attention has been paid to extra-virgin olive oil's content of polyphenols such as hydroxytyrosol, but the main benefit likely comes from another component: the oleic acid fatty acid content of olive oil, which is around 70 percent oleic acid by weight. The oleic acid of olive oil is a great stimulator of *Akkermansia* proliferation.[4] Making a habit of including some extra-virgin olive oil in your day, by cooking with it, dipping in it (with the Herbed Focaccia Bread recipe, page 252, for example), or simply drizzling it over the top of a dish, is a tasty way to stimulate *Akkermansia* and thereby intestinal mucus health, provided you continue a habit of ingesting prebiotic fibers.

AKKERMANSIA AND THE THREE BEARS

Remember how, in the tale of Goldilocks and the Three Bears, Goldilocks enters the bears' home, samples their chairs, porridge, and beds, each time rejecting the biggest and smallest or hottest and coolest, then choosing the middle as "just right"?

That's how it goes with *Akkermansia* too: we don't want too many or too few; we want just the right number.

Include healthy foods such as prebiotic fiber–containing garlic and onions, polyphenol-rich vegetables and fruits, oleic acid from olive oil—all of which cause *Akkermansia* to bloom—and this species can be maintained at around 5 percent of total bowel flora, happily munching on the nutrients you provide and staying away from your mucus. At this "just right" level, *Akkermansia* is a wonderful cultivator of intestinal mucus and exerts substantial benefits such as normalizing insulin responses, reducing blood sugar, reducing triglycerides, preventing fatty liver, strengthening the intestinal barrier, and reducing endotoxemia.[4,5] *Akkermansia* is so crucial to the integrity of the mucus barrier that noted Dutch microbiome researcher Dr. Willem de Vos calls it "the gatekeeper of our mucosa."[6] (*Mucosa* refers to the thin cellular lining of the intestinal tract.)

Deprive them of prebiotic fibers and other nutrients they "prefer," and species such as *Akkermansia* survive by turning to human mucus for sustenance. This leads to intestinal inflammation, increased endotoxemia, and long-term health problems. Like

Goldilocks, we want it "just right" when it comes to *Akkerman-sia*, meaning they make up somewhere around 5 percent of total bowel flora.

Some people have no *Akkermansia* whatsoever, a situation that affects about 5 percent of the population. For these folks, no amount of prebiotic fiber or olive oil can grow *Akkermansia*, just as no amount of water and fertilizer will yield cucumbers in your backyard garden unless you plant them. For people who are miss-ing *Akkermansia*, a probiotic containing this species may be among the strategies to consider. (For a probiotic source of *Akkermansia*, see Appendix A.)

The entire situation therefore hinges on whether or not you eat enough foods that *Akkermansia* prefer: prebiotic fibers, poly-phenols in fruits and vegetables, oleic acid richest in olive oil. You cannot overdo these nutrients, and abundant intakes will not lead to *Akkermansia* overproliferation. It's only when you are deprived of these nutrients that *Akkermansia* is forced to become a mucus consumer.

The balance is not so delicate that you need to monitor your *Akkermansia* populations. But recognize that you can strike a healthy balance by including foods that cultivate this species, such as vegetables, fruits, and olive oil, while continuing to consume prebiotic fibers, also, so that you prevent *Akkermansia* from licking its lips before laying into your mucus lining.

Unexpected dietary factors also have the potential to stimulate intestinal mucus production. Star in this arena are cloves, of all odd things. The oil pressed from cloves is around 80 percent eugenol, an oily compound also present but to a lesser degree in cinnamon oil. Eugenol is a moderately potent antibacterial and antifungal, but further benefit comes from its unique capacity to stimulate the proliferation of several healthy species of Clostridia that, in turn, stimulate intestinal mucus production. The increase in intestinal mucus thickness in the presence of eugenol can be dramatic, in addition to the other potential benefits of enlisting healthy Clostridia.[7]

Another interesting class of plant polyphenols that yields intestinal mucus benefits is the catechins of green tea. They cross-link mucus proteins, which makes the mucus lining thicker, less semiliquid, and more like a gel, and thereby more protective including against infectious microbes and endotoxemia.[8] Among the recipes I provide later is a tasty smoothie that puts highly concentrated matcha green tea to work along with prebiotic fibers for this intestinal mucus–enhancing effect. You will also find a wonderfully healing recipe, Clove Green Tea, that combines the mucus-thickening effect of clove eugenol, the mucus protein cross-linking and gel-generating effect of green tea catechins, and the *Akkermansia*-cultivating effect of prebiotic fructooligosaccharides (FOSs), all to heal your intestinal mucus lining as you sip it throughout the day.

Just as your backyard garden can attract the attention of creatures like raccoons and rabbits, who dig up bulbs and munch on vegetables, so are there factors that break down the mucus lining and reduce its protective properties, a situation associated with real health problems. Erect a fence around your vegetable garden and it keeps out the pests. Maintain a vigorous intestinal mucus lining and it, likewise, keeps the pests away from your intestinal wall.

When the mucus lining is disrupted, the path is paved for motile bacteria, that is, bacterial species that can move independently, to ascend the GI tract. These creatures start out in the colon, climb ten or twelve feet of ileum, eight or nine feet of jejunum, eight inches of duodenum, and then enter the stomach. In other words, a change in mucus composition may be one of the reasons unhealthy bacterial species proliferate, then ascend, the process that leads to fecalization, SIBO, and SIFO. Restoring the vigor and strength of the intestinal mucus lining can therefore be an important part of your effort to rebuild bowel health after reversing dysbiosis, SIBO, SIFO, or any other gastrointestinal condition such as irritable bowel syndrome, celiac disease, ulcerative colitis, and Crohn's disease.

We've discussed how lack of prebiotic fiber intake leads to the proliferation of mucus-consuming species like *Akkermansia* that degrade the protective lining. Common factors in food, prescription and over-the-counter drugs, and even drinking water impact the mucus lining. Just exactly what disrupts the mucus lining, exposing intestinal cells to bacteria and fungi, and permits them to move up the GI tract?

SLIPPERY SLOPE

Have you ever seen an oily film rise to the top of the dishwater as you washed greasy dishes in a sink? You probably noticed that this layer immediately dispersed as soon as you added a few drops of dishwashing liquid to the water. That's what happens to your mucus lining when the wrong things enter your GI tract. You won't get clean dishes, of course, but an intestinal lining that is transiently dispersed exposes intestinal cells to bacteria, food, and digestive components like bile.

Let's talk about emulsifying agents for a minute. Emulsifiers are added to processed foods to keep the ingredients mixed and to prevent separation. Without emulsifiers, peanut butter separates: solids at the bottom, oil on top. In contrast, commercial peanut butters made with emulsifying agents remain smooth and mixed. Emulsifiers also keep ice cream from separating into solids and ice, especially after thawing and refreezing. Who hasn't had the experience of refreezing melted ice cream only to confront an icy mess the next time you dig in? It's hardly the creamy, smooth stuff you want to serve on top of a slice of pie. Most manufacturers add emulsifiers to inhibit this separation.

But the emulsifiers found in foods such as ice cream, salad dressings, and peanut butter are proving to be major culprits in damaged mucus health. The emulsifying agents that keep peanut butter mixed and ice cream creamy also disrupt human mucus because they act like dishwashing liquid, dispersing and thinning the gooey mucus and allowing bacteria to come into close contact with intestinal cells. Although the effect is transient, it is sufficient to cause inflammation of the intestinal wall, endotoxemia, and changes in the bacterial species that comprise bowel flora.

Dr. Benoit Chassaing at the Institute for Biomedical Sciences at Georgia State University in Atlanta is a pioneer in exploring this effect. Chassaing and colleagues have demonstrated that synthetic agents such as polysorbate 80 and carboxymethylcellulose, despite having received the blessing of the FDA as safe food additives, exert potent disruptive effects on the mucus barrier. Transient dissolution of the mucus barrier allows bacteria to contact the intestinal lining and then invade the superficial layer of intestinal cells, which causes inflammation. Emulsifiers also provoke changes in microbial species in the GI tract, increasing populations of Enterobacteriaceae, the organisms of bacterial overgrowth and SIBO. Gut changes introduced by emulsifiers also lead to increased appetite, weight gain, and worsened insulin resistance, prediabetes, and type 2 diabetes.[9]

Think about the implications of these findings: emulsifiers added to processed foods like ice cream contribute to weight gain, obesity, type 2 diabetes, colitis, dysbiosis, and SIBO—it's not the fat or the calories that are problems; *it's the emulsifying agents*. There is also growing suspicion that such food additives may underlie the increasing incidence of inflammatory bowel diseases, ulcerative colitis, and Crohn's disease, the rates of which are now exploding in other countries that have recently adopted a Western diet.[10] Although only polysorbate 80 and carboxymethylcellulose have been studied to date, it is likely that most other, perhaps all, food additives with emulsifying properties, such as carrageenan, dextran sulfate, and propylene glycol, among others, have the same detrimental effects.

I don't think you need me to tell you the bottom line: avoid polysorbate 80, carboxymethylcellulose, and other emulsifiers completely. This means being vigilant in your choices of peanut butter, ice cream, and other fat-containing products, or even better, return to eating foods that don't require labels, like eggs and avocados. It's also simple to make your own foods like ice cream, and I trust you not to add polysorbate 80 or other additives. (Later, I provide several recipes to get you started.) Your bowel flora will thank you.

Modern life includes a number of other mucus-disrupting factors. Similar deleterious effects have been associated with the common food additive maltodextrin, which is found in pastas, frozen meals, sports drinks, and other processed foods.[11] Chlorinated drinking water of the sort that comes out of your kitchen or bathroom faucet disrupts mucus, which, in turn, disrupts intestinal health and encourages growth of intestinal polyps that can lead to colon cancer.[12] Widely consumed nonsteroidal anti-inflammatory drugs, such as ibuprofen, naproxen, indomethacin, and diclofenac, taken by tens of millions of people every year for arthritis pain, menstrual cramps, and headache, are potent disrupters of the mucus lining and microbiome composition.[13] While exercise exerts beneficial effects on intestinal health and bowel flora, extreme exercise of the sort that has people carb-loading ahead of time and running twenty-six miles while suffering cramps, bloating, and diarrhea also disrupts the mucus lining, leading to increased intestinal permeability, endotoxemia, and a rise in inflammation and autoimmune conditions.[14] Suspicion that prolonged emotional stress may also exert harmful health effects via impairment of the mucus lining is also growing.[15] The shift in bacterial species away from healthy species and toward those that proliferate in bacterial overgrowth and SIBO can, by itself, also decrease mucus production and, of course, does so along the entire length of GI tract wherever unhealthy species have taken up residence.[2]

We haven't even tackled the mucus-disruptive effects of antibiotics, the hundreds of other food additives in soft drinks, juices, canned and frozen foods, or the thousands of prescription drugs. I'll remind you that none of these mucus-disruptive factors entered into the lives of hunter-gatherers who hunted and killed or foraged their next meal but are ubiquitous in the lives of those of us who have been persuaded that a meal delivered in a Styrofoam container or microwavable plastic tray, ice cream that never separates, and anti-inflammatory drugs to "treat" psoriatic arthritis are somehow part of a superior lifestyle.

I hope you now appreciate how numerous factors in modern life and diet have set the stage for impairment of our crucial intestinal mucus lining. All of us have been exposed to these many disruptive factors, all of which invite trouble in the form of modern chronic diseases. Avoiding the factors that disrupt the mucus lining and restoring the bacterial species that stimulate intestinal mucus production are therefore crucial to your health and life.

Take care of your mucus lining and it will take care of you. Let's now go on to the serious business of SIBO.

PART II

FRANKENBELLY AND FRIENDS

6

SIBO: FRANKENBELLY

I'LL BET YOU ARE ANXIOUS TO GET TO THE PART OF THE BOOK where I show you how to cultivate microbes that achieve effects such as youthful skin, restoration of youthful muscle, and reduced anxiety and depression. But before we go to the really fun part, we need to clear the way for healthy replacements of the unhealthy microbes most of us have cultivated. We don't want to throw our super microbes into a nasty snake pit.

Right now, you might be intolerant of beans or onions, experiencing excessive gas and bloating after a bowl of chili. Or you have the muscle and joint pains of fibromyalgia that keep you from engaging in simple physical activities like gardening or cleaning your house. Or you suffer the bowel urgency of irritable bowel syndrome that prevents you from venturing more than a few miles from home without having memorized the locations of all public bathrooms. Or you might be overweight, have type 2 diabetes, or suffer with an autoimmune condition like rheumatoid arthritis or Hashimoto's thyroiditis or the numerous other conditions that seem to plague more and more people. Or perhaps you feel fine but are not aware that diet soda, ice cream, and ibuprofen can trigger unhealthy changes in your microbiome. Perhaps you've accepted conventional "solutions" to these chronic conditions—prescriptions from your doctor such as insulin, steroids, and other drugs, or gastric bypass or other surgical or procedural "remedies" for overweight and obesity. Accept solutions offered by conventional health care and just what have you accomplished?

By following the routine advice of medical doctors, you might manage to alleviate the outward phenomena (signs and symptoms) of a disease process yet fail to address the underlying microbial overgrowth that has overtaken your GI tract. You may now begin to appreciate how limited conventional medical solutions are when they do nothing to address the massive disruption of bowel flora that can cause (or worsen) a condition. When you resort to drugs or procedures, they often end up making matters worse. What are the potential consequences of, say, treating fibromyalgia with prescription drugs, which provide temporary relief by blunting pain pathways but do nothing to address the underlying SIBO causing the condition?

The consequences of uncorrected SIBO read like a playbook of deteriorating health that defines modern aging and the common, widespread health conditions that fill the daily schedules of most doctors—who only Band-Aid their patients' health struggles with this or that pharmaceutical. Uncorrected SIBO can permit an autoimmune condition like rheumatoid arthritis or lupus to emerge, increase risk for coronary artery disease, allow insulin resistance to persist or worsen, increase blood sugar, raise blood pressure, contribute to fatty liver, or lead to diverticular disease and even colon cancer. Uncorrected SIBO may even expose you to increased risk for neurodegenerative diseases. In other words, it is downright foolhardy not to take steps to address SIBO and cultivate a return to healthy bowel flora.

Admittedly, the human colon is not a pretty place. It's not flowery or scented with delicate perfumes (quite the opposite in fact!), but it performs several crucial functions for life. It is, for instance, where water is absorbed from the semiliquid mix of partially digested food that flows down from the small intestines. The semisolid waste that results is then retained in the muscular rectum, stored in order to eliminate under purposeful control when the opportunity arises, not to trickle out during a business meeting or while driving in traffic.

The colon is also home to trillions of microbes, some friendly, some not so friendly. Some microbes assist in the digestive process, others yield metabolites that benefit other microbes, and still others produce vitamins that your body can use, and all compete with other species for nutrients and survival. Ideally, friendly microbes dominate the population in your colon, keeping potentially pathogenic species at bay, an around-the-clock Hatfield-versus-McCoy struggle to control this five-foot-long piece of internal real estate.

As we've discussed, numerous factors upset the balance and can allow unhealthy species to dominate. In some people, unhealthy species proliferate as a result of, say, the glyphosate contained in a burrito or an aspartame-sweetened can of diet cola. If these microbes remain in the colon, where they live and die and outcompete useful species, then this is the situation we call colonic dysbiosis. You might also recall that, although the colon is protected by a tough, two-layer mucus lining, proliferating colon-dwelling fecal Enterobacteriaceae and other unhealthy species can weaken it, breaching the intestinal walls and spewing bacterial and fungal breakdown products into the bloodstream. This situation, responsible for such health conditions as ulcerative colitis, diverticular disease, and colon cancer, is bad enough.

But in many people, it gets worse, much worse. Some unhealthy microbes refuse to remain where they belong and instead ascend the five feet of colon into the twenty-four feet or so of ileum, jejunum, duodenum, and stomach—no small feat for microscopic organisms to buck gravity and scurry to places where your body is unprepared for such an onslaught. Imagine I put a ladder in front of you and ask you to climb twenty-four feet higher than your full upright height, which would put you face-to-face with the roof of a three-story building. Shove aside any fear of heights and you might enjoy the view from that vantage point. But how can microbes accomplish such a feat when there is no captivating views of the hills of Tuscany or no alluring scenes of trees and mountains to tempt them but just . . . your GI tract?

Every era of human existence has had a health scourge that defined and shaped life and health during that age. For thousands of years, up until the twentieth century, it was syphilis, so varied in its manifestations— skin sores, enlarged lymph nodes, even dementia—it was called "the Great Pretender." Historically, the cause of this sexually transmitted disease was blamed on everything from tainted water to demonic possession, with useless treatments administered that included arsenic and mercury. Not until the twentieth century did science uncover the bacterium responsible and mostly eradicate it with antibiotics. In other times, scourges included smallpox, tuberculosis, iodine deficiency, and, most recently, coronavirus.

Unlike syphilis or smallpox, or even COVID-19, SIBO is a man-made condition, much like the epidemics of type 2 diabetes and overweight/ obesity that also plague our age. SIBO is caused by the factors that surround you, such as herbicides and pesticides in food and stomach acid–blocking drugs prescribed by doctors. SIBO can also be caused by behaviors, seemingly benign practices such as consumption of sugary or sugar-free soda and even something as familiar and comforting as ice cream or ranch salad dressing.

These factors are, to a great degree, modern phenomena. Nobody in 1950 ate glyphosate-laced corn or was exposed to the polysorbate 80 added to ice cream or took statin drugs to reduce cholesterol. And in no other time has there been more irritable bowel syndrome, type 1 and type 2 diabetes, hypertension, ulcerative colitis and Crohn's disease, autoimmune diseases, skin rashes, food allergies, and neurodegenerative diseases.

Though they may not kill you by next Tuesday, or cause an acute illness necessitating an ICU stay for three weeks, colonic dysbiosis and, even more so, SIBO can result in numerous health conditions that lead to doctor visits, prescriptions, and procedures that bandage over symptoms—but never address the actual cause. We therefore need to redefine so many previously held beliefs about health and disease. Many diseases unique to modern people are *not* best managed using new drugs that block, for instance, some inflammatory pathway or force blood sugar or blood pressure levels down— this is treating the symptoms—but are better managed by getting at the root cause: unhealthy changes in bowel flora.

SIBO is an invasion of your small intestine: unhealthy fecal bacterial species proliferate in the colon, outmuscle beneficial probiotic species, then ascend to take up residence where they don't belong, in the small intestine. These unwanted interlopers degrade the thin single layer of intestinal mucus that lines and protects the upper GI tract. The weakened mucus lining then paves the way for toxic microbial breakdown products to gain entry into the bloodstream for export to other organs.

Just in the few moments it took you to read the last paragraph, billions of microbes lived and died inside your gut. There are, of course, no graveyards for these creatures. They live their brief lives, nonsentient but collaborating and competing with other microbes, then die, releasing the components of their "bodies" into the mix of food, water, enzymes, bile, and other living and dead microbes that fill the intestines. Some of this microbial debris infiltrates the bloodstream. This phenomenon of endotoxemia, substantiated by Dr. Patrice Cani and French colleagues in 2007, provides the crucial missing link that explains how microbes living in the GI tract can cause, for instance, the skin rash of rosacea, the thyroid inflammation of Hashimoto's thyroiditis, or the muscle and joint pain of fibromyalgia, effects far outside the GI tract itself.[1] The dominant toxin transported through the blood is lipopolysaccharide (LPS), a component of the cell walls of Enterobacteriaceae, the main species of fecal bacterial overgrowth and SIBO. In other words, the trillions of microbes in the Enterobacteriaceae family living and dying in the GI tract can exert effects on every other organ and tissue of the body when they die and release the components that make up their cells, namely, LPS, into the bloodstream.

People with SIBO have tenfold higher levels of LPS in the portal circulation, which drains blood from the GI tract and delivers it to the liver. This tells us that the liver is hugely battered by the by-products of bacterial overgrowth, and the onslaught contributes to liver inflammation in fatty liver disease that can progress to cirrhosis (a dangerous type of fibrosis of the liver). They also have two- to fourfold higher levels of LPS in the systemic bloodstream, which effectively exports the consequences of SIBO far and wide to other parts of the body.

Injection of even a microscopic amount of LPS into a laboratory mouse yields an overwhelming inflammatory response, often sufficient to kill the animal. LPS originates in the cell walls of *Escherichia coli* and *Salmonella* and *Pseudomonas* species—yes: the species of SIBO that should only be found in fecal material. (You may recognize the names of these microbes because several related strains cause food poisoning, such as when the kid who failed to wash his hands after using the bathroom prepares your fast-food burger.) You and I are exposed to higher amounts of LPS when fecal bacteria proliferate and claw their way up the thirty feet of permeable GI tract.

It has also become clear that, in addition to their leaked breakdown products, even microbes themselves manage to gain a foothold in the intestinal lining and beyond. Look for microbes in gallstones and you will find them. Look for microbes in pancreatic cancer and they will likely be there. Just how involved microbes are in *causing* such diseases, however, is a story that we're still unfolding. But, just as footprints in the mud outside your bedroom window might be proof of an attempted burglary, the presence of microbes in regions far outside the colon where they originate points toward intestinal bacterial and fungal overgrowth as the source of the disease. How do bacteria like *E. coli*, for instance, get into gallstones when the gallbladder is twenty-four feet away from the colon where *E. coli* normally lives? The colonization of the upper GI by the bacteria of SIBO might explain it. How can bacteria or fungi gain a foothold in the brain? The intestinal invasion by microbes that then erode the intestinal wall and enter the bloodstream is the most likely path. It's a phenomenon so new there is no official label for it: bacterial and fungal species that do not cause outright or overt infection take up residence in various organs and potentially trigger reactions that are expressed as conditions such as pancreatitis and gallstones and dementia.

How do you know if you have allowed such processes to develop? Do specific signs tell you that undesirable microbes have climbed three times the height of your living room ceiling to squat in parts of your GI tract that should be microbial deserts and are now shedding huge amounts of toxic LPS? If there are no footprints or fingerprints to detect their presence, what evidence can you uncover that hints at this microbial invasion?

You can indeed identify the signs of SIBO, what I call "telltale signs." (I shall do the same with SIFO in Chapter 7.) Just as water pooling in your basement signals a problem with water drainage that can end in disaster, so can varied body signs suggest the presence of unhealthy bacteria in the upper GI tract.

One issue, however, is not entirely clear: Where does dysbiosis, that is, disruption of bowel flora composition in the colon, end and where does SIBO begin? In dysbiosis, unhealthy bacterial species have proliferated and suppressed growth of beneficial species but have not ascended into the small bowel. SIBO is a more severe version of colonic dysbiosis in which the same species have proliferated but also ascended.

It is not an all-or-none situation. What if disruptions of bacterial species occur only in the colon, yet lead to diverticular disease and colon cancer? What if the bacterial species of SIBO proliferate in the colon, then ascend only ten feet of the ileum—is that SIBO? Changes in bacterial species composition as well as determining how high up bacteria have migrated are therefore important factors to consider. Obviously, the burden of unhealthy bacteria is greater in SIBO, as there are thirty feet or so of unhealthy bacterial species, as compared to the five feet of colonic dysbiosis. The burden of endotoxemia is greater in SIBO because of the far greater number of bacteria and the small intestines' vulnerability of a thinner mucus lining. Colonic dysbiosis is an abnormal situation with important implications for health, but SIBO presents a worse situation with even greater implications for health.

Dysbiosis confined to the colon generally responds to basic changes in diet, selected nutritional supplements, the addition of advantageous microbiomes from fermented foods, and a few other strategies that shift the composition of bacterial species back to something that better approximates a collection of health-supporting microbes, strategies that I will discuss later. But right now let's discuss how to decide whether a situation worse than dysbiosis is present in which bacteria have migrated northward, taken up residence as high as the duodenum or stomach, and are yielding endotoxemia, thereby necessitating efforts to address SIBO.

Through all this fuss, I want you to know that it's *you* who should be in control. Even if it were only a matter of size, you should be the boss because you are, after all, millions of times larger than the microbes who influence your mind and metabolism. But you should be calling the shots, telling those *Lactobacillus* and Clostridia species who is in charge and kicking those pesky *Klebsiella* and *Salmonella* species to the curb, squashing them with your heel, because it's your body. In a battle between an ant and you, who is likely to win? Unless you are the most acquiescent, passive victim, you should emerge the victor over these teensy-weensy creatures.

THE TELLTALE SIGNS OF SIBO

When you are bitten by a mosquito, do you know it?

Darn right you do: you are plagued by the familiar red, raised mound of skin that itches like mad, repeatedly distracting you, even disrupting sleep.

SIBO, like a mosquito bite, has its own characteristic signs that, when present, signal that you have trillions of rapidly reproducing microbes that have invaded the full length of your GI tract, flooding the bloodstream with their toxic by-products. The upper GI tract is ill equipped to deal with invaders such as *Salmonella* and *Pseudomonas*—bacterial species that your colon is familiar with because they are commonly found in fecal material but are foreigners in the upper reaches of the GI tract. They erode the thin mucus lining of the small intestine, deliver a flood of breakdown products into the bloodstream, and some then invade the intestinal wall and cause inflammation.

So, what are the telltale signs that signal a thirty-foot-long infection and body-wide invasion by the by-products of SIBO? The list is long and includes the following clues:

- **Food intolerances**—Food intolerance presents in a variety of forms: food allergies, intolerance to prebiotic fibers, intolerance to FOD-MAPs (fermentable oligo-, di-, monosaccharides and polyols, essentially all sugars and prebiotic fibers—see the box that discusses this further), intolerance to onions, garlic, and nightshades (eggplant, tomatoes, potatoes, peppers) or histamine-provoking foods (shellfish, aged cheeses, nuts, beans, and many others), intolerance to fructose, sorbitol, eggs, soy, and other foods. It is not uncommon for people to identify long lists of foods they must avoid. The most common experience is to consume any food that contains prebiotic fiber, such as legumes, root vegetables, or inulin-containing foods such as onions, that is followed by excessive gas, bloating, diarrhea, or emotional effects such as anxiety, dark thoughts or depression, or anger within ninety minutes of consumption. (See Part IV for a list of foods containing prebiotic fibers.) These reactions signal the presence of bacteria high up in the GI tract, places that foods can reach within the first ninety minutes of the digestive process, which is not enough time to reach the colon twenty-four feet farther down. Likewise, these sorts of reactions to any sugar strongly suggest SIBO (as well as SIFO). Children can also be plagued by such intolerances, which restrict them to a short list of foods they can tolerate. Avoiding offending food(s) is *not* a solution, although it can serve to reduce symptoms in the near term; addressing the microbial disaster that created the food intolerances in the first place is more likely to yield meaningful long-term solutions. The majority of food intolerances represent SIBO with increased intestinal permeability that leads to entry of microbial and food by-products into the bloodstream that provoke immune responses, which are mistakenly interpreted as food intolerances. This doesn't stop people from advocating all manner of food-avoidance techniques, many of them impossibly restrictive. It also means that many forms of food intolerance testing are really just indirect methods of identifying SIBO. Instead, see most food intolerances for what they really are: SIBO.[2-5]

- **Fat malabsorption**—Although a number of factors can interfere with the ability to digest dietary fats, SIBO is the most common cause in people who are not hospitalized or acutely ill and who have not suffered damage to the pancreas or gallbladder. You can identify fat malabsorption by seeing fat droplets in the toilet after a bowel movement or fat staining around the toilet where water meets porcelain.

- **Persistent or recurrent skin rashes**—You may have consulted a dermatologist for eczema, rosacea, or psoriasis and submitted to their steroid creams or costly biologic drugs that come with life-threatening side effects such as respiratory and fungal skin infections, even lymphoma, as well as huge price tags ($10,000 to $50,000 every three months is not uncommon—no kidding). But you follow their prescription only to have the rash recur or not respond. Time to consider the effects of SIBO (as well as SIFO, discussed in Chapter 7).[6-8]

- **Specific health conditions with high likelihood of SIBO**—Being overweight or obese or having prediabetes or type 2 diabetes, any autoimmune condition, fatty liver, fibromyalgia, irritable bowel syndrome, restless leg syndrome, chronic constipation, rosacea, psoriasis, or presence of a neurodegenerative condition such as Parkinsonism or Alzheimer's dementia signals a high likelihood—as much as 50 percent or more—that SIBO is a prominent player in causing, or at least worsening, the condition.[9-15]

- **Stomach acid–suppressing and anti-inflammatory drugs**—Taking stomach acid–suppressing drugs like omeprazole, pantoprazole, or ranitidine substantially increases likelihood of SIBO, and the longer you've taken one of these drugs, the more likely that SIBO has developed.[16] Likewise, having taken nonsteroidal anti-inflammatory drugs such as ibuprofen, naproxen, or diclofenac, especially for periods of weeks to months, increases the likelihood of SIBO.[17]

- **Lack of stomach acid**—A history of *Helicobacter pylori* infection in the stomach or of hypochlorhydria (lack of stomach acid) is a setup for SIBO. Just as with stomach acid–blocking drugs, lack of stomach acid resulting from *H. pylori* infection or autoimmune gastritis, conditions signaled by prolonged presence of food in the stomach or discomfort upon consuming proteins such as meats, makes bacterial overgrowth much more suspect. SIBO in this situation can be severe, with heavy bacterial infestation of the stomach.[18]

- **History of opioid drug use**—Because opioids slow intestinal activity, they are an open invitation to SIBO.[19] Incidentally, the opioid peptides that derive from the consumption of the gliadin protein of wheat likewise slow intestinal activity and invite SIBO, an issue that I will discuss further.

- **Hypothyroidism**—Because lack of thyroid hormones slows intestinal activity, hypothyroidism also allows proliferation of unhealthy bacterial species. SIBO has been found in more than 50 percent of people with a history of hypothyroidism, even if they have taken thyroid hormones (which likely means that SIBO developed before thyroid hormone correction). Preliminary evidence also points to the fact that simply replacing the T4 thyroid hormone using levothyroxine without addressing the T3 hormone can contribute to the development of SIBO.[20,21]

- **History of abdominal surgery**—Any surgery involving a change in normal anatomy, such as gastric bypass, gastrectomy, cholecystectomy, or colectomy encourages SIBO. Even gallstones and a history of pancreatitis have high-risk associations with SIBO.[22]

This is a partial list of only the most common situations highly associated with SIBO. If none of the above apply to you, you may still have SIBO, as we shall discuss.

FODMAPS: SHOOT THE MESSENGER

Your accountant informs you that your tax bill has increased substantially and the IRS wants its money. You promptly lose control and give your poor accountant a verbal thrashing.

That's called "shooting the messenger." It's not the accountant's fault that your taxes went up—he's just the unfortunate provider of the news.

So, what should we make of people who find that they are intolerant of foods that fall under the categories of fermentable (i.e., fermented by microbes) oligosaccharides, disaccharides, monosaccharides (three types of sugars), and polyols (also called sugar alcohols) known collectively as FODMAPs? They experience excessive gas, bloating, abdominal pain, and diarrhea when exposed to foods containing these sugars that microbes ferment. This can be a problem in people labeled as having irritable bowel syndrome (IBS) and inflammatory bowel diseases such as ulcerative colitis and Crohn's disease. People with these conditions are therefore often advised to avoid eating foods such as fruit, sugars, sorbitol, legumes, and dairy products, all of which contain FODMAPs; these severe limitations can reduce symptoms.

But are these foods the problem or are they just the "messenger"? That is, is something else to blame for the intestinal discomfort? After all, recall that many cases of IBS are really SIBO and that many people with inflammatory bowel diseases have their condition complicated, if not outright caused, by SIBO. I would therefore argue that the problem is not FODMAPs; the problem is the microbes of SIBO residing in the full length of the GI tract or of dysbiosis in the colon that metabolize these foods and thereby cause unpleasant symptoms.

But by avoiding FODMAPs in your diet, you are essentially starving bacteria—good and bad—of their preferred foods. Starving microbes changes the composition of the microbiome as some species die out, with reductions, for instance, in important beneficial species such as *Bifidobacterium longum* (which plays a major role in regulating mood) and *Faecalibacterium prausnitzii* (the most vigorous producer of butyrate, a fatty acid that heals and nourishes the intestinal lining). Whereas reducing the number of SIBO-related species is good, reducing or sometimes even eliminating beneficial species is detrimental.[23] And, if you lose species, as discussed earlier, you cannot grow them back.

Like taking aspirin for a headache, avoiding FODMAPs is only a symptom-limiting strategy and does not address the root cause, and it may even make your microbiome situation worse in the long term. Address the root cause—dysbiosis and SIBO—and you are likely to once again enjoy biting into an apple or having lentils in your soup.

WHO'S GOT SIBO?

SIBO and SIFO are conditions that habits and lifestyle factors have created. They are health conditions indifferent to race, sex, age, and political persuasion. Even following an otherwise healthy lifestyle may not have protected you either because the factors creating bacterial and fungal overgrowth are so widespread.

SIBO is so common that, in any classroom, office, or social situation, you are likely to encounter several people, if not the majority, with this condition. And, of course, it could also include you. Whereas plenty of headlines publicize the epidemics of overweight and obesity, the epidemic of SIBO is at least as large and affects as many, if not more, people but is hardly talked about. You can see signs of SIBO in the people around you: the facial rash of rosacea, the abdominal fat of obesity, and the gnarled and swollen joints of rheumatoid arthritis. But its signs and symptoms are also often hidden, experienced privately as the bowel urgency of irritable bowel syndrome or the inability to eat common foods without an unpleasant reaction.

Let's therefore discuss which health conditions suggest the underlying presence of SIBO. Clinical studies correlate various conditions with SIBO, though research results have varied given the evolution of testing methods (older methods of detection tend to underestimate SIBO). Conditions associated with SIBO include the following:

- **Obesity**—SIBO has been documented in 23–88.9 percent of obese people. This alone suggests a potentially huge number of people with SIBO considering that 70 million Americans are obese, meaning somewhere between 16 and 62 million people with obesity have SIBO.[24] This doesn't even factor in the additional 60 million Americans who are overweight, but not obese.
- **Diabetes**—The likelihood of SIBO in type 1 and type 2 diabetes is in the range of 11 percent to 60 percent.[25] With 34 million people with type 2 diabetes and 1.3 million people with type 1 diabetes, we can tally up at least several million people with diabetes who also have SIBO.
- **Irritable bowel syndrome (IBS)**—Estimates vary, but generally 35 percent to 84 percent of people with IBS test positive for SIBO.[26] Thirty to 35 million Americans have been diagnosed with IBS, and an equal number are believed to have the condition without a formal diagnosis. Of the total 60 to 70 million people with IBS, this adds another 21 to 50 million Americans with SIBO to the tally.
- **Inflammatory bowel disease**—Around 22 percent of the 3 million people with ulcerative colitis or Crohn's disease also have SIBO.[27]
- **Fatty liver**—Nonalcoholic fatty liver disease, a condition estimated to now affect nearly half the US population, carries a 40–60 percent likelihood of SIBO.[28] This means that around 75 million American adults with fatty liver also have SIBO.
- **Autoimmune diseases**—Each disease in this disparate collection of conditions, which includes systemic sclerosis, rheumatoid arthritis, psoriatic arthritis, and type 1 diabetes, has a varying association with SIBO. Preliminary studies suggest that around 40 percent of people with an autoimmune condition have SIBO.[28]
- **Skin rashes**—Rosacea, psoriasis, and eczema have been associated with SIBO in about 40–50 percent of people with these conditions, meaning that another 6 million Americans have SIBO.[29] People with rosacea, in particular, have a tenfold greater likelihood of having SIBO.[30]
- **Parkinson's disease**—Of the 1 million people in the United States with this incapacitating neurodegenerative condition, 25 percent to 67 percent have SIBO.[31]

- **Alzheimer's dementia**—The evidence is preliminary, but people with Alzheimer's have a fivefold increased likelihood of also having SIBO.[31]
- **Restless leg syndrome**—This condition prevents deep sleep with consequent substantial effects on mental, emotional, and metabolic health, and it is accompanied by SIBO in up to 100 percent of sufferers.[32]
- **Depression and anxiety**—Emerging evidence demonstrates that many of the 60 million Americans struggling with these psychological issues have dramatically higher blood levels of LPS, along with measures of increased intestinal permeability, pointing to SIBO.[33]

It's tough to come up with an exact figure of just how many Americans might be affected by SIBO not only because estimates vary depending on the testing method used to identify SIBO but also because there is overlap between groups: for example, some obese people also have type 2 diabetes, fatty liver, and psoriasis. But from the figures above, I believe that you can still appreciate that SIBO is far from an uncommon condition. It is certainly not an "orphan" condition like Kasabach-Merritt syndrome (a rare disease in infants) or Whipple's disease (a rare infectious disease) that could elude even the best doctors. In fact, I believe that a back-of-the-envelope calculation tells us that the number of people walking around with SIBO is staggering. Even if we use the low end of SIBO incidence in obese people, 23 percent, it means that 16 million people have SIBO (and are likely unaware of it). Of the 60 to 70 million people with IBS, using the low end of 35 percent with SIBO translates to 21 million people with SIBO. If half the 200 million adults in the United States with fatty liver disease also have SIBO, then that's at least another 40 million. Keep on tallying up the numbers and you will see that the sum easily exceeds 100 million people in the United States with SIBO, or approximately one in every three people.

Add to that number the many people who have silent SIBO, that is, they have bacterial overgrowth but do not (yet) have symptoms. We see silent bacterial overgrowth playing out in nearly every clinical study in which people with some health condition are compared to "healthy controls," or people presumed to be healthy. In one clinical study of people with irritable bowel syndrome, for instance, 30 percent of 150 participants in the healthy control group proved positive for SIBO.[34]

From a practical standpoint, you may also appreciate that some conditions are so consistently associated with SIBO that, if someone has any of these conditions, the likelihood of SIBO having either caused that health condition or worsened it is very high, and therefore these conditions serve as a virtual red flag for SIBO. Irritable bowel syndrome, fibromyalgia, restless leg syndrome, and fatty liver are among these red flag conditions. But expanding evidence reveals that the universe of health conditions caused or worsened by SIBO includes autoimmune, neurodegenerative, metabolic, and atherosclerotic conditions.

It is not uncommon for people with SIBO to suffer undiagnosed with various health conditions for years, even decades, enduring pain, disability, frustrating doctors' appointments that yield only partially effective or ineffective pharmaceutical solutions. Despite the flood of evidence, most practicing physicians remain unaware of this widespread and profound disruption of human health. Most conventional medical solutions fail to address the underlying cause: proliferation of unhealthy microbial species that export their inflammatory effects to other parts of the body.

IS THAT HYDROGEN I SMELL ON YOUR BREATH?

To chart the location of bacteria in the GI tract, we don't use a map, compass, or GPS. Step one in confirming whether SIBO is present is determining whether hordes of bacteria are living in the upper GI tract. This was previously a cumbersome and difficult process. But it has recently become as easy as turning on your smartphone and texting a friend.

Not everyone, of course, has SIBO. Many simply have some version of dysbiosis, that is, the situation in which undesirable microbial and fungal species have proliferated, outmuscled desirable species, disrupted the mucus lining, and caused endotoxemia, but remain confined to the fecal material of the colon. Because disruptions of the modern microbiome are so common, it is safe to assume that *everyone* begins with some degree of dysbiosis. You could submit a stool sample for analysis to document the proliferation of Enterobacteriaceae species such as *E. coli* and *Salmonella* and *Campylobacter* species (though such analyses do not map out *where* in the GI tract these fecal bacteria are located). But, if there are no telltale signs of SIBO or you test negative (discussed below) for SIBO, then the basic efforts I shall lay out that include a high-potency, multispecies probiotic (or a probiotic you make yourself; I will show you how), fermented foods, prebiotic fibers, and some other simple methods will almost always help you chart your way back to a healthier microbiome.

If SIBO is present, however, additional efforts will be necessary. In SIBO, microbes have, of course, ascended the GI tract. A gastroenterologist can insert an endoscope and obtain a sample of upper intestinal contents to examine for bacteria, but this represents a flawed method because it is invasive, is subject to difficulties in sampling fluid without contamination, and identifies only severe cases of SIBO in which bacteria have ascended high up in the GI tract, not the cases in which bacteria lodge deeper in the small intestine, beyond the reach of the endoscope. In most instances, the aspirate is then cultured, but most of the species that contribute to SIBO cannot be cultured because typically they are anaerobic and die on contact with oxygen. This means that earlier studies (studies up until the last few years) have underestimated the incidence of SIBO because they yielded negative results even when fecal bacterial proliferation was present. Although gastroenterologists prefer this endoscopy method, given the economics of medical procedures, it is not the most user-friendly or reliable because it is subject to plenty of "false negatives," showing negative results even when SIBO is present.

Other, less-invasive methods take advantage of the ability of bacteria to produce hydrogen (H_2) gas, something that humans are not very good at doing. If plentiful H_2 gas is detected in the breath rapidly after consuming a sugar or prebiotic fiber (you cannot smell it; I was just kidding in this section's heading), it suggests that bacteria have proliferated outside the colon. We can therefore use this phenomenon as a sounding device: the faster H_2 gas is produced after a person consumes a food that bacteria convert to hydrogen, the higher up the bacterial invasion of the upper GI tract must be. Not all foods are converted to H_2 gas, but sugars and prebiotic fibers are.

To sample how high bacteria have ascended, you consume a sugar or prebiotic fiber that bacteria gobble up, such as glucose, lactulose, inulin, legumes such as black beans, or a raw white potato (raw white potatoes are virtually pure fiber and water, unlike cooked potatoes), then measure

H_2 gas in the breath. H_2 breath tests are usually performed in a laboratory or clinic. Breath samples are taken at the start and then every 30 minutes after you've consumed the test food. The sooner high levels of H_2 gas are detected, the higher up the GI tract bacteria have moved. A big uptick in H_2 gas within the first 90 minutes is diagnostic of SIBO. Because more time is required for the sugar or fiber to reach the colon—"transit time"—down twenty-four feet of intestine from the stomach, H_2 gas generated at 90 to 180 minutes is equivocal because it may represent H_2 gas emitted by bacteria farther down the small intestine or it may simply represent H_2 gas produced by microbes in the colon, where they are welcome residents and thereby represent a normal response.

Your doctor can order an H_2 breath test for you. This diagnostic technique requires a doctor who knows what he or she is looking for, as well as experienced staff adept at capturing your breath samples (which is uncommon, unfortunately). Ask your doctor about SIBO, but don't be surprised if you encounter ignorance, indifference, or resistance. "Hey, Doc, I have gas and bloating after I eat. Do you think I might have SIBO?" Typical response: "I don't know what that is." "Don't waste my time." "There is no such thing." "Did you consult Dr. Google again?" Or worse, your primary care doctor sends you to a gastroenterologist, who performs the obligatory upper endoscopy and colonoscopy, then declares, "Good news: you don't have a stomach ulcer or colon cancer." You ask, "What about my question about SIBO?" Once again: "I don't know what that is." "Don't waste my time." "There is no such thing." At best, a doctor might prescribe a conventional antibiotic with 40 percent to 60 percent efficacy while not discussing how or why you developed this condition, how to increase the efficacy of the antibiotic, whether fungal overgrowth accompanies SIBO, how to restore a healthy mucus lining that enhances healing, or how to prevent recurrences that plague SIBO management efforts, likely resigning you to your weight loss plateau, autoimmune condition, chronic pain, or even endless rounds of antibiotics.

No question: H_2 breath testing is cumbersome to perform. It requires several hours in a lab or clinic with repeated breath samples obtained. After the initial test, the entire process is often repeated following antibiotics to assess success or failure, then again later if recurrences are suspected. Each bout of testing involves several hours of time and costs hundreds of dollars.

You can also perform H_2 breath testing on your own using a kit provided by a lab. The same cumbersome nature of the test applies, however, with multiple breath samples obtained over several hours and with test kits available for around $150 to $250. (See Appendix A for resources.)

SIBO: THERE'S AN APP FOR THAT

Thankfully, the process of detecting SIBO by H_2 on the breath has recently become enormously easier and less costly. One innovation that has taken diagnosis of SIBO out of the doctor's office is a new consumer device called AIRE. Originally conceived by the engineer-inventor Dr. Aonghus Shortt of Dublin, Ireland, as a device to navigate a low-FODMAPs diet for people with irritable bowel syndrome, it is really a device that, by detecting H_2 gas in the breath, can be used to identify SIBO. (I've had several conversations with Dr. Shortt, who now recognizes the full usefulness of the wonderful device he invented; he and his company, FoodMarble, are adjusting to this insight.) Blow into the AIRE device, and breath H_2 gas level on a scale of 0 to 10 registers on your smartphone via Bluetooth. Although you need to purchase the device (around $200; links in Appendix A), you can use the device over and over again, representing a substantial cost savings over performing the H_2 breath test in a lab, which incurs hundreds of dollars each time. You can also share the device with members of your family. An updated version of the device has the added ability to measure hydrogen sulfide (H_2S) and methane, additional gases that, if released early after consumption of a sugar or prebiotic fiber reveal the presence of other unwanted microbes high up in the GI tract. (Measurement of H_2S, in particular, is largely uncharted territory but will likely prove to uncover an even greater number of people who have SIBO but test negative for H_2 gas, a very exciting development.[35])

When the AIRE device first became available to consumers in 2019 and I asked people to assess their breath H_2, the results were shocking: As our prior calculations suggest, SIBO is everywhere. The AIRE detected abnormal breath hydrogen in women and men, in young, middle-aged, and older people. Rather than excessive breath H_2 representing the exception, as I used to believe, it became clear that abnormal breath H_2 was the rule, as common as blue jeans or acne on teenage faces.

For those of you who remember what the management of diabetes was like before the 1980s and the availability of fingerstick checks for blood glucose, you may recall seeing people with type 1 diabetes succumb to kidney failure, blindness, and amputations before age thirty because management of their insulin was based on dipping urine to indirectly gauge blood glucose levels, a crude method that suffered from enormous imprecision. Imagine how dangerous it was to have a three-year-old diabetic child lose consciousness and not to know whether the blood sugar was way too high and the child was going into life-threatening diabetic ketoacidosis or the blood sugar was way too low and the little one was going to die of brain damage in the next few minutes—until you dipped the urine. How awful the experience was without fingerstick glucose measures. Once fingerstick glucose-measuring devices became available, they were a game-changer for diabetes.

At-home detection of breath hydrogen is likewise a game-changer for intestinal health. It is a bacterial mapping process used to determine whether bacteria have invaded the upper GI tract. It can also help you document success or failure of efforts to eradicate SIBO and detect recurrences. And, just as glucose monitoring has evolved, with devices now providing, for instance, continuous glucose monitoring without sticking your finger, so will detection of breath H_2 gas and other measures, all empowering us in managing our bowel flora. But, because the AIRE device was originally intended only to help people navigate a low-FODMAPs diet, with its full potential not recognized, I will provide the simple protocol that puts the device to full use in detecting breath H_2 and other gases for management of SIBO later in the book. (The instructions currently provided with the device do not detail this application for SIBO.)

For many people, the case for SIBO is so likely that you do not need to confirm high levels of H_2 gas and you can proceed with an effort to eradicate SIBO, as well as SIFO, based on your best judgment. If you have, for instance, fibromyalgia or fat malabsorption evident every time you have a bowel movement, you likely do not need to measure breath H_2 but can proceed with efforts to eradicate SIBO. I discuss later when such empiric efforts—that is, efforts based on your best informed judgment—are appropriate and can still lead you down the path of restoring magnificent health by building your Super Gut.

In the near future, other methods to detect SIBO and endotoxemia will be recognized. Direct measurement of LPS blood levels, for instance, which is currently used only as a research tool, holds enormous promise as a simple way to gauge whether increased intestinal permeability to LPS is present and needs to be addressed.

WANT SOME PREDNISONE WITH THAT SUGAR DOUGHNUT?

Here are some lethal combinations: Bonnie and Clyde, Thelma and Louise, the gliadin protein in wheat and LPS endotoxemia.

Combine the endotoxemia of SIBO with the increased intestinal permeability triggered by the gliadin protein in wheat products and 2 + 2 = 7. (I discuss the destructive health consequences of wheat and grain consumption in Part IV.) Each situation alone opens the door to intestinal permeability and leads to increased body-wide inflammation. Put them together and you have an especially potent way to provoke numerous common health conditions.

It is well established that the gliadin protein of wheat, along with related proteins in rye (secalin), barley (hordein), and corn (zein), is on the short list of factors in the human diet that abnormally increase intestinal permeability, which is when the undigested components of food and bacterial breakdown products cross the intestinal wall to gain entry to the bloodstream. This is not a phenomenon unique to people with celiac disease or gluten sensitivity; it is a process that occurs in everyone who allows a bagel, a pretzel, or breadcrumbs to cross their lips. We now know that this effect is responsible for initiating autoimmune diseases such as rheumatoid arthritis, type 1 diabetes, and others.[36,37]

Whereas each process on its own—bacterial endotoxemia and consumption of gliadin protein—is a potent inflammation-producing factor, the combination is an especially lethal duo responsible for an impressive amount of human disease, weight struggles, and even accelerated aging.

While the LPS of endotoxemia cannot yet be measured clin-
ically, you are able to measure the zonulin protein (in blood and
stool) that increases with consumption of wheat and grains and
that reflects greater intestinal permeability.

On the bright side: if increased intestinal permeability of
wheat + SIBO + the endotoxemia of SIBO results from such a
frightening combination, think how powerful it will be when you
reverse all of them.

THE MYSTERIOUS CASE OF METHANE

People with irritable bowel syndrome with diarrhea (IBS-D) are no strangers to bowel urgency. Sufferers often describe how they cannot go anywhere
without knowing the location of the nearest toilet. It interrupts activities as
mundane as going to the post office or having a meal at a restaurant. Conventional prescription drugs for IBS-D therefore force intestinal motion to
slow and reduce diarrhea frequency—but fail to target the SIBO that drives
the process. Of every one hundred people with IBS, 90 percent have the
form usually associated with loose bowel movements that is detectable by
increased levels of breath H_2 (or H_2S). But there is another form of IBS and
SIBO defined by constipation; these are labeled IBS-C or methanogenic
SIBO or intestinal methanogen overgrowth and they affect the remaining
10 percent of people with IBS. These forms are not typically associated
with increased H_2 or H_2S in the breath but are associated with increased
levels of methane gas on the breath.

IBS-C and methanogenic SIBO are associated with a curious nonbacte-
rial collection of microbes called Archaea. Because Archaea species do not
grow when standard culturing methods are used, the ubiquitous nature of
these creatures, which live in the ocean and soil, was enormously underestimated until recently. Microbiologist Gary Olsen from the University
of Illinois remarked that "overlooking the Archaea has been equivalent to
surveying one square kilometre of the African savanna and missing over
300 elephants."[38] The same holds true for Archaea in the human GI tract.

The species of Archaea are ancient, predating mammals, predating dinosaurs, even predating bacteria on the evolutionary timeline. Archaea are also called "extremophiles," given their ability to survive in extreme environments, including boiling hot water in the geysers of Yellowstone National Park, at extreme pressures at the bottom of the ocean, and in the high salinity of the Dead Sea—and in the human GI tract.

In IBS-C, an overgrowth of Archaea, such as *Methanobrevibacter smithii*, has been identified. This microbe produces methane gas that slows intestinal motion (peristalsis, the propulsive action of the intestines), resulting in constipation. Eradication or reduction of these microbes reverses constipation.

Our understanding of these peculiar creatures is still evolving. Just as with bacteria, there are "good" Archaea and "bad" Archaea species. While some species are associated with constipation and may worsen inflammatory bowel disease, others may be beneficial to the human microbiome. The compound trimethylamine (TMA), for instance, produced by bacteria, has been associated with increased risk for cardiovascular disease (when the liver converts it to trimethylamine oxide, or TMAO; see discussion in Chapter 4). Archaea species have been found to consume TMA, thereby likely reducing cardiovascular risk from this compound.[39] Just as changes in bacterial composition have occurred in modern humans compared to hunter-gatherer populations, so have changes occurred in archaeal populations, with Westerners harboring fewer numbers.[40] The implications of this reduction are not yet understood.

To produce methane gas, archaeal species *consume* H_2 gas and can thereby conceal the presence of the bacterial species of H_2-producing SIBO organisms. For this reason, when we detect methane gas in the breath that reveals overgrowth of archaeal species, we often assume it accompanies H_2-producing SIBO; that is, *both* H_2-producing bacteria and Archaea have proliferated. (This can be true in overgrowth of H_2S-producing microbial overgrowth, as well.)

Methane can be measured in the breath of people with the overgrowth of Archaea in their gut. Methane can be detected through conventional testing or with the AIRE device. If high levels of methane are detected, it is therefore likely that SIBO complicated by Archaea overgrowth is present, even if high H_2 levels are not detected.

Thankfully, one of the herbal antibiotic regimens that we use for IBS-D and SIBO (the CandiBactin regimen) is also effective for IBS-C and methanogenic SIBO. The *Lactobacillus reuteri* that we use to make yogurt can also help suppress methanogenic species. More on that later.

H$_2$S: SEWERS, ROTTEN EGGS, AND THE HUMAN GI TRACT?

In addition to H$_2$ and methane, a third gas is measurable in the breath that reveals the presence of undesirable microbial species: hydrogen sulfide, or H$_2$S.

H$_2$S is a curious thing: It is the gas that sewers emit, giving sewage its characteristic offensive smell, the gas that makes sewer workers ill when they're overexposed. H$_2$S is also produced by rotting eggs and meat. And it's produced by select microbes that, when allowed to overproliferate in the human GI tract, create yet another form of dysbiosis and SIBO. When a similar odor is emitted from bowel movements or in gas, it can suggest an unhealthy proliferation of sulfur-producing microbes.

Because testing for H$_2$S was not widely available, hydrogen sulfide remained only a research curiosity for many years, with little appreciation for its role in human disease. But preliminary evidence now suggests that many people with all the signs and symptoms of SIBO—diarrhea, abdominal discomfort, IBS, inflammatory diseases, and other health conditions—who test negative for H$_2$ gas in the breath really have a type of SIBO that is dominated by microbes that produce H$_2$S.[41]

Problem: Other health conditions such as emphysema and bronchitis can involve overproduction of H$_2$S. Even bad breath caused by sulfur-producing microbes in the mouth can raise breath levels of H$_2$S.[42] The "rules" for measuring H$_2$S and determining its source are therefore evolving and remain preliminary. But the recent availability of a commercial test for H$_2$S developed by SIBO expert Dr. Mark Pimentel (see Appendix A) and a new version of the AIRE device that tests for H_2, methane, and H_2S will open the door to many new insights into this recently recognized form of SIBO.

Because we're just beginning to recognize this form of dysbiosis and SIBO and have little experience with it, there is no agreement on how best to manage or eradicate microbes such as *Desulfovibrio* that produce H_2S. Having a new consumer device that tracks this gas, however, means that our crowdsourced experience is likely to yield effective solutions faster than the science will. Stay tuned to my online conversations for the latest.

HUNT DOWN THE MONSTER

We have a monster on the rampage in the thirty feet of our GI tracts. The microbial equivalent of Dr. Frankenstein's monster is marauding through your village, killing livestock, terrorizing villagers. I won't kid you: just like cornering a monster, healing this mess won't be all fun and games.

Beating back undesirable species and replacing them with species that support your health means eradicating trillions of unwanted microbes. Killing off trillions of microbes yields a flood of debris that can transiently affect your emotional and physical health as dying microbes release their toxic components. But the end result can be a return to magnificent health, slenderness, even youthfulness as you build your Super Gut and cultivate various microbial species that produce often spectacular health effects.

If you are lucky enough to only have dysbiosis that is confined to the colon, this situation nearly always responds to the basic efforts that I shall detail later. Not having SIBO is good news, but it does not mean that dysbiosis confined to the colon is benign. It still leaves you at risk for conditions such as diverticular disease and colon cancer and can bloom into SIBO in the future if uncorrected. If you are absolutely convinced that SIBO and SIFO do not apply to you, feel free to skip ahead to Chapter 9.

If SIBO is present, however, it means a drastic change in bowel flora composition is necessary. This process of deleting unhealthy bacterial species conventionally begins with antibiotics. The antibiotic of choice to reduce the Enterobacteriaceae species of SIBO is rifaximin, a prescription drug with about 40–60 percent efficacy that is costly and typically not covered by health-care insurance. I believe there is a better choice: herbal antibiotics.

I was initially skeptical about herbal antibiotics because they are concocted in a haphazard, unscientific way. Choose an herbal agent, say, oil of oregano, known to be effective against *Staphylococcus aureus*, *E. coli*, and *Klebsiella* (common species that overgrow in SIBO), combine it with berberine, a plant-sourced compound used in Ayurvedic medicine known to suppress SIBO microbes like *Pseudomonas* species, and several other herbal components with varied antibacterial effects and call it an herbal antibiotic—this seemingly arbitrary process is not how herbal antibiotics should be created.

It therefore came as a surprise to me when evidence emerged out of Johns Hopkins University showing that two herbal antibiotic regimens were not as effective but *more* effective than rifaximin, the conventional drug of choice for SIBO.[43] In this study, the success rate in eradicating SIBO for rifaximin was 34 percent, while success with herbal antibiotics was 46 percent (i.e., the percentage of participants who tested negative for H_2 gas in their breath). Herbal antibiotics were also effective in participants who failed to respond to rifaximin. The overall success rate with rifaximin in this study was lower than in most other studies, highlighting how difficult it is to eradicate SIBO by any method. The two herbal antibiotic regimens that generated successful results were a combination of the proprietary herbal blends of CandiBactin-AR with CandiBactin-BR, and FC-Cidal with Dysbiocide. (See Appendix A.) Although you can choose to have your doctor prescribe rifaximin (or another conventional antibiotic), you also have the option of choosing one of these herbal antibiotic regimens, which are available over the counter, have efficacy rates likely superior to rifaximin's, and cost 90 percent less.

NO FUNERAL NECESSARY

In the late nineteenth century, European doctors Adolf Jarisch and Karl Herxheimer described a syndrome of fever, chills, racing heart, emotional distress, and even shock that develops after administering a drug that kills the microbes causing syphilis, a phenomenon that has become known as the "Jarisch-Herxheimer reaction." This response is not unique to syphilis die-off and can occur with eradication of any major infection, such as pneumococcal pneumonia or *E. coli* pyelonephritis (kidney infection).

Killing off the many trillions of unhealthy microbes in SIBO and SIFO in order to cultivate your Super Gut can produce a less severe version of the Jarisch-Herxheimer reaction, one not as dramatic or life-threatening, that reflects a "die-off" reaction. It represents a form of endotoxemia, a result of the flood of bacterial and fungal breakdown products released upon microbe death, some of which enters the bloodstream. You may recall the clinical studies I mentioned in Chapter 1 in which nondepressed volunteers were administered LPS endotoxin that promptly made them exhibit the symptoms of depression—the die-off reaction you create by killing off unhealthy microbes is much the same. Killing off SIBO- and SIFO-causing microbes such as *E. coli*, *Klebsiella*, and *Candida albicans* can yield transient and unpleasant reactions such as anxiety, depression, achiness, low-grade fever, and anger.

Should you experience such phenomena during SIBO and SIFO correction efforts, don't panic: It means that you are indeed eradicating microbes that have overproliferated and that have been churning out endotoxin. Soon, they'll be gone and so will their negative effects.

The microbial die-off reaction can be a challenge. But don't let fear of it stop you from taking the important steps to empower your health and optimize your weight and appearance. Later in the book, I shall detail several steps you can take to minimize this reaction.

You can also choose to use a specific probiotic yogurt you can make (I will show you how) to eradicate SIBO, what I call Super Gut SIBO Yogurt. (See box on page 88.) Our experience with this yogurt is preliminary, but a growing number of people have been reversing high breath H_2 levels by making this yogurt that includes the microbe *Lactobacillus gasseri*, specifically the BNR17 strain, fermented to high bacterial counts in a special process I will share later in the book. *L. gasseri* is unique in that it takes up residence in the upper GI tract (where SIBO occurs) and produces up to seven bacteriocins (natural antibiotics produced by bacteria, as you will recall). *L. gasseri* is a virtual bacteriocin powerhouse, producing natural antibiotics effective against many of the species of SIBO. Super Gut SIBO Yogurt can further stack the odds in favor of reversing SIBO and potentially is a nicer, softer, friendlier way to do it. Just recognize that our experience with the results is preliminary. (I am planning a clinical trial to formally document the effects.)

One of the hurdles we need to overcome in correcting SIBO and SIFO is that bacteria and fungi have the ability to manufacture a mucus-like film, or "biofilm," in which they can hide and become invisible to the human body's immune response and less susceptible to antibiotics, herbal or conventional. There is therefore advantage in disrupting this biofilm in order to make unhealthy bacterial species more susceptible to antibiotics. In the protocol I outline in Appendix B, I include a biofilm disrupter, N-acetyl cysteine (NAC), a form of the amino acid cysteine. NAC has a long track record of efficacy and safety in the world of cystic fibrosis and pneumonia, in which aerosolized NAC is administered to break up thick sputum in the airways. It also has a history of increasing the success of antibiotic regimens used to treat *Helicobacter pylori* infestation of the stomach: it can improve the likelihood of successful eradication by about 10 percent, improving efforts from around 60 percent to 70 percent successful.

Biofilm disruption is, however, an unhealthy practice outside the few days it's used in purposeful eradication of SIBO. I cringe when I hear that some people are taking NAC as part of an effort, for instance, to preserve brain health because of NAC's ability to enhance the brain antioxidant glutathione—all the while they are also disrupting the mucus lining of their GI tract, a potentially dangerous practice over the long term (just as we learned with the polysorbate 80/carboxymethylcellulose emulsifier experience, as discussed in Chapter 5).

I recognize that this sounds like it is becoming a bit complicated, but bear with me. I will lay out the prescriptive part of the program in simple steps. A stepwise approach, I believe, can readily be put into practice. I am explaining all these details so that you can appreciate the logic behind this approach.

SUPER GUT SIBO YOGURT

Let's explore the Super Gut SIBO Yogurt option for eradicating SIBO. A growing number of people have reversed high breath H_2 levels—meaning, they've pushed hydrogen-producing bacteria from the upper GI tract back to where they belong—with this strategy. The results are preliminary and not fully tested, but let's discuss the rationale and I believe you will see the wisdom in it.

First of all, how are conventional commercial probiotics concocted? Manufacturers that formulate probiotics choose this or that species based on evidence that each bacterial species exerts some beneficial effect in humans, such as relief from diarrhea after a course of antibiotics. They do not choose species that specifically stack the odds in favor of addressing SIBO. Also, recall that most commercial probiotics do not specify which bacterial strains they include, and you therefore have no idea whether the microbes in the product will exert *any* benefits. (Strains of microbes are subtypes of microbial species; the species is the larger group to which various strains belong, and different strains in the same species have different characteristics that can, in some instances, literally make life-and-death differences. I shall discuss this issue of strain specificity further later in the book.) For this reason, standard commercial probiotics have been a disappointment in managing SIBO and in achieving substantial benefits in health.

What if instead, in crafting a probiotic explicitly to fight SIBO, we carefully curated species and strains that have specific helpful characteristics such as the following:

- The ability to colonize the upper GI tract—that is, after all, where SIBO species reside: in the upper GI tract
- The ability to form a biofilm of their own, thereby enabling them to reside long term in the upper GI tract and to interact with SIBO species over a longer timeframe
- The ability to produce bacteriocins, natural peptide antibiotics that suppress or eliminate the Enterobacteriaceae species of SIBO

Surprisingly, this relatively obvious strategy has not yet been explored. So let's explore it ourselves.

Followers of my program have been combining the following species and strains:

1. *Lactobacillus gasseri* (strain BNR17), which colonizes the upper GI tract and produces up to seven bacteriocins
2. *Lactobacillus reuteri* (strains DSM 17938 and ATCC PTA 6475), which colonizes the upper GI tract, forms a biofilm, and produces several potent bacteriocins
3. *Bacillus coagulans* (strain GBI-30,6086), which also produces a bacteriocin and has been shown to reduce the symptoms of IBS (which, you will recall, is virtually synonymous with SIBO)

We source each strain separately because there is no single source for the combination, then make yogurt with it (by fermenting all three together). Making yogurt is our way of amplifying bacterial counts so that they are higher than what is in the original probiotic products. We then consume one-half cup per day and track H_2 gas in our breath: we measure the value at the start and then after consuming yogurt for four or more weeks. We follow this regimen for a longer time than most antibiotics require.

Preliminary experience suggests that Super Gut SIBO Yogurt is a viable option for eradicating H_2-positive SIBO. If you are nervous about diving into the world of antibiotics, herbal or conventional, this might be worth trying. (The recipe is in Part III.) As with use of any antibiotic, anticipate several days of a die-off reaction, which might manifest as anxiety, dark moods, fatigue, or disrupted sleep. These effects reflect the flood of toxic substances like LPS that is being flushed out of your system as you eradicate unhealthy bacterial species in the GI tract.

Is it worth it? Is it worth the effort, the emotional roller-coaster ride of microbial die-off, the physical challenges to restore something resembling a healthy intestinal microbiome? How about the additional efforts I discuss later about cultivating super microbes like *L. reuteri* that can restore youthful skin and *Bacillus coagulans* that reduces arthritis pain and accelerates muscle recovery after strenuous work or exercise, further steps we can take to create a Super Gut?

It absolutely is. A life without being overweight or obese, without type 2 diabetes or hypertension, without irritable bowel syndrome or fibromyalgia, without dependence on prescription after prescription from the doctor to "treat" this or that condition, a life in which you can enjoy slenderness, lower potential for conditions like colon cancer, magnificent health, accelerated healing, deeper sleep, and higher levels of day-to-day functioning—isn't that what life is about all along? Once you reverse dysbiosis and SIBO, then you can embark on all the fascinating fermentation projects that can help you reduce skin wrinkles, restore youthful muscle and strength, and cultivate empathy.

DON'T FORGET ABOUT THE FUNGI

Because so many people with SIBO also have SIFO—small intestinal fungal overgrowth—and because eradication of SIBO can transiently disrupt the microbial balance in a way that encourages fungal proliferation, it is worth considering antifungal efforts along with SIBO-eradicating efforts. It is my personal view that we should always include at least some antifungal efforts with any SIBO-eradicating effort. The presence of any signs of fungal overgrowth as discussed in the next chapter should cause you to consider including antifungal efforts with your SIBO management efforts.

In some people, SIFO is the dominant process and then a more serious antifungal effort may be required.

So let's next discuss this other class of microorganism that, although present in the guts of indigenous people, has proliferated, ascended the GI tract like unhealthy bacterial species do, and invaded other parts of the body. These microbes are ubiquitous, found in air, water, soil, and virtually all surfaces, including those in all the nooks and crannies of the human body. And several species have evolved to inhabit the special environment of the human GI tract. So let's now discuss fungi.

SIBO = small intestinal bacterial over-growth
(upper G.I)

SIFO = small intestinal Fungal overgrowth

7

SIFO: FUNGAL JUNGLE

BACTERIA ARE, BY A LONG STRETCH, THE DOMINANT CLASS OF microbes that live in your GI tract. But there's another group of microorganisms that, although they can also dwell in the GI tract quietly and mind their own business, can proliferate as bacteria do and terrorize your GI tract: fungi. *Like Hamas!*

Fungi are everywhere: in the air, water, and soil; on surfaces in your house; on kitchen utensils. After a spring rain, toadstools might appear overnight in your yard, a visible form of the fungi that live in the soil. Fungi can appear as mold on stale bread or on the walls of a wet basement. You can consume them as white button mushrooms on a salad or as cremini mushrooms in a tasty sauce. And you can find them in the various nooks, crevices, and organs of the human body, from airways to beneath fingernails. In the GI tract, fungi inhabit the mouth, tongue, and throat on down, all the way to the rectum. Despite their ubiquity, fungi normally comprise less than 1 percent of all microbes in the human body.

Up until recently, it was believed that the human GI tract was home to only a few fungal species. As with bacteria, newer methods that rely on DNA mapping have revealed a surprisingly rich variety of fungal species occupying the entire length of the GI tract. The latest count has revealed that nearly two hundred fungal species—what I call a "fungal jungle," a complex system of fungal microbes in your gut—interact with one another,

93

Fungus Among us

bacteria, and you.[1] Fungal microorganisms are a hundred-fold larger than bacteria; they are relative giants among tiny microbes.

A number of fungal species are normal inhabitants, residing there since your childhood, perhaps even playing a beneficial role in the complex web of GI microbes. Although the number and species vary from person to person, everyone has fungi living in them. As with their bacterial neighbors, when the normal microbial order is disrupted, fungi can overproliferate in the GI tract, ascend, export their toxic by-products, and spread to other body parts when the opportunity presents itself. Antibiotic use is, in particular, known to trigger fungal proliferation.[2] Fungi such as *Candida albicans* and *Candida glabrata* can multiply unchecked in numerous body sites after, say, a course of azithromycin for a sore throat or sinus infection. Fungal proliferation is commonly experienced as red, itchy fungal rashes in the armpits, throat, groin, or vagina. Fungal proliferation in the GI tract virtually always accompanies such outward symptoms.

Fungi are known to cause serious infections of artificial devices implanted in the body, such as prosthetic knees and heart valves or indwelling catheters, and they cause infections in people who have compromised immune systems. In these situations, fungal infections are catastrophic, necessitating prolonged administration of potent intravenous antifungal drugs. The mortality rate of people with such fungal infections approaches a horrifying 30 percent because of both the destructive nature of out-of-control fungi and the toxic nature of the intravenous antifungal drugs, such as amphotericin B (what doctors call "amphoterrible"). Fungal infections are serious business.

C. albicans is the most common fungal opportunist in the human body. Given a chance, it will proliferate, form its own protective biofilm (i.e., a film of mucus and other elements), and cause some of the toughest infections to eradicate because the gooey biofilm makes the organism less susceptible to antifungal agents. This explains, for instance, why *Candida* infections of artificial heart valves or prosthetic hips are almost impossible to eradicate with antifungal drugs. (For this reason, the device almost always has to be surgically removed.)

Fungi and bacteria can also work together, with colonization by one encouraging infection by the other. This is seen, for instance, in urinary tract infections in which *Escherichia coli* colonizes the bladder and sets the

E. Coli

stage for fungal infection. Pneumonia in people on ventilatory support can begin with candidal species that allow the *Pseudomonas* bacterial species to join in.[3] There are also instances in which fungi "collaborate" with bacteria such as streptococcal and staphylococcal species that, in combination, can be particularly fierce in causing devastating infections.[4]

Let's put aside such serious candidal infections treated in hospitals and instead focus on more common, but less severe, forms of fungal overgrowth. After all, fungal species normally colonize infants within the first few weeks after birth, then stay with us to varying degrees for the rest of our lives. Like death, taxes, and marital spats, fungi are an inevitable part of human life.

It's not necessary to have a prosthetic device for fungi to begin the fireworks. Fungal species occupying our GI tracts and other nooks and crannies of our bodies live quietly, without causing health problems, until a course of antibiotics, steroids, overconsumption of sugars, excessive alcohol intake, or stomach acid–suppressing drugs—many of the same factors that enable SIBO to develop—allow fungi to proliferate.[2,5,6] Any situation in which the intestinal lining becomes inflamed, such as in dysbiosis, SIBO, Crohn's disease, ulcerative colitis, and probably irritable bowel syndrome, also creates an environment favorable for fungal proliferation.

Overgrowth of fungi is most commonly experienced as increased numbers of *C. albicans* in the colon. One of the biggest challenges in deciding whether fungi are simply happy residents or are contributing to health problems is deciding just how many fungi need to be present to be associated with health problems. Because about 50 percent of healthy people have up to 10,000 CFUs of *C. albicans* per milliliter of stool, some have argued that fungal infestation requires more than 100,000 CFUs per milliliter in a fecal specimen. (CFUs stands for "colony-forming units" and represents the number of living microorganisms in a sample.) This or similar measures are reported when you submit a stool sample for analysis. Such measures reopen the question, however, of whether the fungal counts found in healthy people are a reliable yardstick because "normal" people in the twenty-first century no longer have a truly healthy microbiome. Just as unhealthy bacterial species can ascend and invade the entire length of the GI tract, so can fungal species. If a sample of contents from the upper GI tract is examined, such as fluid from the duodenum obtained via endoscopy,

CFUs = Colony-Forming units

then a threshold of more than 1,000 CFUs/ml (much lower than numbers expected in stool) is typically used to identify small intestinal fungal overgrowth.[7]

　Habitual overconsumption of sugars, a phenomenon unique to the last one hundred years, is an especially common factor that invites fungal species to proliferate and ascend the GI tract. Fungal species are enthusiastic consumers of sugars delivered to them through soft drinks, fruit juices, sugary snacks, and breakfast cereals, and they bloom with consumption of these sweet foods. Yes, that fast-food special-deal hamburger with bun, french fries, and sixteen-ounce soft drink is an open invitation to fungal proliferation, as is a breakfast of high-fiber cereal with orange juice. Fungi also thrive in people with high blood sugar and thereby high tissue levels of sugar, which accounts for the increased trouble with fungal infections people with diabetes struggle with; that is, people with high body-wide levels of sugar not uncommonly can experience several simultaneous fungal infections in various parts of the body. People with diabetes and those who are obese also host different fungi than slender, nondiabetic people.[8] The poorer a person's blood sugar control, the higher their blood and tissue sugars, the more their weight ranges out of control, and the more widespread and troublesome their fungal infections.[9] Combine high sugar with disruptions of bacterial communities, and fungi, of course, are likely to rampage through your intestinal microbiome.

MISERY LOVES COMPANY

As we've discussed, intestinal overgrowth of bacteria, SIBO, is surprisingly common. You may see your primary care doctor regularly, undergo colonoscopies every few years, and have Pap smears and blood pressure checks to screen for common health conditions like precancerous polyps, cervical cancer, and hypertension. As common as these conditions may be, SIBO is more common than colon cancer, cervical cancer, and hypertension combined. But I would be shocked if your doctor screened you for SIBO, even if you have conditions virtually synonymous with SIBO, such as IBS or fibromyalgia, and even if you complain of symptoms like bloating, bowel urgency, or restless legs. You might have even undergone a colonoscopy and no mention was made about bacterial or fungal overgrowth because

(margin note: No McWendy King !!)

these conditions cannot be seen with a scope. But they're everywhere, right under the nose of your unsuspecting doctor.

Just as identification of SIBO is woefully neglected in conventional health care, so it goes with SIFO. It is uncommon for a conventional doctor to suspect that eczema, daytime fatigue, joint pain, or even cognitive impairment might be due to fungal overgrowth in the GI tract. Although it is not as common as SIBO, we are still talking about tens of millions of people with this condition expressing itself in a variety of ways that goes unrecognized.

Disentangling bacterial from fungal overgrowth on the basis of symptoms alone can be tricky, often impossible, because there is overlap in the effects of the two classes of microbes, despite the much greater bacterial numbers. In a recent study of people with unexplained abdominal pain, for instance, if SIBO was present, there was a 36 percent likelihood that SIFO was also present and another 24 percent likelihood that SIFO alone was present to account for symptoms.[10] As you can imagine, the potential for wreaking havoc on the health of the host is considerable when SIBO is combined with SIFO—then you're dealing with hordes of bacterial and fungal species inhabiting all thirty feet of the human GI tract, continuously reproducing and dying, releasing their toxic by-products at a dizzying pace. It is also often not clear whether fungal overgrowth is a cause of a health condition or a result. Regardless of this chicken-or-egg situation, excessive proliferation of fungal species, whether alone or in combination with SIBO, can pose substantial health troubles.

Fungal overgrowth is associated with many of the same symptoms and health consequences as SIBO, such as the following:

- **Skin rashes**, especially atopic dermatitis and eczema, that are unresponsive or poorly responsive to steroid creams and other treatments
- **Allergies** of the skin, airways, sinuses, and other mucous membranes, at least some of which are due to the release of fungal proteins
- **Triggering or worsening of autoimmune diseases**. Children with type 1 diabetes, for instance, are much more likely to have fungal intestinal colonization.
- **Abdominal discomfort, bloating, and diarrhea**; these are irritable bowel syndrome–like symptoms.

The G.I. tract is 30 Ft long!

- **Fatigue, mood swings**. If you suffer from fatigue you cannot explain or wide swings in mood that make no sense or follow no pattern, these are reasons to suspect fungal overgrowth.[6]

- Sugar cravings, an insatiable around-the-clock desire for sweet foods in any form, are another peculiar signature symptom of SIFO. Because fungi thrive on sugar, whether provided through diet or by tissues body-wide as in diabetes, it has to make you wonder: How do fungi manage to drive human behavior to serve their own purposes? Creepy but fascinating to consider.

With these signs of fungal overgrowth present, you can either proceed to strategies that reduce fungal populations or have a stool analysis performed to confirm whether excessive fungal populations are indeed present. (See Appendix A for testing choices.)

Fungi that proliferate in the GI tract are destructive inhabitants, aggressively degrading the protective mucus lining and damaging intestinal cells.[11] As with bacterial overgrowth, the full implications of fungal overgrowth are not just related to the fungi themselves. Fungi are also responsible for the toxic release of the components of their cell walls (e.g., beta-glucans) into the bloodstream, a process similar to the bacterial endotoxemia of SIBO. This has been found to be an important phenomenon in conditions such as lupus, ulcerative colitis, and other health conditions.[12–15] You can begin to appreciate that the common combination of SIBO and SIFO dumps a tsunami of toxic breakdown products into your system, much of which gains entry into the bloodstream to export inflammatory effects to distant organs. As mentioned, this storm of toxins explains how overproliferation of bacteria and fungi in the GI tract can be experienced as rosacea and eczema rashes on the skin, joint and muscle pain in fibromyalgia, and the crippling disability of Alzheimer's disease in the brain.

Fungi inhabiting the GI tract and elsewhere tend to be more troublesome to reduce than bacteria because they can mount extraordinary resistance to eradication efforts. They are, after all, naturally adapted to survive in all sorts of extreme environments, from the undersurface of rocks in a river to the grout in your shower. Fungi have the ability to form spores and biofilms that make them impervious to antifungal agents, and they can shift between single-cell forms and communities of hyphal, or string-like, forms that spread more aggressively. All this means that, in order to reduce fungal populations, we need to outsmart them by using several agents at the same time and employing these agents for several weeks, sometimes months, much longer than efforts to eradicate SIBO. Thankfully, the new tidal wave of effective antifungal agents are benign and inexpensive, making them relatively accessible remedies for a SIFO-eradicating effort.

Just as bacteria themselves, not just their by-products, can escape the bounds of the GI tract and take up residence in other organs, so can fungi—they are now being uncovered in the most unexpected places, from the skin to the airways, vagina, and cerebrospinal fluid that bathes the brain. The mouth and sinuses are loaded with fungi. But when does a harmless resident transform into a disease-causing agent, including in the brain?

BRAINSTORM

One of the most disturbing examples of human fungal infestations comes from observations of fungi found in the human brain. Investigations conducted by Dr. Ruth Alonso and colleagues at the Autonomous University of Madrid have revealed that the brains of young people who die in car accidents or other traumatic incidences contain no fungi. The brains of elderly people without evidence of dementia reveal a moderate quantity of fungi. The brains of people with dementia reveal dense populations of fungi that fill every part of the brain. Examine the blood and cerebrospinal fluid (which bathes the brain) of people with dementia, and you will encounter high levels of fungal proteins and DNA. Inject a small quantity of fungi into the bloodstream of a mouse and it will develop all the hallmarks of dementia in the brain.[16–19]

Let's continue to connect the fungal dots. Research into Alzheimer's dementia has focused on the beta-amyloid plaque that accumulates in the brains of people with this condition. Pharmaceutical companies have therefore developed drugs that block formation of beta-amyloid plaque. But, when these drugs are administered to human subjects, beta-amyloid plaque is reduced but progression of dementia is *accelerated*, with faster deterioration of memory and other mental faculties than if they had not taken the drug. It has therefore become clear that blocking beta-amyloid plaque accumulation is not the solution to Alzheimer's.

If we reinterpret these phenomena, we can surmise that beta-amyloid plaque is more likely a *response* and not the cause of dementia, a realization that has dashed decades of work and caused the beta-amyloid plaque theory of dementia to be discarded. Recent research by a team in Boston at Massachusetts General Hospital and Boston University uncovered the fact that beta-amyloid plaque has potent antifungal properties—could the accumulation of beta-amyloid plaque be the body's *response* to fungal infection in the brain? Is the solution to dementia to address (earlier in life, preferably) sources of fungal infestation?[20]

Beyond Alzheimer's disease, emerging evidence associates fungal infestation of the GI tract and brain with multiple sclerosis and Lou Gehrig's disease. There are even preliminary reports of multiple sclerosis going into remission after fecal transplantation—the Power of Normal?[21] Why would a condition involving the central nervous system reverse after altering bowel flora? Fungi are everywhere, including in the brain for many of us.

But where did these fungi originate? Is there a central source of fungal species that seeds the skin, groin, vagina, sinuses, scalp, airways, mouth, throat, and brain? While these issues are just beginning to be sorted out, my bet is on the GI tract, consistent with these early favorable experiences with fecal transplantation. It raises some unsavory questions, such as how and why fungi residing in the GI tract manage to be exported to all these other body sites. We know, for instance, that consuming foods or probiotic supplements containing *Lactobacillus* species can reach the vagina and reduce fungal colonization there.[22] But how? How do *Lactobacillus* species ingested orally travel through the GI tract to the vagina, because there is no direct connection between the two? These sites are contiguous, but not directly connected. I believe that it is a small leap to propose that microbes dwelling in the intestines, passed to the exterior via bowel movements, spread by that route. Alternatively, given the recent discovery that fungi can take up residence in various organs like the brain, could they spread first by exiting the GI tract through the intestinal wall, then travel via the bloodstream to other organs? It seems a virtual certainty.

If so, it potentially means that fungi inhabiting the upper and lower GI tract many years earlier may set the stage for fungal infestation of the brain that manifests as dementia and other neurodegenerative conditions. Could eradication of intestinal fungal overgrowth thereby be one key to preventing the cognitive decline, loss of memory, and helplessness of Alzheimer's and the progressive disability of multiple sclerosis? Obviously, more research is needed, but bottoms up: my prediction is that this line of work will yield some exciting solutions.

BEATING BACK JUNGLE OVERGROWTH

The program that I lay out in Part IV of this book contains safe and effective strategies that discourage overgrowth of fungal species. But, when fungal overgrowth is identified, you can add a number of herbal and probiotic preparations, all natural, that pack more of an antifungal punch. There are, of course, antifungal prescription drugs that kill fungi. However, I am going to focus on antifungal agents that are readily available without prescription, that are relatively benign, yet reduce fungal numbers throughout the entire length of the GI tract. That, by the way, may be among the greatest challenges: ensuring that the agents we choose work not just in the stomach and duodenum, but twenty-some feet farther down in the ileum and colon. We therefore choose natural agents that are more likely to reduce fungal numbers throughout the length of GI tract. I will detail how to choose among the various agents in Part IV of this book. Here I will give you an overview of these agents.

Curcumin

Curcumin, a component of the spice turmeric, is an antifungal champion because it is benign (even at very high doses) yet effective against multiple fungal species. Because it is minimally absorbed, about 99 percent of any amount ingested remains within the GI tract to exert antifungal effects before it is then passed out into the toilet. Ironically, intensive efforts have been devoted to increasing absorption of curcumin by adding ingredients such as piperine (an alkaloid found in black pepper) and bioperine (an extract of black pepper) or creating nanoparticle or liposomal forms of curcumin. But, for our antifungal purposes, we actually *do not want absorption* and want curcumin to stay within the GI tract. We therefore seek preparations, listed in Appendix A, that do *not* have added ingredients to increase absorption.

Poor absorption also caused critics not to take curcumin seriously because it cannot be taken orally to treat fungal or bacterial infections of the

See Apendix A   FoodMarble.com Aire device

bladder or skin, for instance. But those critics did not recognize that lack of absorption may be the reason curcumin is such a wonderful intraintestinal antimicrobial agent, and why curcumin has been shown to induce remission of conditions like ulcerative colitis and to provide relief from irritable bowel symptoms despite minimal absorption.[23,24] The many people who have experienced relief from inflammatory conditions such as knee arthritis and skin rashes are therefore likely inadvertently treating SIBO and SIFO, the probable causes of their inflammatory condition, even when they take forms of curcumin that are minimally or not absorbed.

Because it possesses antibacterial and antifungal properties, curcumin is not an agent you want to take for extended periods but only during the period when you are working to reduce fungal numbers—fungal *eradication* is not the goal; a rebalancing of fungal and bacterial populations is the goal.

CAN YOU CURCUMIN?

Solve this little riddle and you may gain a useful insight into health.

When ingested orally, almost no curcumin is absorbed. Take 100 milligrams, for instance, and you will pass around 99 milligrams into the toilet. The minor quantity that is absorbed is rapidly processed by the liver, then returned to the GI tract for excretion in the stool. If 99 percent of orally ingested curcumin simply passes through your system without absorption, why would it have such noticeable effects as reduction in inflammatory blood markers and reduced arthritis joint pain and swelling? Given several clinical trials studying the effects of curcumin, there is little doubt that it does indeed exert such inflammation-subduing effects.[25]

But why? Why would the swelling and pain of knee arthritis, for instance, be reduced by an agent that never even makes it out of the GI tract and therefore cannot act at the knee joint? Some speculate that a metabolite of curcumin may make its way into the bloodstream, but it remains simply that: a speculation.

Let me add another speculation, one that I believe makes more sense: Curcumin does not exert its anti-inflammatory effects by leaving the bloodstream and entering the knee joint, liver, or other organ, and it does not exert most of its beneficial effects via some metabolite. Instead, curcumin stays within the GI tract and exerts antibacterial and antifungal effects in people with dysbiosis, SIBO, and SIFO, reducing the associated endotoxemia and thereby reducing inflammation throughout the body. We know, for instance, that curcumin produces moderate antibacterial and antifungal effects within the GI tract. Curcumin has also demonstrated other potent effects in the intestines: strengthening the intestinal barrier by doubling the activity of the lipopolysaccharide-detoxifying enzyme alkaline phosphatase along the intestinal lining, maintaining the integrity of the mucus lining, decreasing "leakiness" between intestinal cells, and increasing production of peptides with antimicrobial properties.[26] In other words, the benefits of curcumin for, say, the knee, hip, or skin result because it reduces the bacterial and fungal endotoxemia that causes inflammation in those parts of the body.

You might view taking curcumin as a therapeutic test: If you respond positively to curcumin, it likely means that you have reduced the endotoxemia of SIBO, SIFO, or both that leads to reduced inflammation. It means that you need to address the SIBO and SIFO for full relief from the consequences of inflammation and bacterial and fungal overgrowth, not simply take curcumin.

Future research may lead to modifications of curcumin or its metabolites to make it more effective, but we are going to take advantage of its lack of absorption in order to put its intestinal effects to best use. Curcumin is one of the components of the Super Gut program; we will discuss it further in Part IV.

Berberine

The traditional Chinese plant extract berberine has been shown to produce a number of health benefits, including reduced blood sugar and reduced measures of inflammation. But, like curcumin, it is poorly absorbed, yielding only minor rises in blood levels with ingestion. In other words, berberine's negligible absorption rate suggests that it has a bowel flora and/or intestinal barrier effect that may explain why this nutritional supplement provides such outsized benefits—not through absorption. Also like curcumin, berberine has antibiotic effects on common SIBO species, including *Staphylococcus*, *Streptococcus*, *Salmonella*, *Klebsiella*, *Pseudomonas* species, and antifungal effects on SIFO species such as *C. albicans*. Berberine also increases the population of *Akkermansia*, improves intestinal barrier function, increases butyrate production, and reduces the level of bacterial endotoxemia.[27,28] Berberine can therefore be helpful while eradicating SIBO and SIFO, and it is a component of one of the herbal antibiotic regimens we use. Like curcumin, it is unclear, given its antibiotic effects, whether berberine is safe to consume outside a SIBO/SIFO-eradicating effort.

Essential Oils

Essential oils are concentrated phytochemicals sourced from plants that have become popular for a variety of applications. We focus on essential oils sourced from food, that is, derived from foods that we commonly consume such as cinnamon with proven safety records. Having heard many wild claims surrounding essential oils over the years, I was initially skeptical of their use. But the science has advanced and shows that essential oils are among the most potent antifungal agents available.

Essential oils contain a mixture of naturally occurring terpenes and terpenoids (natural plant chemicals) with unique scents that are responsible for many of their effects. For example, curcumin, above, is rich in terpenes. In addition, essential oils are fat-soluble and thereby are able to disrupt the cell walls of fungi. They also disrupt the biofilm that fungal species so effectively create to protect themselves. This combination of effects means that essential oils are proving to be among the most effective and accessible agents available to us in our antifungal campaign.

Among the most effective are food-sourced essential oils from cinnamon bark, clove, oregano, and peppermint. At least in experimental settings, these oils have proven to be more potent antifungal agents than the conventional antifungal drugs amphotericin B and fluconazole. Of the oils, cinnamon oil possesses the most potent antifungal effect while clove oil is rich in a compound called eugenol that increases the thickness of the protective intestinal mucus barrier, an effect that helps intestinal healing proceed. The essential oils can be useful in small quantities, for example, 1 to 6 drops (approximately 33–200 micrograms) diluted in one tablespoon of olive, avocado, fish, or another healthy oil (oils only, not water). (In Part IV, I detail how to start low, then build up the dose gradually to minimize adverse effects.) Because they can also be caustic and burn the sensitive lining of your mouth and GI tract, *never* take essential oils directly. Dilute very small quantities in an edible oil instead. These essential oils are not appropriate to treat systemic infection, nor have they been adequately tested for vaginal use.[29]

Saccharomyces boulardii ☑

The fungal species *S. boulardii*, a strain of *Saccharomyces cerevisiae* used in winemaking, bread making, and brewing beer, is available as a probiotic supplement and suppresses intestinal fungi by competing with them. Five billion colony-forming units (CFUs) per day is the dose most commonly used. *S. boulardii* does not colonize the gastrointestinal tract and is gone within days, but its presence discourages proliferation of other fungal species.[30]

Bacterial Probiotics

Although the precise composition of the ideal probiotic to suppress *Candida* has not been determined, several preparations have been shown to reduce this fungus. The results are slow to develop, requiring up to one year of probiotic use. *Lactobacillus* species, strains of *Lactobacillus rhamnosus*, in particular the GG strain, may be especially effective against *Candida*.[31,32]

Of the herbal antibiotic regimens we use to manage SIBO, CandiBactin-AR and CandiBactin-BR have some antifungal effects because the AR version of this product provides oil of oregano and the BR version provides berberine, both of which have antifungal properties. The FC-Cidal and Dysbiocide combination provides carvacrol from oregano, thyme, and dill that also has some antifungal effects. (More on this in Chapter 8, where I lay out precisely how we manage SIBO and SIFO.)

Even though they are usually present in far fewer numbers than bacteria, fungi are tough to deal with and typically require that more than one agent be used over a longer time period to reduce their numbers, typically

four or more weeks. With SIBO and SIFO combined, it is not uncommon
to take a two-week course of herbal antibiotics for the SIBO component,
followed by four to eight weeks of antifungal agents to obtain relief from,
say, skin rashes or sugar cravings and perhaps to even impact your long-
term risk for Alzheimer's dementia.

ⓔ Many people describe a constellation of fatigue, low-grade fever, and
malaise when they tackle fungal overgrowth. These effects are presump-
tively due to die-off, the death of fungi that releases their toxic components.
This phenomenon appears to develop regardless of which antifungal regimen you use and therefore likely cannot be attributed to being a side effect
of the treatment agents but a consequence of fungal die-off. Should you
decide to proceed with an antifungal program, I will show you how to go
"long and slow" to minimize such die-off effects. Mainly, we add antifungal
agents one at a time, building up to taking three agents simultaneously to
circumvent the fungi's ability to develop resistance. Of all the measures we
take to restore a healthy microbiome, reducing fungal numbers may be the
toughest step of all.

I encourage anyone embarking on a SIBO-eradicating effort to include
at least some tactics aimed at discouraging fungi because the disruption of
bacterial populations that is a necessary part of SIBO eradication can sometimes provide an invitation for fungal overgrowth. Alternatively, if you have
made efforts to reverse SIBO and have had only partial success, then it's
time to consider whether you have fungal overgrowth. You can submit a
stool sample to quantify *Candida* or other fungal species using the lab services listed in Appendix A. However, as time goes on and experience with
these issues grows, I am coming to the conclusion that the best approach is
to always combine efforts of reducing fungal and bacterial numbers whenever a SIBO management program is initiated. In other words, because the
antifungal agents we now can choose from are relatively benign and accessible, and because SIBO management efforts can sometimes invite fungal
proliferation, I believe it is advisable to always include antifungal efforts in
SIBO eradication.

The ups and downs of microbiome management efforts may seem a bit
complicated. Want to feel really smart about what you've learned so far in
Super Gut? Just go to your primary care doctor's office and start a conver-

sation about, say, H_2 gas detection in the breath, or how you are intrigued by the intraintestinal antifungal potential of curcumin, or whether the eugenol terpene of clove oil provides any benefits to the intestinal mucus barrier. When you encounter a blank stare, stuttering responses, or something like "Oh, did you consult Dr. Google again?" you will know just how far you have come in your microbiome journey.

8

CONQUERING YOUR FRANKENBELLY: MANAGING SIBO AND SIFO

NO ANGRY FARMERS WILL BRANDISH PITCHFORKS HERE TO DEfeat this monster. We are instead going to take concrete steps to manage this enormously disempowering epidemic of SIBO and SIFO so that we can regain magnificent control over health, weight, and youth. In this chapter, I describe the rationale behind the Super Gut method to manage SIBO and SIFO. (The actual step-by-step protocols are laid out in Appendix B.)

It's a given that virtually everyone living a modern life has some degree of dysbiosis. How many of us can claim to never have taken a prescribed antibiotic, never indulged in diet sodas sweetened with aspartame or ice cream softened with polysorbate 80? How many of us can still claim to be normal weight and to have never taken an anti-inflammatory drug? We have, as a society, experienced enormous changes in bowel flora composition. But if you are among the one in three people with signs of the more serious disruptions of bowel flora composition and location that are characteristic of SIBO and SIFO, then this is where you want to be.

Some good news: The information and technology to help you achieve success in reversing SIBO and SIFO have taken several leaps forward in just the past few years. Even if your doctor fails to answer your questions about why you have a long list of unexplained health problems, you now have direct access to many of the tools you require to fix these problems—even if doctors don't understand what you are trying to accomplish.

You have access to the newest insights into bacterial and fungal overgrowth with the book you presently hold in your hands. You are able to obtain herbal antibiotics that are at least as effective, perhaps more effective, than conventional antibiotics and that are also safer and more cost effective. You have the added choice of making your own mix of probiotics in yogurt, what I call Super Gut SIBO Yogurt, to use in place of antibiotics as a potential means of beating back SIBO. You have access to a breath-testing device that can confirm where bacteria are located and whether they produce H_2, H_2S, or methane. And you have the option of making a variety of fermented foods that yield spectacular health benefits once you are through your SIBO- and SIFO-eradicating efforts.

Let's first lay down some ground rules on dealing with SIBO and SIFO. Although this is a work in progress, we can be confident of the following:

- Regardless of whether you choose conventional or herbal antibiotics, good choices are available. If you cringe at the thought of antibiotics, conventional or herbal, you can choose to make my Super Gut SIBO Yogurt that, in preliminary experience, has reversed SIBO for some people, as evidenced by normalization of H_2 breath levels.
- You have the ability to gauge the success or failure of your efforts by tracking telltale signs, tolerance to prebiotic fiber, and H_2, H_2S, and methane levels in your breath.
- It is often worth dealing with fungal overgrowth at the same time you eradicate SIBO because the two occur together in about a third of people who have SIBO. For this reason, we include curcumin with its antifungal properties during both SIBO and SIFO efforts. If you are convinced that fungal overgrowth is present, it is best to first address SIBO, then continue with at least a four-week additional effort at SIFO eradication with curcumin combined with diluted essential oils. You could address both SIBO and SIFO fully and concurrently, but that can be difficult for many people, given the die-off reactions that many experience.
- You can help prevent frequent recurrences of SIBO by including *Lactobacillus reuteri* (which we make yogurt with) in your diet after SIBO

eradication, taking advantage of its upper-GI-colonizing ability coupled with its production of bacteriocins.

* You now can identify SIBO recurrences with breath testing and awareness of the telltale signs.
* As exciting and fun as the fermentation projects can be, you are best served by delaying their introduction until you complete your SIBO- and SIFO-eradicating efforts. There's no harm in conducting these projects during SIBO/SIFO eradication, but you won't experience the sorts of benefits you're after until the SIBO/SIFO process is completed.

Because much of this information is so new to so many people, let's once again run through how you can decide whether or not SIBO and SIFO are issues you need to address. There are three ways to begin this journey that suggest or prove that SIBO is present:

1. The presence of telltale signs reveals that the population of bacterial species in your gut has changed and some have ascended from the colon to infest the length of your GI tract. These signs include seeing fat droplets in the toilet, intolerance to prebiotic fiber–containing foods such as legumes and inulin, other food intolerances, conditions such as irritable bowel syndrome, fibromyalgia, or any autoimmune or inflammatory conditions. See the full list in Chapter 6.
2. Have your doctor order an H_2 breath test, ideally with H_2S and methane testing also.
3. Test yourself using the AIRE device. This is the best choice of all because the newest version of the device tests H_2, H_2S, and methane.

It is indeed reasonable to embark on a SIBO-eradicating effort based on the presence of one or more telltale signs without confirmatory testing. It is an advantage to test for excess H_2, H_2S, and methane to gauge response to your efforts and to assess for possible recurrences, but many people do indeed manifest such reliable and perceptible signs and symptoms that an empiric approach, that is, making decisions based on evidence using your best informed judgment, is reasonable. However, if it fits into your budget, owning and using the AIRE device can be truly helpful.

Recall that, with SIBO, there is a 36 percent chance that it is accompanied by fungal overgrowth. The presence of SIFO is further suggested by fungal skin rashes (face, scalp, forehead, neck, throat, under breasts, groin, toenails, etc.), skin rashes that are recurrent or persistent, sugar cravings, and unexplained wide mood swings. You can determine whether SIFO is present with formal stool analysis, but I find that most people do well following their best judgment, particularly given the relatively benign nature of the antifungal choices we now have available.

HOW TO USE THE AIRE DEVICE

As I mentioned earlier, the inventor of this wonderfully empowering device intended it to help people suffering with irritable bowel syndrome navigate a low-FODMAPs diet to reduce symptoms of bloating and bowel urgency. But this device really has the potential to assess H_2, H_2S, and methane gases in the breath to detect the numerous forms of food intolerances caused by SIBO. A person's intolerance might be to nightshades, nuts, legumes, fructose, or histamine-containing foods, or their intolerances might be identified by blood tests (e.g., IgG antibody testing). But nearly all people with food intolerances produce these gases upon consumption of a triggering food because of SIBO. The solution is therefore not to just eliminate the food but to *address the SIBO causing the intolerance.* Don't make the mistake of eliminating culprit foods without addressing the SIBO that leaves you at risk for its long-term complications, such as diverticular disease and colon cancer. The AIRE device can also detect increased levels of these gases even if you have no symptoms of SIBO, a situation that is surprisingly common.

Admittedly, formal breath testing can be a hassle—the day-before prep, collecting breath samples every thirty minutes for several hours, waiting for results. If you obtain samples directly without a doctor, you collect the gas samples yourself and mail them to a lab. Each test kit costs between $150 and $250. If you go through a doctor, additional charges are typically added. Each test kit is useful for only one round of tests. If you want to verify, for instance, that SIBO has been eradicated after a course of antibiotics, then you have to purchase another test kit and go through the process again. The same is true when assessing for all-too-common recurrences: another test kit, another round of testing.

The AIRE device is therefore a game-changer because it is reusable over and over again. At around $200 per device, it can save you money over time, as well as cut down considerably on the hassle of breath testing. The AIRE device is exceptionally easy to use: turn it on and open the app on your smartphone. After a brief warm-up, the device tells you to blow into the mouthpiece for about five seconds and then provides H_2, H_2S, and methane readings within a few seconds.

The real usefulness of this device is to generate a time course of gas release. In other words, you obtain a baseline measure prior to eating, consume a food that contains prebiotic fiber, then test again every thirty to forty-five minutes for up to three hours; you can stop testing if you obtain a positive reading. This method of testing helps you assess whether prebiotic fibers are converted to H_2 gas by bacteria high up in the stomach, duodenum, jejunum, or ileum. If you test positive for hydrogen gas within 90 minutes of eating the fiber, you have SIBO. A positive test between 90 and 180 minutes is not definitive for SIBO because it is difficult to distinguish mild SIBO in the ileum (nine or so feet down from the stomach) from colonic fermentation, especially in people with rapid transit time, when food is rapidly digested and transported to the colon. Judgment may be required in interpreting your response in this situation. Likewise, release of H_2S and methane within the first 90 minutes suggests that abnormal bacteria are present high up in the GI tract; however, the "rules" for H_2S assessment (what level is abnormal? should we challenge with proteins instead of fibers since proteins are the source of hydrogen sulfide gas? and so forth) have not yet been fully worked out.

The AIRE device is also useful for assessing response to a course of treatment. During a course of antibiotics, for example, you may see consistently high H_2 levels after ingesting a prebiotic fiber, then reduced levels on day 6 or day 7. This suggests a positive response to the chosen antibiotic regimen, which is reducing the numbers of gas-producing bacteria in the small intestine. After you have successfully treated SIBO, you can use the AIRE device to assess for recurrence. This is important because recurrences do not always echo original symptoms. For example, if your original sign of SIBO was restless leg syndrome, which dissipated upon SIBO eradication, but you experience insomnia and anxiety six months later, test with the device to assess whether SIBO recurrence is to blame.

TESTING WITH THE AIRE DEVICE

To use the AIRE device for breath testing, follow these steps.

Day Prior

For at least twelve hours prior to breath testing, consume only foods that contain no prebiotic fibers or sugars. You should therefore avoid legumes, hummus, any foods that contain inulin and acacia fiber, fruit, starchy or root vegetables, onions, garlic, sugars or fructose, and all dairy products. Also avoid any alcohol. Limit your diet to fat- and protein-rich foods such as eggs, beef, poultry, fish, leafy greens, oils such as olive oil, and nonstarchy vegetables (e.g., spinach, kale, lettuce, green peppers, cucumbers, green beans, zucchini).

Day of Testing

1. Turn on the AIRE device.
2. Activate the AIRE/FoodMarble app on your smartphone, then follow the instructions in the app.
3. Blow into the device when prompted by the app—this is your baseline value.
4. Consume some food that contains prebiotic fiber, for example, 2 teaspoons of inulin or acacia fiber in coffee or yogurt or ¼ cup of legumes. You can eat other foods of your choosing, also, such as eggs, bacon, sausage, and so forth.
5. Test every thirty to forty-five minutes for up to three hours and record your results.

Interpreting the Readings

Each unit of measure on the AIRE device, from 0 to 10, corresponds to an increase in hydrogen gas of 5 parts per million (ppm) obtained by formal H_2 breath testing. A reading of 4 therefore equals 20 ppm H_2, a reading of 8 equals 40 ppm, and 10 corresponds to 50 ppm and above.

After you have consumed prebiotic fiber, interpret the readings as follows:

- A reading of 4–6 is suggestive of SIBO.
- A rise of 4 units above baseline is also suggestive of SIBO, for example, a baseline of 2.0 increasing to 6.0.
- Any value above 6 confidently suggests that SIBO is present. The higher the value, the greater the likelihood that SIBO is present.

In the majority of people with SIBO, the results will be obvious, such as a rise from 1.2 at the start to 9.8 at the thirty- or forty-five-minute mark. (The rules for interpreting H_2S and methane testing on this device are not yet available.)

As elegant as the device is, there are a few downsides:

1. The information provided with the device describes this technology as useful only for identifying intolerance to FODMAPs foods. In other words, if you eat an apple (which is considered a high-FODMAP food because it contains fructose) and thirty minutes later you test positive for H_2, FoodMarble says to stop eating apples. You can see the problem with this and all similar conversations about FODMAPs: they do not address the cause, that is, the SIBO or severe dysbiosis that is behind the reaction to the food. This is why I advise people that a low-FODMAPS diet is nothing more than a symptom-reducing maneuver that does not correct the underlying cause or restore a healthy microbiome or remove a potent source of inflammation (SIBO). Follow the directions on how to operate the device, but ignore the advice on avoiding FODMAPs.
2. This device is for the personal use of one person or family— the mouthpiece is not disposable but can be wiped off with a moist cloth or paper towel. The company urges you not to use alcohol because it can damage the silicone mouthpiece. You can share the device, of course, with someone you are intimate with or family members, but it's a bad idea to share

with, say, coworkers or neighbors. Purchase one device for each person or family who wants to engage in testing.

Here are the tools of SIBO and SIFO management and descriptions of how and why these strategies are useful. The exact protocol for putting all this to use is laid out in Appendix B.

HERBAL ANTIBIOTICS

Although many herbal preparations are promoted as being effective for SIBO and SIFO, only two regimens possess formal evidence of efficacy: CandiBactin-AR + CandiBactin-BR and FC-Cidal + Dysbiocide.[1] The other products may work, but you'd have to take it on faith, not on evidence. On our eradication program, you can choose to take either regimen for fourteen days or until a prebiotic fiber challenge yields lower values on the AIRE device (H_2 readings below 4) for at least two successive days.

You can choose from

CandiBactin-AR: 1–2 capsules twice per day, and
CandiBactin-BR: 2 capsules twice per day

Or

FC-Cidal: 1 capsule twice per day, and
Dysbiocide: 2 capsules twice per day

See Appendix A for sources of herbal antibiotics.

MANAGING BACTERIAL AND FUNGAL DIE-OFF

The age of antibiotics also brought to light a curious reaction called the Jarisch-Herxheimer reaction, first observed with antibiotic treatment of syphilis over a century ago. It is commonly called "die-off." It includes the fever, chills, skin rash, and emotional turbulence that result when an antimicrobial agent is administered and the offending microbes die. Because SIBO and SIFO manifest as proliferation of microbes along thirty feet of GI tract, when you take an agent to eradicate them, the same sort of reaction can occur. The experience can be especially unpleasant with SIFO-eradicating efforts.

The die-off reaction typically occurs during the first few days of antibiotics or antifungals. Should you experience such a reaction, don't panic but recognize the following:

- Microbial die-off is a natural consequence of pushing back this infectious process.
- You have the option of reducing the number or dose of agents you are taking. For instance, if you successfully navigated two weeks of herbal antibiotics and are now embarking on an antifungal regimen of curcumin, oil of oregano, and oil of cinnamon and experience anxiety and dark moods, reduce the regimen to just curcumin and a low dose of oil of oregano, such as three drops diluted in one tablespoon of olive oil. You then can increase the dose of oil of oregano and add back the cinnamon oil after a couple of weeks, once again starting with a low dose of two to three drops per tablespoon, building up to five or six drops over time, and stretching out your efforts for another several weeks. (We discuss these antifungal strategies further in a bit.) This way, the die-off reaction is softer and spread out over time.
- Another option is to take activated charcoal (available in most health food stores) to reduce the die-off reaction. Take 1,000 milligrams in capsule form or ½ teaspoon mixed into eight ounces of water, twice per day. It typically works within fifteen minutes to reduce die-off symptoms.

Unfortunately, no antibiotic or antifungal is 100 percent effective. Rifaximin, the conventional antibiotic of choice for SIBO, for instance, has only a 40–60 percent efficacy. Although the herbal antibiotic regimens have a somewhat better track record, they still fall short of ensured eradication.

For this reason, we can add strategies that increase the likelihood of a successful response. These strategies fall into three categories: strengthening the intestinal barrier, disrupting microbial biofilms, and providing prebiotic fibers.

Strengthening the Intestinal Barrier

Recall that curcumin strengthens the intestinal barrier in a variety of ways, which helps to reduce endotoxemia and even favorably influence bowel flora composition, both bacterial and fungal. I therefore advise anyone taking antibiotics or antifungals to take curcumin concurrently, 300 milligrams twice per day to start, increasing to a maximum of 600 milligrams twice per day, for as long as they take antibiotics or antifungals. Recall that we choose curcumin preparations that do not have additives to enhance absorption because *we do not want absorption*. The basic supplements, vitamin D and omega-3 fatty acids from fish oil, will also be part of your program, as discussed in Part IV, and these supplements likewise strengthen the intestinal barrier.

Clove Green Tea (recipe on page 247) provides eugenol from cloves that increases intestinal mucus, green tea catechins that cross-link mucus proteins and create a gel-like consistency, and fructooligosaccharides (FOS; short-chain fructose polymers or chains) that stimulate the gut microbe *Akkermansia*, which increases mucus production. It is another wonderful and tasty way to strengthen the intestinal barrier.

Disrupting Biofilms

You can add the biofilm-disrupting properties of N-acetyl cysteine (NAC), 600–1,200 milligrams, twice per day, to your antibiotic regimen. N-acetyl cysteine has a proven track record as an aerosolized agent administered in hospitals to people struggling with thick airway secretions, such as in cystic fibrosis. It is also added to antibiotics used to eradicate *Helicobacter pylori* (the ulcer-causing microbe), increasing the efficacy of treatment by disrupting this microbe's biofilm. I do not recommend, however, that anyone take this agent continually (as advised by some for brain health and other benefits) because biofilm disruption is not a healthy practice outside our efforts to eradicate SIBO and SIFO.

Providing Prebiotic Fibers to Prevent Sporulation

Some bacteria and fungi can enter spore-forming mode and thereby become impervious to antibiotics. This process of sporulation especially occurs when microbes are deprived of prebiotic fibers. Adding prebiotic fibers to your SIBO and/or SIFO management therefore tips the scales in favor of blocking sporulation, keeping microbes active and more susceptible to your antibiotic and antifungal efforts. Even if you were previously intolerant of prebiotic fibers because of SIBO, after several days of antibiotics you should be able to add them back to your diet. Prebiotic fibers also provide food for the health-promoting bacteria in your colon, helping them to thrive and outcompete the pathogenic microbes you are in the process of eradicating.

Increase prebiotic fiber intake, as tolerated, up to a target of 20 or more grams per day from sources such as legumes, garlic, asparagus, leeks, dandelion greens, jicama, raw white potato, green unripe banana, inulin powder, pectin, and acacia fiber.

WHAT IF I JUST IGNORE MY SIBO?

It's important to know that you have enormous control in identifying and confirming the presence of SIBO and SIFO. And you can manage it on your own even when the doctor's eyes glaze over.

But what if you say, "This is simply too much. I'll just live with it"? Not a good idea. We know with confidence that burying your head in the sand and enduring uncorrected SIBO/SIFO over time leads to higher risks for

- Type 2 diabetes
- Obesity
- Fibromyalgia

- Irritable bowel syndrome
- Worsened symptoms of ulcerative colitis, Crohn's disease, celiac disease
- Autoimmune conditions
- Depression, anxiety
- Fatty liver
- Diverticular disease, diverticulitis
- Colorectal cancer
- Neurodegenerative disorders—Alzheimer's disease, Parkinsonism, multiple sclerosis

Yes, correcting SIBO and SIFO involves some effort. Yes, you may have to tangle with a few days of die-off reactions, and, yes, there's a little cost involved. But the power you have to seize control over your health is enormous, with implications that stretch out over your lifetime.

CAN WE CURATE AN EFFECTIVE PROBIOTIC TO MANAGE SIBO?

Let's talk a bit further about this notion of creating a probiotic effective against SIBO.

We cannot rely on conventional probiotic formulations to eradicate SIBO because they have only limited effects and do not typically reverse SIBO. High H_2 breath readings, food intolerances, and fibromyalgia, for instance, usually persist despite regular consumption of probiotics. This should come as no surprise because conventional probiotics are prepared without attention to choosing species and strains that have specific SIBO-eradicating effects.

Could we instead choose specific microbial species and strains that can yield SIBO-eradicating effects, then increase their numbers by making yogurt with them? We're searching for microbes that can do the following:

- Colonize the upper GI tract because SIBO means that colonic species have moved up to dominate the small intestine, the process called fecalization.
- Produce bacteriocins. A good candidate produces natural peptide antibiotics, especially those effective against the Enterobacteriaceae species that dominate in SIBO, as well as other species such as *Streptococcus* and *Enterococcus*.
- Support the proliferation of other healthy bacterial species.
- Suppress methane-producing Archaea.

Would such microbes thereby increase the effectiveness of a probiotic effort to eradicate SIBO? Could they also exert suppressive effects on methanogenic SIBO? Can we thereby avoid the use of antibiotics?

TENTATIVE COMPOSITION OF A SUPER GUT SIBO YOGURT

Let me warn you: This is a work in progress with results that I shall be reporting in future. But a growing number of people have reported success in reversing high breath H_2 levels by eating this yogurt. (There is insufficient experience with the newly available H_2S testing to make any determinations on the yogurt's efficacy with it.) The following species and strains hold promise as candidates to include in our first-line effort to reduce and eradicate the species of SIBO:

- *Lactobacillus reuteri* DSM 17938 and ATCC PTA 6475 (the strains contained in the BioGaia Gastrus product): *L. reuteri* colonizes the upper GI tract and produces bacteriocins effective against the species of SIBO. By itself, *L. reuteri* is unlikely to overcome SIBO or SIFO, but it may exert greater effects in the presence of other bacteriocin-producing species. *L. reuteri* has also been shown to reduce the Archaea species that dominate in methanogenic SIBO.[2,3]
- *Lactobacillus gasseri* BNR17: *L. gasseri* strains colonize the upper GI tract and have been shown to be bacteriocin powerhouses, producing as many as seven different bacteriocins, and to reduce the symptoms of irritable bowel syndrome, which is virtually synonymous with SIBO.[4]

- *Bacillus coagulans* GBI-30,6086: Several strains of *B. coagulans* have been shown to reduce the symptoms of irritable bowel syndrome. *B. coagulans* also produces a bacteriocin.[5]

Through our yogurt fermenting projects, we can commonly increase total numbers to two hundred billion (per half-cup serving) and higher, for enhanced efficacy, potentially increasing a ferment's potential for SIBO-suppressing effects. Note that we ferment the four strains of all three species together.

It is likely that four weeks or so of consuming SIBO yogurt will be necessary because probiotics are not as potent as antibiotics. Nonetheless, be aware that Super Gut SIBO Yogurt can also generate presumptive die-off effects, just like antibiotics.

Note this odd twist: After four weeks of consuming SIBO yogurt, delay retesting H_2 for two weeks to assess eradication. *L. reuteri*, like undesirable species, can convert prebiotic fibers to H_2 gas in the small intestine. We therefore need to allow the *L. reuteri* to recede from the upper GI tract before retesting. Once you confirm a negative H_2 value, then resume the *L. reuteri* yogurt to reap its magnificent benefits.

Find the recipe for making Super Gut SIBO Yogurt on page 240, which includes sources for each microbe.

After completing your four-week course of SIBO probiotic, it would be wise to resume taking a high-potency multispecies probiotic (or yogurt fermented from a multispecies kefir or probiotic, per the recipe in Part IV) and eating fermented foods and prebiotic fibers, to maintain basic bowel flora health.

REDUCING FUNGAL OVERGROWTH

Bacterial overgrowth, SIBO, is the dominant condition for most people with intestinal overgrowth of microbes. But, for a significant number of people, SIFO accompanies SIBO. It is also probable that anyone with fungal overgrowth likely has some degree of disrupted bacterial populations that permitted fungal overgrowth in the first place. In other words, we can view SIFO as evidence of disturbed bacterial populations that would ordinarily have helped keep fungal species in check, allowing the fungi to range out of control, much as Archaea, *Clostridium difficile*, and other pathogens emerge when healthy bacterial species are no longer in charge.

Over the last few years, a number of effective, yet fairly benign, supplements with moderate to potent antifungal properties have emerged. There are, of course, antifungal prescription drugs that we know suppress fungal species such as the *Candida* species. But there are now effective natural agents available with antifungal properties.

The herbal antibiotic regimens we use to manage SIBO exert modest antifungal effects, in addition to their antibacterial effects. I also believe that, because of its advantageous antifungal and intestinal barrier properties, we should always include curcumin during any effort to reduce fungal populations. Berberine is another good choice that can be used in place of curcumin, with similar antifungal and intestinal barrier effects.

Fungal reduction requires a longer course of treatment than SIBO, typically a total of four or more weeks, because fungal species tend to form a protective biofilm and have the ability to enter a quiescent mode that is less susceptible to antifungal agents. Because it is cumbersome and costly to perform repeated stool analyses for fungal counts, it really helps if you have a telltale sign or symptom of SIFO to track, such as a skin rash, sugar cravings, or moodiness, to help you gauge your response to the treatment. The total duration of your antifungal efforts depends on how severe SIFO is at the start, but you should anticipate at least a four-week effort.

Here are my suggested regimens to choose from when tackling both SIBO and SIFO combined:

- Two weeks of the CandiBactin regimen + curcumin, or two weeks of the FC-Cidal/Dysbiocide regimen + curcumin.
- Instead of herbal antibiotics, consume the Super Gut SIBO Yogurt for four weeks along with curcumin.
- Once you have completed either a course of herbal antibiotics or the Super Gut SIBO Yogurt, continue four or more weeks of curcumin combined with one or two food-sourced essential oils (to be discussed further).

If you are tackling only SIFO, then four weeks of a combination of curcumin and food-sourced essential oils is a good regimen. For best results, add at least two food-sourced essential oils, building up dosage over time, to circumvent fungal resistance.

Among our choices for antifungal agents are the following:

Curcumin: In addition to antibacterial effects, curcumin shines as an effective antifungal agent against numerous species and strains of *Candida*.[6] It has even shown efficacy against species that are resistant to conventional antifungal drugs. Curcumin has the added advantages of being both safe and virtually nonabsorbable, so it remains in the GI tract for concentrated effect. For this reason, avoid brands that boast added ingredients or any manipulation that increases absorbability, such as the addition of black pepper, piperine, bioperine, or nanoparticles. Curcumin also helps strengthen the intestinal barrier, a major advantage as you heal from the inflammation of microbial overgrowth. As with all antifungal strategies, it is wise to start with a lower dose to minimize die-off symptoms, for example, start with 300 milligrams twice per day and increase to a maximum dose of 600 milligrams twice per day.

Berberine: Like curcumin, this poorly absorbed botanical is among our top choices of safe and effective antifungal agents.[7] Doses range from 300 to 500 milligrams two to three times per day. As with curcumin, if you purchase a product that can be divided, you can reduce the dose during the first few days to weeks to soften the die-off effect. Curcumin and berberine are approximately equal in antifungal efficacy, so you are able to choose one or the other.

Food-sourced essential oils: Essential oils, concentrated phytochemicals sourced from plants, are proving to be potent antifungal agents. The mixture of terpenes and terpenoids in these oils are fat-soluble and thereby have the ability to disrupt the cell walls of fungi (obviating the need for an added biofilm-disrupting agent). Among the most effective are cinnamon oil, clove oil, peppermint oil, and oil of oregano, oils sourced from foods that we know are safe for consumption. These oils have proven more potent than even conventional antifungal drugs amphotericin B and fluconazole, drugs with serious side effects.[8] Of the oils mentioned, cinnamon oil is the most potent. Each oil is effective in small quantities diluted in a tablespoon of olive, avocado, fish, or other healthy oil for reducing intestinal fungal colonization. *Never* take an essential oil directly without diluting it first. Capsule preparations are also available. (They are not appropriate for treating systemic infection, nor have the oils been adequately tested for vaginal use.) One or more essential oils should be at the top of your list to deal with fungal overgrowth. I have had good results adding one oil at a time to an anti-SIFO regimen, starting with small quantities, such as one to two drops in a tablespoon of oil, and building up to four to six drops (a maximum of approximately 200 micrograms if you choose capsules), twice per day. Go slow at first to minimize die-off reactions and then continue for a minimum of two weeks, likely longer. Once at full dose, add one or even two more essential oils, once again starting slow with each one and increasing the dose over time. You can also add essential oils to foods; for example, add one to two drops of cinnamon bark oil to Gingerbread Coffee (recipe on page 249). The NOW brand, Plant Therapy, and DoTerra have proven to be reliable sources of quality oils.

Saccharomyces boulardii: The fungal species *S. boulardii*, a strain of *Saccharomyces cerevisiae* used in winemaking, bread making, and beer brewing, can be taken as a probiotic supplement to suppress intestinal *Candida* through competition. A dose of five billion CFUs per day can work. *S. boulardii* does not colonize the gastrointestinal tract and is gone within days of stopping supplementation.[9]

Bacterial probiotics: Although the precise composition of the ideal probiotic to suppress *Candida* has not been established, several different preparations have been shown to reduce *Candida*, an effect that requires up to one year to develop. Strains of *Lactobacillus rhamnosus* (GG strain) may be especially effective.

After a several-week effort to reduce fungi such as *Candida*, you can re-peat a stool test to quantify how many fungi persist. Alternatively, you can make that judgment based on the reversal of any symptoms.

Many people describe a constellation of fatigue, low-grade fever, anx-iety, and malaise when they address fungal overgrowth. These effects are presumptively(due to fungal die-off,)when the death of microbes results in release of their numerous potentially toxic components into the blood-stream, similar to the die-off experienced during SIBO management ef-forts. This phenomenon appears to develop regardless of which antifungal regimen you use and therefore likely cannot be attributed to being a side effect of the treatment agents but a consequence of fungal die-off.

Long term, you can stack the odds in your favor of not experiencing a recurrence of fungal overgrowth by including these foods in your diet. All have been shown to exert antifungal effects:

- Cloves
- Oregano
- Thyme
- Cinnamon
- Cumin
- Rosemary
- Coriander
- Peppermint

The essential oils extracted from these spices and herbs are more po-tent than the oils when they are intact in the plant, so using these plants as herbs and spices in your food is a way to ingest their essential oils but in a less-potent form. This is helpful for long-term prophylaxis.[10]

DÉJÀ VU ALL OVER AGAIN: PREVENTING SIBO RECURRENCES

Imagine you address your SIBO with the strategies we've discussed and are enjoying relief from years of muscle and joint pain, disability, and help-lessness. But then, six months later, a body-wide recurrence coupled with feelings of anxiety and panic hits you.

For reasons that are not clear, once you've had SIBO, there is potential for its recurrence, when unhealthy Enterobacteriaceae species once again overproliferate and ascend the GI tract. In people who use conventional (pharmaceutical) efforts, about half will experience a recurrence over the subsequent few months if they do not take steps to prevent it. This is especially true when a conventional antibiotic has been prescribed, which is almost never accompanied by advice on how to prevent SIBO recurrences. We are therefore going to discuss a number of strategies that stack the odds in favor of reducing or eliminating recurrences.

Because of the enormous variety of bacterial, fungal, and archaeal species that can repopulate the GI tract, the symptoms of SIBO recurrence can be different from your original symptoms simply because different species can proliferate. If you originally experienced joint pain and Hashimoto's thyroiditis, for example, recurrence could be signaled by bloating and anxiety. This is where measuring breath H_2 can also be useful (and H_2S and methane, if available). If, however, the very same symptoms you originally attributed to SIBO recur, it would be reasonable to proceed to another round of antibacterial efforts without confirmation, that is, empirically, based on your best informed judgment.

You can increase chances of long-term success and prevent recurrences by doing the following:

- Continuing to avoid the factors that disrupt the microbiome. These factors, discussed in Chapter 10, include genetically modified food with glyphosate, stomach acid–blocking and anti-inflammatory drugs, sugars, synthetic sweeteners like aspartame, emulsifying agents, and other microbe-unfriendly substances. These factors disrupted bowel flora in the first place and they can do it again if you don't avoid them.
- Adding a high-potency multispecies probiotic that includes at least some of the keystone species and strains discussed in Part IV. (My current recommended list of commercial products can be found in Appendix A.) Probiotics inhibit unhealthy species from proliferating, encourage mucus production, and provide species and strains that produce bacteriocins that suppress the species of SIBO and SIFO.

⊘ Enthusiastically consuming daily at least one, if not several, fermented foods, which increase intestinal mucus production, encourage proliferation of other healthy species, and discourage unhealthy species.

- Including prebiotic fibers in your daily routine. Aim for a minimum intake of 20 grams per day from the choices listed in Part IV and preferably include some in every meal. Take care of your healthy bacteria by feeding them, and they take care of you.
- Making the *L. reuteri* yogurt. Ferment *L. reuteri* alone or as part of a mixed-culture yogurt. The unique characteristics of *L. reuteri*, including its ability to colonize the upper GI tract (where SIBO and SIFO occur) and produce bacteriocins, help prevent resurgence of undesirable microbes.

These prevention measures are, without a doubt, a work in progress. But these simple moves have still accomplished huge successes in reversing fibromyalgia, IBS, many autoimmune diseases, and weight gain, over and above any results achieved by basic dietary and nutritional supplementation efforts.

CAUSES OF RECURRENT SIBO

Can you do everything right and still experience recurrent SIBO/SIFO?

Yes, absolutely. Most people do indeed enjoy long periods of freedom from bacterial and fungal overgrowth. But the occasional person is plagued by frequent recurrences. Should you find yourself in this situation, here are issues to consider as the underlying cause:

- **Hypochlorhydria:** Lack of stomach acid resulting from infection with *H. pylori*, autoimmune gastritis, or stomach acid–blocking drugs is among the most common reasons for recurrent SIBO. A doctor knowledgeable in these questions, for example, a functional medicine practitioner, can help untangle this situation by testing you, for instance, for levels of gastrin in the blood or testing your stomach pH before they resort to acidification strategies such as betaine HCL, various vinegars, and seltzers.

- **H. pylori**: This microbe is present in around 15 percent of Americans and in as many as 50 percent of the population outside the United States. Its presence contributes to disruptions of bowel flora composition.[11] Identification via blood, breath, or stool testing is readily accomplished, followed by eradication with antibacterial agents. (See Appendix C for a regimen using natural preparations that has been successful in eradicating *H. pylori* without prescription agents.)

- **Hypothyroidism:** Iodine is a basic supplement that we will discuss in Part IV. Long-standing iodine deficiency slows intestinal activity and encourages SIBO. Hypothyroidism from other causes, such as autoimmune thyroid inflammation, can also permit SIBO to recur. We also suspect that taking the thyroid hormone T4 (levothyroxine) alone without addressing hormone levels of T3 can encourage SIBO.[12]

- **Poorly controlled diabetes:** As you might recall, bacteria and fungi love when you have high tissue levels of sugar. Long-standing diabetes (type 1 or type 2) can also lead to gastroparesis, when stomach emptying is slowed, and it's another contributor to SIBO recurrences.

- **Inadequate bile or pancreatic enzyme production:** These conditions are uncommon but frequently cited as causes of recurrent SIBO. In my experience, wheat and grain elimination addresses low enzyme production in the majority of people because it removes the blocker of cholecystokinin, wheat germ agglutinin, which blocks bile and pancreatic enzyme release. Look for evidence of low elastase enzyme or undigested fats in a stool test.

- **Slowed peristalsis:** Once again, in my experience this issue is uncommon in people who have banished wheat and grains from their diet and thereby gliadin-derived opioids that impair intestinal action. If you suspect you have slow motility despite wheat and grain elimination, several agents can help drive peristalsis such as low-dose naltrexone, low-dose erythromycin, and ginger root.

- **Immune system dysfunction:** Genetic inability to produce intestinal immunoglobulin A (IgA; an antibody that plays a crucial role in the immune function of mucous membranes) antibodies occurs in the occasional person and predisposes to SIBO.
- **Chronic stress:** Profound stress such as death of a loved one, acting as caretaker for someone with cognitive impairment, and other prolonged periods of stress readily lead to recurrent SIBO.
- **Anatomic variants:** Abnormalities in the structure of the GI tract, such as blind sacs or abnormal connections, prior gastric bypass, colectomy (colon removal), and other surgical alterations can affect the balance of your microbiome. Anatomic variability is something that can only be identified through formal testing by a gastroenterologist or general surgeon.

As you can appreciate, some of these issues have no quick and easy answer. The best solution is to find a capable practitioner, such as someone in functional medicine or integrative health, to help you explore these questions should you be plagued by SIBO/SIFO recurrences.

MASTER OF THE UNIVERSE

Well, maybe you won't become master of *the* universe, but perhaps you will be master of *your* universe of microbes in the thirty feet of your GI tract and thereby master of your health. Surely, you, armed with a 5G-enabled smartphone, millions of apps, and instant access to the information of the world, can prevail over creatures smaller than a pinhead. Don't pooh-pooh the incredible power you have over numerous health conditions, from hypertension to ulcerative colitis, as well as the way you feel, your mood, and your internal dialogue, by being mindful of the microbial lives you carry within.

Everything in human life—the food you eat, your exposure to light and darkness, the company you keep, the life stresses you experience, the water you drink—*everything* has consequences for the microbes that inhabit your body and where they live in your GI tract. Paying attention to the details of life therefore can pay off big in how you influence your personal microbiome.

In the next chapter, we consider many of the strategies you can adopt to begin rebuilding your microbiome and start down the road toward a Super Gut.

PART III

GUT REACTION

9

TAKE A WALK ON THE WILD SIDE

CAN WE UNDO ALL THE EFFECTS INFLICTED ON OUR INTERNAL microbial landscape, from birth by C-section to consumption of unnecessary antibiotics and processed foods, and rebuild a microbiome that works with us rather than against us? And will such changes restore health and slenderness and free us from modern diseases? Could we regain health of the sort enjoyed by people who hunt and gather their meals, breastfeed their children for two or more years after birth, and congregate around a fire to share the bounty of the day's hunt? Though indigenous people suffer from injuries and infectious diseases like malaria and Dengue fever and lack modern medical care, they do not succumb to the hundreds of common chronic health conditions that plague people in the developed world. I believe that there are important lessons to learn from this.

Modern people have done something fundamentally wrong with our intestinal microbes and in the process have created an awful, fiendish monster within that terrorizes our health. SIBO or not, modern people have decimated the diversity of bacterial species that used to inhabit our GI tracts and thus have lost advantageous species while allowing unhealthy opportunists to proliferate. Thankfully, most of us have not yet reached a point of no return—but we've come close.

Granted, we don't know everything about the microbiome. But we can still craft an approach to restoring it that, for example, banishes fibromyalgia symptoms, frees you from the bowel urgency and bloating of irritable bowel syndrome, reverses many of the phenomena of premature aging, and even pulls back some of the symptoms of neurodegenerative disease, while also achieving Super Gut benefits such as accelerated weight loss, deeper dream-filled sleep, smoother and more supple skin with reduced wrinkles, improved mood, increased energy, and happier relationships.

Let's begin this part of the book with some background on the steps you can take to rebuild a healthy microbiome by bringing back your inner primate—you know, that creature whose needs are programmed into your genetic code.

PLANT YOUR GARDEN OF BOWEL FLORA

What does a healthy microbiome look like?

Should we mimic the bowel flora of the Tanzanian Hadza or Amazonian Yanomami, hunter-gatherers unaffected by modern microbiome disruptions? Never prescribed antibiotics, never having consumed grains laced with glyphosate, or a bowl of Rocky Road ice cream thickened with polysorbate 80, they have bacterial species that we lack while we have acquired species that they almost entirely lack. Are these differences disadvantageous for us, or does the modern microbiome reflect adaptations necessary to navigate a world that is not forest, jungle, or mountains?

In other words, some of the changes that have evolved in microbiome composition may be positive adaptations that help us respond to the demands of our modern world, but others may reflect adverse effects from, say, herbicides and antibiotics. But how do we tell the difference?

No one has all the answers. But we can nonetheless adopt a number of strategies that help us craft a healthier microbiome, one that is in better shape than our current disastrous situation. First we will discuss strategies that minimize modern microbiome-disruptive factors, then drill down to specific strategies that eradicate overproliferated unhealthy species and cultivate healthier species in their place. We will dive deeper into the worlds of SIBO, SIFO, and endotoxemia, adopting efforts that can lead to life- and health-transforming experiences.

To help get our arms around these ideas, I compare our efforts in cultivating a healthy intestinal microbiome to starting a backyard garden in springtime. Say it's May and you want to plant a garden. You begin by preparing the soil: pick out weeds, sticks, and stones. Next, you plant seeds for peas, carrots, zucchini, cucumbers, and tomatoes. You then water and fertilize throughout the growing season and guard against critters like raccoons and rabbits, who would like to gobble up your precious vegetables. Give it a couple of months or so and, with proper care, voilà, you've got a bounty of vegetables to harvest, delicious salads and healthy accompaniments to your meals.

Efforts to cultivate an intestinal "garden" of microbes are very similar. We are going to prepare the "soil," plant "seeds," then "water and fertilize" our inner garden. In the garden we call bowel flora, of course, we won't be harvesting zucchini but simply keeping up efforts to propagate the microbes we have cultivated for health.

Let's talk about preparing the soil, or how to remove factors that have disrupted your garden of bowel flora, much like removing the sticks and stones in your backyard garden in early spring that makes room for a thriving vegetable garden.

GO GET YOUR SHOVEL

As modern people, we have so disrupted our intestinal microbiome that we may need the biological equivalents of shovels, pickaxes, and a backhoe to get this garden going. You may have to figuratively engage in digging out deep taproots and carting away wheelbarrows full of weeds and stones.

What are the "roots," "weeds," and "stones" of your microbiome? Let's run through them, one by one, focusing on the factors that you can change. In other words, if you or someone you care about was delivered by C-section forty years ago, you cannot obviously undo not being delivered vaginally. If a baby formula manufacturer persuaded your mom that synthetic formula was preferable to human breast milk when you were an infant, you can hardly go back and undo this tragic mistake of marketing.

Or if you were given ten courses of antibiotics over the years for a variety of infections, there's nothing you can do now to undo having taken the drugs. And if you were an ice cream aficionado, consuming bowls or cones of emulsifier-rich French vanilla, you cannot go back and un-eat the ice cream.

Which factors can you correct or change now to prepare your garden of bowel flora?

- **Avoid sugars:** Sugars are to bowel flora as breadcrumbs are to birds and ducks: they will take the bait. Consume, say, sugary soft drinks or snacks, and you are delivering bacteria and fungi an invitation to ascend and proliferate. Lots of sugar in your diet is a virtually guaranteed setup for both SIBO and SIFO.
- **Avoid synthetic noncaloric sweeteners:** Avoid all foods sweetened with aspartame, sucralose, or saccharine. These include sugar-free sodas, ice creams, frozen yogurts, chewing gum, and other processed foods containing these ingredients.
- **Banish processed foods that contain emulsifying agents:** We've discussed how polysorbate 80 and carboxymethylcellulose not only degrade the mucus lining but also provoke unhealthy changes in bowel flora species and increase intestinal permeability that leads to increased appetite, weight gain, and inflammation and sets us up for autoimmune conditions. We do not yet know how far and wide this applies to other less-potent emulsifiers such as carrageenan, propylene glycol, and lecithin. Until the details are sorted out, we follow a commonsense rule: choose natural whole foods such as avocados, eggs, green vegetables, and others that have no added synthetic ingredients. When buying processed foods, look for brands with the shortest list of ingredients that you can recognize by name. Choose, for instance, salad dressings with olive oil, vinegar, salt, and herbs, but no thickeners, gums, or mixing agents. Look for ice creams with nothing but cream, berries, cocoa, or other natural flavorings and safe sweeteners such as monk fruit or stevia (I discuss which sweeteners are safe and do not disrupt bowel flora or cause weight gain later), or make ice cream yourself. (I'll show you a shortcut to making ice cream without the need for unhealthy additives.)

- **Choose organic:** Whenever possible, as permitted by budget and availability, choose organically grown foods. Organic vegetables and fruits are less likely to contain herbicides and pesticides that, even in small quantities, can exert unhealthy effects on bowel flora, not to mention effects on our endocrine and hormonal systems. Choosing organic also means you're minimizing exposure to glyphosate, the herbicide with antibiotic properties that is in genetically modified foods such as corn and soy. Eating organically grown foods is especially important if you regularly consume the skin or exteriors of the foods, such as berries or apples with their skin on, and less important when you discard the skin, as with bananas and avocados. Also choose organic meats whenever possible so as to avoid the antibiotic residues frequently found in conventionally raised poultry, beef, pork, and farm-raised fish.

- **Filter drinking water:** Municipal drinking water is treated with chlorine (or, even worse, chloramine, which cannot be boiled off) and fluoride, both of which have adverse effects on the mucus lining of the intestines. A charcoal or reverse osmosis filtration system can remove most water contaminants. Countertop pitcher water filters have lately also expanded their list of filtered contaminants and have become a viable choice.

- **Avoid or minimize wheat and grains:** We know with confidence, given recent scientific research, that the gliadin protein of wheat and related proteins of other grains increase intestinal permeability so that undigested food components, microbes, and toxic breakdown products can seep into the bloodstream. This is the process that initiates many, if not most, autoimmune diseases, including type 1 diabetes and rheumatoid arthritis. The combination of wheat or grain consumption with the endotoxemia of SIBO and SIFO is therefore a lethal process that opens the door for numerous health conditions because of intestinal permeability. The solution? Eat no wheat or grains. (This is the message in my Wheat Belly series of books, which alone has transformed the health and lives of millions of people.) Avoiding wheat and grains (a list that includes rye, barley, corn, oats, millet, sorghum, and rice) and soy products also hugely reduces your exposure to glyphosate.

- **Go light on alcohol:** Alcoholic beverages are a mixed bag: some good components (polyphenols and flavonoids that confer color and flavor), some bad components (alcohol and sugars) that cultivate unhealthy bacterial species, but especially fungal overgrowth.
- **Get off NSAIDs and stomach acid–suppressing drugs:** Start by challenging your doctor to help you accomplish this. Sadly, more than 90 percent of doctors will fail to help, claiming that once you are prescribed these drugs, there is no way to get off them. This is simply not true. The basic strategies articulated in this book may be sufficient to enable many, if not most, people to avoid nonsteroidal anti-inflammatory drugs like ibuprofen and naproxen. But getting off stomach acid–blocking drugs such as Protonix (pantoprazole) and Prilosec (omeprazole) can be more complicated, but not impossible, and will require you and your doctor to explore issues such as hypochlorhydria (low stomach acid), SIBO, and other contributing factors.

If this list seems daunting, just remember that a return to real, whole foods is key. Choose foods that are, as often as possible, in their original state, such as eggs, meats, vegetables, fruit, and legumes rather than processed packaged foods that come with labels listing dozens of additives, emulsifiers, mixing agents, sweeteners, and other chemicals.

You should also, of course, minimize exposure to antibiotics, accepting a prescription only when truly necessary. If you have been exposed to the flu or another respiratory virus like the common cold, for instance, and are handed a prescription "just in case" your condition converts to a bacterial infection, this is *not* a good reason to take an antibiotic. Undoubtedly, antibiotics are truly beneficial in certain situations, but view these drugs as an occasionally necessary evil and question their need each and every time.

A complicated landscape of factors has decimated the microbiome of modern humans. Not all disruptive factors have been identified. But if you follow the limited list above, you will have eliminated or reduced the most disruptive factors of all. Only then can we even begin to consider planting the seeds of the microbes you have been deprived of while also eliminating or reducing the microbes that are responsible for making you gain weight, increasing your blood pressure, or disrupting your emotional and mental health.

PLANT THE SEEDS

The best way to seed your gastrointestinal tract is to have been delivered vaginally as a baby, breastfed for at least the first two years of your life, and exposed to a mother and family with their own rich and healthy microbiomes. Alas, we cannot undo the harmful consequences of decisions made in early life and the other myriad factors in your past. Let's instead focus on practices that you can manage in the here and now to reseed your microbiome.

Probiotics and fermented foods are the cornerstone of our reseeding program. Let's first tackle the world of probiotics.

Commercial probiotics are products that contain collections of live microbes believed to be beneficial. Typically sold in capsule form, they contain millions to billions of microbes, or colony-forming units (CFUs). (One live bacterium equals 1 CFU in the language of microbiology.) Whereas most of the microbes in commercial probiotic preparations are bacteria, beneficial fungal species such as *Saccharomyces boulardii* are sometimes included. Some probiotics contain spore-forming or soil-based microbes.

Unfortunately, we are still in the Dark Ages when it comes to commercial probiotic formulations. Most products are haphazard collections of species that are believed to be beneficial, but these formulations are not typically designed to achieve a specific purpose. Most preparations on the market today fail to specify which bacterial strains they contain, a major oversight. We simply cannot know whether a probiotic provides specific benefits unless we know the strain. (See box: Choose Your Friends Carefully on page 143.) Taking a probiotic that does not specify strain is little better than choosing a random drug to treat a specific disorder—you might inadvertently pick out a stomach acid–blocking drug, anti-inflammatory steroid, antipsychotic, or chemotherapy agent because that is how different the effects different strains of the same species can be. Without knowing the strain, you are therefore unlikely to choose a product that yields the effects you desire. Yet you can pay a lot of money for a probiotic preparation that fails to mention the strains.

There's another fundamental dilemma with commercial probiotics. If your mom gave you, for instance, the microbe *Bifidobacterium infantis* through breastfeeding, it would likely take up residence for years, perhaps a lifetime, in your GI tract, provided you didn't unintentionally eradicate it with a course of antibiotics or other microbiome-disruptive agent. If you were to take the same microorganism as a probiotic, it might live in your gut for a few weeks or months, then it's gone—but why? Why do species and strains delivered to your microbiome as a probiotic not take up long-term or permanent residence as do those given to you by your mother or acquired through the environment?

No one yet has the answer to this fundamental question. But it means that, when you take a commercial probiotic, a useful species or strain takes up residence and provides benefits for the short period of a few hours or days it sticks around. Encouraging long-term residence of good microbes is one of our goals, but not always possible with commercial probiotics.

The good news is, even in their transient passage, we can experience the beneficial effects of these microbes. Even if the bacteria in the probiotic you took on Monday have passed into the toilet by Thursday, they still yield a number of benefits, including the following:

- Stimulating production of intestinal mucus. Many *Bifidobacterium* species are champions at this, especially when "fed" prebiotic fibers that they convert to fatty acids such as butyrate and propionate that, in turn, trigger enthusiastic mucus production by intestinal cells.[1]
- Converting dietary components such as flavonoids and polyphenols (phytonutrients from vegetables and fruits) into metabolites that are beneficial[2]
- Inhibiting growth of pathogenic species
- Producing nutrients, especially B vitamins like B_1, B_2, B_6, folate (B_9), and B_{12}[3]

Taking a commercial probiotic can therefore provide benefits, but not the full range of benefits that you'd hope they would provide. My suspicion is that current probiotic formulations fail to provide the "keystone" species and strains that our Super Gut requires, that is, the handful of microbes that, absent from the modern microbiome, support the proliferation of other beneficial microbes. I predict that the probiotic of the future will not be composed of some slap-dash collection of microbes haphazardly assembled in the hopes that it yields benefits but will be a purposeful collection of keystone species and strains that cultivate an environment conducive to the proliferation of hundreds of other beneficial species and strains. Future probiotics may take advantage of what my friend and famed microbiologist Dr. Raul Cano calls "guild" or "consortium" effects in which microbe A produces a metabolite beneficial to microbe B, which in turn produces a metabolite beneficial to microbe C, which then produces a metabolite beneficial to microbes A and B—they collaborate and thereby generate bigger benefits for their host. In other words, if we restore keystone or collaborative species, dozens or hundreds of other beneficial species will follow. A limited number of such preparations on the market have moved in that direction (listed in Appendix A). You can appreciate that crafting a list of keystone and collaborative species may therefore be the Holy Grail of rebuilding bowel flora. Seeding the right mix of foundational species potentially explains the extravagant benefits of, for instance, fecal transplant, as well as some of the surprisingly beneficial results from the fermentation projects discussed later.

Although emerging evidence does indeed suggest some benefits to seeding spore-forming and soil-based microbes, we do not yet know what role they should play in rebuilding the microbiome and whether they provide further advantages—yes, there's plenty of marketing, but not a lot of real evidence. We do know that some spore-forming species, such as *Bacillus coagulans* (one of the species included in my Super Gut SIBO Yogurt recipe), provide substantial health benefits, such as reduced pain and swelling of arthritis, reduced abdominal bloating and swelling, and accelerated recovery from strenuous exercise, an advantage for athletes. I will show you later how to make yogurt or other fermented foods with this species.

CHOOSE YOUR FRIENDS CAREFULLY

Remember the issue of strain specificity we discussed earlier? Take *Escherichia coli:* You have *E. coli* naturally occurring in your gut. Most of your friends and family have *E. coli*. Even that nice guy or gal you may be eyeing at work has *E. coli*. But consume romaine lettuce contaminated with *E. coli* from the cow manure in the pasture next door to where it was grown and you can experience diarrhea that lasts for days or even die of kidney failure—same species: *E. coli*, but a different strain. Differences in strain within a single species— strain specificity—can literally make a life-and-death difference.

This may seem painfully tedious, but this conversation will help you become more savvy about probiotics so that you can tell the difference between helpful and not-so-helpful microbes.

Problem: The majority of commercial probiotics fail to specify the bacterial strains they include. Clinical studies demonstrate that *Lactobacillus rhamnosus* GG (i.e., the GG strain), for example, hastens recovery from diarrhea after a course of antibiotics, but other *L. rhamnosus* strains do not. It means that the great majority of commercial probiotics containing *L. rhamnosus* are virtually worthless for this purpose because manufacturers often choose strains that are less costly rather than specific strains that yield a known benefit, which are often more costly. It would be like choosing a dress or pair of pants off the rack without regard to the size, color, or style, but just blindly buying what you randomly choose—you'd hardly make a fashion splash, and perhaps would be unable to even pull the dress or pants on. Likewise, accepting a commercial probiotic formulation slapped together with no knowledge of strain is a recipe for failure.

As you can imagine, having to choose among a multitude of strains complicates the world of probiotics. I therefore do my best to make it easy for you by specifying in Appendix A the short list of commercial products that recognize this issue. The yogurt fermentation projects also make use of only specific strains to ensure greater likelihood of benefits. As commercial products improve and incorporate, for instance, strains with keystone and collaborative effects, better and more effective products with greater health benefits will become available. When critics make statements like "Probiotics have not been proven to yield any health benefits," they are partly correct— but that is likely to change in coming years. I shall also detail how we can obtain benefits way beyond those provided by commercial probiotics by fermenting specific species and strains to high counts. Using modified methods of fermentation allows us to obtain extravagant results—and purposeful probiotic application yields *extraordinary* benefits, contrary to such blanket statements.

Do we need to replace each and every bacterial species and strain that might be beneficial? No, I don't believe so. As we learn which are among the keystone species and strains, replacing these microbes, which perform functions crucial to the proliferation and survival of other beneficial species, may be the solution. Much as plankton in the ocean supports the survival of other ocean creatures, from jellyfish to whales, so do keystone bacterial species in our intestinal ecosystems support numerous other microbes. *Bifidobacterium infantis* in newborns is a good example. If *B. infantis* is passed from mother to child, the child is better able to metabolize the milk oligosaccharides (sugars) in breast milk that, in turn, nourish other bacterial species in the child's microbiome.[4] Without *B. infantis*, the infant's ability to digest the components of breast milk is impaired, growth is slowed, and overall microbiome composition is compromised because fewer beneficial species survive. Replacing or restoring keystone species like *B. infantis* is therefore preferable to a shotgun approach to probiotics.

We do not yet have a full list of every keystone species that, by their mere presence, supports the entire complex web of microbiome species and thereby your health. Given current knowledge, however, I list the following as among the most important species and strains, as suggested by the evidence:[5-14]

- *Bifidobacterium infantis* ATCC 15697, M-63, and ECV001
- *Lactobacillus reuteri* DSM 17938, ATCC PTA 6475, and NCIMB 30242
- *Lactobacillus gasseri*—multiple strains including BNR17 and CP2305
- *Lactobacillus rhamnosus* GG and HN001
- *Lactobacillus plantarum* 299v and P-F
- *Faecalibacterium prausnitzii* A2-165 and L2-6. This species is responsible for as much as 25 percent of all intestinal production of butyrate, which yields health benefits for the human host.
- *Bifidobacterium longum* BB536

- *Akkermansia muciniphila* ATCC BAA-835
- *Bacillus coagulans* GBI-30,6086 and MTCC 5856. The presence of this microbe supports the proliferation of other healthy strains, including *F. prausnitzii*. These strains are not included in most commercial probiotics.

This is, by no means, a complete list but a work in progress. Replacing keystone species is a better strategy than trying to obtain each and every bacterial strain shown to offer benefits. In other words, cultivate keystone species and they then become the "farmer" that helps you maintain dozens, even hundreds, of beneficial bacterial species that will provide you benefits.

There's no need to memorize this list or work to restore each and every strain listed because I share the names of the commercially available probiotics that include some of these species and strains and show you how to ferment yogurt and other foods with them.

How long should you take a commercial probiotic? They are, after all, costly. Nobody has a firm answer to this question, but my view is that commercial probiotics are helpful at the start of your program and until you have achieved relief from whatever bothersome conditions or markers you are following, such as bloating, diarrhea, or skin rash or breath H_2. There's no harm in continuing to take a probiotic, but you can likely obtain similar or superior benefits just by engaging in all the other strategies I discuss, such as including fermented foods in your daily routine, including pre-biotic fibers in your diet frequently, and making various yogurts to replace important bacterial species.

Fermented foods are another way to "seed" your GI tract with healthy microbes. Although fermented foods suffer from the same drawbacks as most commercial probiotic products in that the helpful species and strains do not take up residence in the human GI tract for long, there are still benefits to their consumption. Humans have enjoyed fermenting foods for centuries as a food-processing technique that can improve taste and nutrition and prevent spoilage: prosciutto in Italy, olives in Greece, gochujang in Korea, umeboshi in Japan, among many others, made according to recipes handed down over generations. For current purposes, we are mostly interested in microbial fermentation that yields the natural preservative lactic acid, not fungal fermentation that converts sugars to alcohol such as in beers and wines (filtration usually removes microbes from alcoholic beverages). Fermented grain products, such as sourdough bread, are heated during baking, which kills any potentially beneficial microbes. We are interested in fermented foods that yield live microbes that, upon ingestion, exert beneficial effects during their brief adventure through the human GI tract.

Fermented foods are as rich and varied as the starting food, the hundreds of different fermenting microbes, and the ambient conditions in which the food is fermented. Indulging in foods such as kimchi, kombucha, traditional sauerkraut, fermented pickles, kefir, yogurt, home-fermented veggies, and the numerous traditional fermented foods unique to various cultures around the world is another way to augment your intake of *Lactobacillus*, *Bifidobacterium*, *Pediococcus*, and *Leuconostoc* bacterial species, as well as friendly fungal species (especially in kefir and kombucha). While some people make a hobby out of fermenting vegetables like radishes, asparagus, cucumbers, and beets—almost any food can be fermented—and making their own kefir, kombucha, and yogurt, there is also an increasing number of commercial products available. Just be sure that the product is labeled with "live cultures," "live and active," "fermented," or another indication that live microbes are indeed present. Pickles in brine and vinegar or products that have been heat inactivated for shelf stability do not contain live microbial cultures. One reassuring sign that bacteria are still alive: cloudy, milky liquid indicates swarms of live bacteria. And, yes, you can drink that soupy mix once the pickles or sauerkraut have been consumed.

PROBIOTICS VERSUS PREBIOTICS: EAT OR BE EATEN

People sometimes get confused with the terminology of probiotics and prebiotics, but it's really quite simple.

Probiotics are the microbes themselves. They are microscopic creatures that are presumed to exert beneficial effects on their human host. *Lactobacillus* and *Bifidobacterium* are among the most common groups of bacteria that we regard as probiotics. Probiotics "eat"—incorporate and metabolize—prebiotics that you ingest as part of your diet.

Prebiotics are nutritional constituents of plants that microbes themselves consume and process. Prebiotics include various fibers such as inulin, the galactooligosaccharides in lentils and kidney beans, and sugars such as lactose in dairy products. Unlike humans, microbes don't convert their prebiotic foods into fecal material, but they do turn them into metabolites that are important for human health, such as the fatty acid butyrate and vitamins such as folate and vitamin B_{12}.

I elaborate on the very important topic of prebiotic fibers later in the book.

Because the microbial composition of fermented products depends on the species present in the starting food (microbes on the surface of a vegetable or the mix of bacteria and fungi in a batch of kefir), we cannot be specific in choosing species and strains. Such foods might have many varieties of microbes present in the billions, or sometimes even in the trillions.[15] Species present in fermented foods that we eat typically do not take up residence in the gut for more than a few days or weeks; sometimes they pass through the GI tract in hours. Microbes from fermented foods can, nonetheless, provide benefits similar to those of commercial probiotics such as protection against pathogens like *Salmonella*, production of beneficial metabolites and vitamins, and conversion of inactive nutrients into active forms.

The evidence showing that fermented foods improve human health is limited but does suggest that constipation is improved, risk for type 2 diabetes is reduced, inflammatory markers are reduced, and a modest effect on preventing weight gain is recognized.[15,16] The wide variety of microbes in kefir, in particular, may even provide some protection against proliferation of Enterobacteriaceae, the species most prevalent in SIBO.[17]

DOUBLING UP ON BENEFITS

In the yogurt recipes using specific bacterial species and strains that I provide later in the book, I introduce specific changes to the traditional process of fermentation that are responsible for generating far greater effects than you'd expect. Let me explain.

Remember the kids' trick question that asks, "Would you rather have a million dollars or a penny that doubles each day for a month?"

Kids invariably choose the $1 million. But the penny that doubles every day—$0.01, $0.02, $0.04, $0.08—nothing to get excited about at the start—ends up totaling over $5 million! $5,368,709.12 to be exact after thirty days. Hard to believe, but that is the power of doubling or, as they say in financial circles, "compound interest." We put this principle to work in making our yogurts to obtain huge numbers of bacteria that yield greater health effects.

If graphed, the growth of money starting with a penny looks like this:

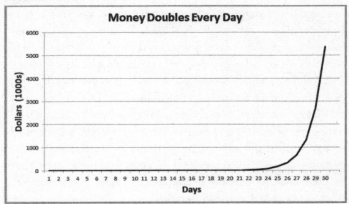

You can see that there is only a trivial increase in money up until day 25 or 26, but then growth explodes with huge increases over the last few days.

The same mathematical phenomenon applies to bacterial reproduction: the more time that passes, the greater the increase in bacterial numbers: 1, 2, 4, 8, etc. (Bacteria reproduce by one bacterium becoming two, two becoming four, and so on. For simplicity, we assume that bacteria don't die. This is not true, of course, but the basic principle of increasing numbers over time still applies.)

L. reuteri, a bacterial species that we put to work to make a high-potency fermented yogurt, doubles every three hours at 100°F. Replace "Days" on the *x* axis with increments of three hours (i.e., 12 doublings over 36 hours) and you have the graph for bacterial doubling time. From the trajectory of this curve, you can surmise the following:

- There is very little increase in bacterial numbers during the first thirty hours of fermentation, the period along the horizontal part of the curve. (Hour 30 with *L. reuteri* coincides with day 25 of money.)
- There is explosive growth in bacterial numbers starting at hour 30, with the greatest increases from 30 to 36 hours.

This means that commercial yogurt manufacturers, which typically ferment for only 4 hours (one doubling) to hasten production, and home yogurt makers, who typically ferment for 12 hours (four doublings), achieve minimal bacterial numbers. We ferment for a minimum of 30 hours, preferably 36 hours, to achieve the big numbers we are after that generate substantial biological effects. This doubling phenomenon explains why yogurt you buy in the supermarket provides almost no health benefits: brief fermentation times and microbial species that yield little benefit add up to no noticeable effects. It also explains why commercial yogurt nearly always requires the addition of synthetic thickeners like xanthan gum or gellan gum to achieve a thick end result because there are few bacteria and minimal bacterial metabolites, which naturally thicken the milk during fermentation.

Why do we not ferment longer than 36 hours? At some point, available resources (lactose, prebiotic fiber, etc.) for the microbes are exhausted and die-off exceeds doublings. My team and I have run flow cytometry studies to determine bacterial counts, and bacterial counts appear to plateau at 36 hours—longer, and the rate of die-off exceeds the rate of reproduction. Longer fermentation time also risks fungal contamination because fungi in the air and on utensils inevitably seed the yogurt, given the chance. At 36 hours, we have measured bacterial counts of 200–260 billion in the *L. reuteri* yogurt per half-cup serving—far higher counts than contained in a commercial probiotic and enough to generate big benefits.

By using my unique method of prolonged fermentation time combined with feeding your yogurts prebiotic fibers, not only do you cultivate hundreds of billions of bacteria that yield real and substantial health benefits, but you also will enjoy a thicker, richer, more delicious end product that goes great with a handful of berries, no thickening agents required.

IN DEFENSE OF ROT

All throughout human history, if you killed an animal and harvested its meat and organs, stumbled upon a bounty of wild berries, or managed to squeeze some milk from the mammary glands of a goat, you would allow the food to ferment in order to keep it from becoming inedible or poisonous through spoiling.

Fermentation is controlled rotting: the production of lactic acid by bacteria, the production of ethanol by fungi. Early people buried meat, fish, and eggs in the ground and allowed them to ferment and then retrieved them a few weeks or months later when fresh food was in short supply. They stored milk in the stomach of an animal they had killed, the rennet (an enzyme produced by the stomach lining) in the stomach assisting in its fermentation into cheese, or they buried urns filled with juice pressed from grapes, recovered months later as wine. Managed rotting has been a part of the human experience for thousands of generations.

Then came refrigeration. At first only a commercial process, refrigeration became available to consumers in 1927, then got a big boost when Frigidaire developed the refrigerant freon. It popularized the notion of always having fresh foods on hand while demonizing foods that were fermented and thereby riddled with microbes. In less than a century, the long-standing practice of consuming foods teeming with bacteria and fungi essentially ended in many Western countries.

Refrigeration meant that food could be stored for extended periods, delaying fermentation. People came to view fermented food with distrust because it seemed just a step away from being rotten (the exceptions being products of fungal fermentation such as beer and wine). Most people, upon viewing the cloudy, slimy bacterial soup that develops when veggies are submerged in water and salt, for instance, would promptly toss the whole lot in the trash, not recognizing it as edible and an actually healthy food. As a result of this widespread disdain for fermented foods, our intake of friendly bacterial and fungal species dropped to nearly nothing. Even common modern fermented foods like yogurt contain minimal, if any, live bacteria because the fermentation process is abbreviated for the sake of hastening production. And traditionally fermented foods such as pickles and sauerkraut are no longer fermented but just bottled in brine and vinegar, with no bacteria or fungi in the mix.

Combine our near-century-long failure to consume fermented bacteria- and fungi-filled foods with the other modern factors that disrupt bowel flora, and we have a surefire way to create dysbiosis—massive disruption of bowel flora and the wide collection of health conditions that result.

Part of the solution is to return to eating the foods that humans consumed for millennia before refrigeration made us squeamish. I shall therefore discuss how you can ferment your own vegetables and other foods, make yogurts with high bacterial counts, and buy foods that are already fermented and alive.

Super Gut Success: Michael, 59, Colorado

"I've gained significant benefits over the past few months from two yogurts made with *L. gasseri* BNR-17 and *B. coagulans* GBI30,6086 at age fifty-nine.

"My workout results have increased significantly. For many years, I've trained very hard in the weight room three times a week. For the past ten years, I've basically just maintained my strength and conditioning. Over a nine-week period with the two new yogurts, I experienced an increase in upper body strength of 10 percent or more. For example, my bench press increased from 225 pounds to 250 plus pounds. I've also added four to five pounds of lean body mass without changing my diet or calorie consumption.

"I've noticed a significant increase in endurance while skiing. I've been a mogul skier for many years. For as long as I can remember, after seven or eight runs my legs would become weak noodles with pain from lactic acid buildup. I'd stop and fall more frequently and eventually quit after nine or ten runs. Recently, with the yogurts I skied eleven nonstop runs, with no weakness or lactic acid pain.

"I recently conducted an impromptu experiment on myself. I embarked on a business trip for seven days without my yogurts. Instead, I took small doses of each probiotic in capsule form—1 million CFUs or less for each. I thought this would be enough to get me through the yogurt-free week. Unfortunately, it wasn't. After about two days, I felt like I had aged: my energy level dropped especially at the end of the day, my body was achy and stiff, and I became moody. When I returned from the trip, I immediately resumed eating the yogurts. After about 1-½ days, I was back to normal. In the future I'll pack the yogurts in my suitcase.

"Although I didn't really have significant SIBO/SIFO symptoms aside from some mild bloating after meals, every time I used the AIRE device it registered 10. I began a regimen of the antifungal and antibacterial supplements as you suggested. Since then I've noticed that some nagging problems I had experienced for years had disappeared: bloating, rosacea, blepharitis, and mild toenail fungus."

WATER AND FERTILIZE YOUR "GARDEN"

We've discussed how we prepare the soil to plant our garden, how we plant the seeds of probiotics and fermented foods. Let's now talk about the equivalent of water and fertilizer for your garden.

Much of this conversation centers around fiber. Humans simply do not possess the digestive enzymes to break down the fibers from vegetables, mushrooms, legumes, nuts, and fruits into sugars. Although you may not recognize fiber as a form of sugar, fiber is indeed a long chain of sugar molecules. Unlike humans, bacteria possess the enzymes to metabolize the many forms of fiber (the exception being cellulose fiber, which is a structural component in plants; few bacteria in our microbiome can digest this type of fiber, unlike those in grazing creatures like cows, horses, and goats, which can). Sure, you can navigate your way around the internet, file pages of tax forms, maybe even do trigonometry with your teenager—but you cannot digest fiber.

Bacteria are enthusiastic consumers of fiber. This is a wonderful example of the interdependence of humans and bacteria: feed your microbiome the fiber it needs and your microbial partners will convert it into nutrients and metabolites that you and your intestinal tract need. It's also a reflection of the fundamental human need for plant matter. Despite dietary fads that reduce or eliminate vegetables, fruits, and legumes from the diet, the fact remains that your bacteria cannot thrive on a diet of only animal matter. Neglect intake of the fibers that feed bacteria and odd things happen, as we shall discuss. Fibers digestible by bacteria are therefore labeled "prebiotic" fibers. They are essential, and without them you cannot enjoy a bounty of healthy microbes.

A healthy microbiome therefore requires prebiotic fibers, fibers that humans ingest but cannot digest. They are crucial to health success and more important than probiotics for long-term health. Not only do prebiotic fibers cause beneficial bacterial species to proliferate, they also provide the nutrition necessary for bacteria to produce healthy fatty acids and other metabolites that nourish and support the intestinal lining.

As mentioned, neglect prebiotic fiber intake, as most Americans do, and the mucus lining of your gastrointestinal tract thins out, opening the door to intestinal inflammation, autoimmune diseases, and unhealthy changes in bowel flora populations. A diet lacking in prebiotic fibers triggers changes in microbiome composition that sometimes cannot be reversed simply by resuming intake of prebiotic fibers, changes so profound that they can even be passed on to offspring.[18,19] Minding our prebiotic fiber intake is therefore crucial, teaching us new lessons on how to construct a healthy human diet. (See box below: Bacterial Hunger Strike.)

It is not uncommon for people living the hunter-gatherer lifestyle to take in 100 grams or more of prebiotic fibers per day, which they obtain largely from the roots and tubers they dig out of the ground. The average modern person obtains no more than 12 grams of fiber per day, of which 5–8 grams are of the prebiotic variety. Peak benefit develops with a daily prebiotic fiber intake of 20 grams or more per day. (It has not yet been demonstrated that we need to mimic the intake of a hunter-gatherer and obtain 100 or more grams.) By eating this much fiber, you are not only contributing to maintaining a healthy intestinal mucus lining but also can begin to experience the health benefits of plentiful bacteria-produced butyrate, a fatty acid that offers better weight control, improved response to insulin, lower blood sugar and blood pressure, lower blood triglycerides, and lower potential for developing fatty liver.[20,21] Which is better: achieving normal blood pressure by taking two or three blood pressure drugs with multiple side effects or normalizing blood pressure by cultivating healthy intestinal bacteria that help you maintain normal blood pressure with no side effects, only side benefits?

BACTERIAL HUNGER STRIKE

It's a peculiar reality of human behavior.

Because "official" dietary guidelines, such as those provided by the USDA and the US Department of Health and Human Services that advocate cutting fat and increasing grain consumption, have been such an unmitigated disaster—to a substantial degree, they are responsible for the modern epidemics of obesity, type 2 diabetes, fatty liver, and autoimmune diseases—many people have rejected guidelines and have gone to the opposite extreme and eliminated all carbohydrates. Although there is no question that, to undo our modern dietary disaster, restricting carbohydrates, especially grains (whole and white—there's virtually no difference in glycemic potential or in many other effects) and sugars, makes sense, but *eliminating* carbohydrates is a really bad idea. Yet there are millions of people who have embraced ketogenic, carnivorous, or other variations of extreme low-carb diets. (When carbohydrate intake is slashed to around 10 grams per meal, metabolism of fat stores causes the release of a by-product called ketones, thus the label "ketogenic diet.")

Because prebiotic fibers that nourish microbes come only from plants—there are zero animal sources of prebiotic fibers (except for consumption of the contents of raw stomach and intestines)—slashing plant matter too far means that prebiotic fiber intake suffers. Some people who are mindful of this mistake maintain an intake of low-carb prebiotic fiber sources such as asparagus, garlic, and leeks, but they are the exception. Most people on such extreme diets rely on largely nonstarchy greens like spinach, kale, and broccoli, with generous servings of beef, pork, poultry, and fish but with no awareness of the injustice they are inflicting on their bowel microbes.

What happens when you follow one or another of these strict low-carb diets without maintaining generous intake of the fibers that nourish microbes? In addition to degradation of the mucus barrier that I discussed in Chapter 5, with plenty of science to guide us, we know that slashing carbs without compensating by maintaining prebiotic fiber intake has been shown to have the following consequences:[22-28]

- Reduces bacterial species diversity. The healthiest people have the widest species diversity, that is, the greatest variety of bacterial species, while the unhealthiest people have the least species diversity with proliferation of undesirable species, especially fecal Enterobacteriaceae like *E. coli*, *Salmonella*, and *Desulfovibrio*, this last microbe being an especially nasty player that causes intestinal inflammation via increased levels of H_2S. Fail to feed your microbiome and some species are reduced or lost entirely.

- Reduces bacterial species believed to be beneficial, such as *Prevotella* (species present in substantial numbers in the microbiomes of the Hadza, Malawi, and Yanomami), *Bifidobacterium*, and *Faecalibacterium prausnitzii*, the most important intestinal butyrate-producing microbe.
- Triggers proliferation of bile acid–tolerant species that lead to an increase in production of potentially carcinogenic forms of bile ("secondary" bile acids such as lithocolic and deoxycholic acids).
- Triggers overproliferation of bacterial species such as *Akkermansia* that consume human mucus in the absence of prebiotic fibers.
- Causes 50–75 percent lower production of intestinal butyrate, which nourishes the intestinal lining. Less butyrate means less protection from colon cancer and less suppression of Enterobacteriaceae.

We have the benefit of plenty of clinical observations of the results of ketogenic diets because thousands of children with epilepsy have been put on these diets to reduce the frequency of grand mal seizures that are poorly responsive to antiseizure drugs. Ketogenic diets have been used for this purpose since the 1920s and can reduce seizures by as much as 50 percent or more—no question: they work. Earlier experiences, unfortunately, upped the children's fat intake that is required to maintain ketosis by supplementing with substantial quantities of corn oil, which, by itself, results in unhealthy consequences (e.g., increased intestinal "leakiness" to bacterial breakdown products, excessive oxidation upon heating). That practice has been abandoned, however, and kids now obtain higher fat intake with medium-chain triglycerides (MCTs), coconut oil, fatty meats, olive oil, and butter.

Many of these children on the ketogenic diet have been studied, and it's been observed that they develop kidney stones (which children otherwise rarely experience), osteopenia (bone thinning), impaired growth, and cardiomyopathies (impaired heart muscle that can lead to heart failure).[28,29] The same sorts of changes in bowel flora occur in both children and adults on strict low-carb diets, and these changes are associated with constipation and increased potential for diverticular disease.

The lack of prebiotic fiber has been shown to trigger proliferation of bacterial species such as *Akkermansia muciniphila* and others, as discussed in Chapter 5, that have the unique ability to exist exclusively on human mucus. In other words, when deprived of prebiotic fibers, many bacterial species die or diminish in numbers, while *Akkermansia* thrives and overproliferates by consuming human mucus. This deteriorates the mucus lining of the intestines, allowing entry of bacteria into the intestinal wall along with intestinal inflammation and increased endotoxemia that then exports inflammation to other parts of the body. People typically experience the consequences of inadequate prebiotic fiber intake as increased levels of triglycerides, increased insulin resistance and high blood sugar, and increased blood pressure, changes that undo the initial beneficial effects of a low-carb diet.

Bottom line: Sure, limit your carbs, especially the most offensive to health of all: wheat, grains, and sugars. But be mindful of your prebiotic fiber intake to ensure that you are feeding your garden of happy microbes. (You can find a list of common sources of prebiotic fibers in Part IV.)

Don't worry. Although this may all seem painfully complicated, once we get to the part of the book where we discuss how to incorporate these concepts into day-to-day life, I give you simple step-by-step actions that take advantage of the insights we have into probiotics, the microbes of fermented foods, prebiotic fibers, and the fascinating and powerful fermentation projects we will tackle that will help you achieve smoother skin, look and feel younger, like other people better, and be free of many common health conditions.

10

BOWEL POWER

Before we get to the nitty-gritty of the four-week Super Gut program, let's dive a little deeper into why a number of strategies provide real advantage in rebuilding a healthy microbiome. You've heard of horsepower and girl power, so let's now focus on "bowel power." We are not just aiming for pedestrian goals like bowel regularity, or relief from common complaints such as loose stools or hemorrhoids. We are seeking magnificent health, smoother skin, deeper sleep, improved mood, increased strength—in other words, effects you may have never associated with your bowels or the microbes they contain. In the next section, I discuss how we use diet, replace crucial nutrients missing from modern life, and rebuild healthy bowel flora. But before we get to that, in this chapter I'd like to detail the reasons why some additional efforts are important.

You may notice that the efforts discussed in this and the next part of the book bring you closer to the way humans lived before factors like antibiotics, prescription drugs, and dietary guidelines got in the way. On the Super Gut program, we will, as much as possible in the twenty-first-century world, revert to the way early cultures conducted their lives, sans loincloth and spear. We avoid foods that dietary guidelines tell us should dominate the modern diet but that were never present in the diets of people who hunted and gathered their meals, people like our ancestral predecessors whose dietary habits helped write our genetic code. We restore vitamin D that people living outdoors would have enjoyed simply by getting plentiful sun exposure over large surface areas of their skin, augmented by consuming the organs of animals, especially liver, and meats, fish, shellfish, and birds' eggs. We restore omega-3 fatty acids that our predecessors obtained by consuming the brain matter of animals along with fish and shellfish and that we can obtain by consuming fish occasionally and fish oil supplements regularly because these types of fats restore the integrity of the intestinal lining and reduce endotoxemia. We restore microbial species that modern people have lost. We also reverse the abnormal situation one in three of us shares in which unhealthy bacteria and fungi have proliferated and climbed up into the upper GI tract—SIBO and SIFO. Only then can we proceed to adding in the magnificent super microbes we cultivate in the unique yogurt recipes I provide.

Because our microbiome has drifted so far off course, just following a healthy diet and life practices is no longer sufficient to regain control over our disrupted microbial universe. You might choose healthy foods, not smoke cigarettes, exercise regularly, vote in every election, yet still find yourself in the midst of a microbiome disaster that causes unpredictable bowel urgency or unrelenting skin rashes. The additional strategies discussed in this chapter, such as supplementing with curcumin, berberine, cloves, and green tea, can help reverse the unnatural situation we've created, with an overabundance of Enterobacteriaceae, lack of healthy bacterial species, and disrupted intestinal mucus barrier.

Let's explore the whys and hows of various strategies (in no particular order) so that, by the time you get to the next section, you understand the details of the Super Gut program.

VITAMIN D

You may already know that the majority of people in our world are deficient in vitamin D as a result of modern lifestyle habits that include living and working indoors and wearing clothes that cover most of the body's surface area, both of which limit sun exposure on our skin that activates vitamin D. Although sunscreen is helpful to avoid sunburn and skin damage, its overuse adds to vitamin D deficiency. As we age, we lose the ability to activate vitamin D production in the skin, especially after age forty. You can have a deep tan at age sixty-five, for instance, yet remain severely deficient.

We can obtain only minor amounts of vitamin D through diet. We therefore need to add a vitamin D supplement.

● Vitamin D deficiency has been associated with weakening of the intestinal mucus barrier, an effect most prominent in the far reaches of the ileum that impairs the protective immune response of intestinal cells, tilts microbiome composition toward unhealthy Enterobacteriaceae stool species, and allows unhealthy species such as toxic strains of *Escherichia coli* to ascend—SIBO.[1,2] In other words, deficiency of vitamin D paves the way for colonic bacteria to gain entry to the small intestine. The combination of SIBO and vitamin D deficiency is particularly destructive, with impaired mucus production, increased intestinal permeability, and a marked increase in endotoxemia.[3-5] This is a problem of particular importance in people prone to inflammatory bowel diseases, ulcerative colitis, and Crohn's disease because vitamin D deficiency amplifies intestinal inflammation. Correction of vitamin D deficiency leads to substantial health benefits that include; reversal of insulin resistance, decreased risk for autoimmune diseases, and decreased risk for various cancers. Vitamin D also plays a crucial role in shaping your microbiome.

The Super Gut program therefore features the restoration of healthy vitamin D levels as a way to help restore a healthy microbiome and improve overall health. Getting this right, all by itself, provides a huge advantage for health. I have witnessed people successfully restoring their blood vitamin D levels (25-OH vitamin D) to what I believe is the ideal level of 60–70 nanograms per milliliter, a level associated with maximum benefit and no toxicity. Replenishing vitamin D is, for many of us, not as easy as obtaining fifteen minutes of sun because of our impaired ability to produce this factor with sun exposure resulting from reduced sun intensity in northern climates, reduced ability to activate vitamin D as we age, and other factors. Given our modern lifestyle, the majority of us fare better by supplementing vitamin D.

● OLIVE OIL

Numerous benefits have been associated with increased consumption of olive oil, from reduction in cardiovascular risk to reduction in some forms of cancer and various forms of inflammation.

Oleic acid comprises 70 percent or more of the fatty acids in olive oil, among the richest sources of this monounsaturated oil, which we obtain in lesser quantities from meats, organ meats, eggs, and avocados. Many of the benefits of consuming olive oil are due to oleic acid's ability to shape the microbiome.

Now stick with me here: Oleic acid is converted to the endocannabinoid oleoylethanolamide (OEA), which, in turn, increases *Akkermansia*. OEA is among the several natural agents that emerged from research into tetrahydrocannabinol, or THC, the psychoactive element in cannabis, that led to the cannabidiol (CBD) explosion.[6] OEA is a non-THC, non-CBD endocannabinoid that regulates inflammation and energy consumption and exerts microbiome effects. And you will recall that having more *Akkermansia* around exerts powerful effects in reducing insulin resistance and blood sugar. It therefore logically follows that enthusiastic consumption of olive oil reduces blood sugar and all the other phenomena associated with insulin resistance, such as high blood pressure. Generous consumption of olive oil yields a broad panel of health benefits via OEA and *Akkermansia*, both of which also help heal the intestinal cellular and mucus barrier while also supporting proliferation of healthy bacterial species.

Extra-virgin olive oil (but not "light" olive oil) also contains polyphenols such as hydroxytyrosol that contribute to creating a healthier environment for bowel flora. Olive oil polyphenols are actually moderately potent antibiotics against bacteria like *E. coli* and *Salmonella*, the Enterobacteriaceae species of dysbiosis and SIBO.[7-9]

The *Akkermansia*-cultivating effects of oleic acid and the antibacterial effects of hydroxytyrosol put extra-virgin olive oil at the top of our list for preferred oils to include in generous quantities in our diet. Ideally, include generous quantities of extra-virgin olive oil in your diet every day by making it your preferred oil for salad dressings, cooking, and drizzling over various dishes. Don't worry: you cannot overdo consumption of olive oil.

OMEGA-3 FATTY ACIDS

The omega-3 fatty acids EPA and DHA are examples of nutrients the need for which is programmed into your genetic code. Without omega-3s, you can die of a deficiency syndrome. Plentiful omega-3s, which our ancestors obtained by consuming the brain matter of animals as well as fish and shell-fish, provide advantages in intestinal health along with protecting cardio-vascular and brain health.

- Omega-3s have the wonderful effect of increasing the expression of an enzyme called intestinal alkaline phosphatase that disables the toxic lipo-polysaccharides (LPS) produced by Enterobacteriaceae. By disabling LPS, endotoxemia is reduced, explaining why omega-3s have been associated with reductions in inflammation body-wide, in joints, skin, liver, and brain. The diet of most modern Americans is woefully deficient in omega-3 fatty acids and is overloaded with omega-6-rich oils, such as corn oil, which *increase* endotoxemia. In addition to disabling LPS, plentiful omega-3 fatty acids help repair a disrupted intestinal barrier and shift intestinal flora toward healthier species, including decreases in Enterobacteriaceae and increases in the numbers of *Akkermansia* and *Bifidobacterium*.[10] Emerging evidence suggests that infants who obtain plentiful omega-3s may be par-tially protected from the microbiome-disrupting effects of antibiotics.[11]

In an ideal world, we would obtain omega-3 fatty acids by consuming plentiful fish. But our world has contaminated the oceans with mercury and other chemicals so that we must rely on purified fish oil supplements to obtain healthful intakes of omega-3 fatty acids in addition to occasionally consuming fish.

IODINE

Iodine is a trace mineral all humans require. Just as lack of vitamin C leads to joint disintegration, loss of teeth, and open skin sores—scurvy—a situa-tion remedied *only* by vitamin C and not the best orthopedic surgeon, den-tist, or plastic surgeon, so too is iodine deficiency remedied only by iodine. At least 20 percent of Americans are deficient in iodine, but the numbers are likely worse than that, given the lax definition of iodine deficiency.

Iodine deficiency was a huge worldwide public health problem un-til the early twentieth century. Before 1924, when the FDA encouraged table salt manufacturers to add iodine to their product, hypothyroidism and goiters (enlarged thyroid glands on the neck from lack of iodine) were epidemic, and not uncommonly led to heart failure, compression of the blood vessels of the neck, or suffocation from collapse of the airway.

If you could ask your great-grandmother about goiters, she would likely share horror stories involving friends and neighbors who died from this condition. The introduction of iodized salt was therefore hailed as a huge public health success.

Fast-forward sixty years and, because some people proved salt-sensitive, the FDA advised Americans to stop using so much salt, forgetting that this was how most people obtained iodine. (It also failed to recognize that the US Dietary Guidelines advocated unrestrained consumption of grains that, coupled with proliferation of sugary snacks and soft drinks, *caused* sodium retention via insulin resistance, which led to much of the difficulties with salt.)

Predictably, iodine deficiency and goiters are therefore making a comeback with the recommended lower consumption of salt, and, with it, hypothyroidism, slowed intestinal peristalsis, and—yes, you guessed it—SIBO and SIFO.[12] I shall therefore show you how to supplement iodine early in your program.

FLAVONOIDS AND POLYPHENOLS

You've likely heard that brightly colored vegetables and fruits yield many health benefits that have been attributed to their vitamin C, fiber, and phytonutrient content. Similar effects have been observed with foods such as green tea, red wine, and coffee. These foods are all rich in compounds called flavonoids and polyphenols, which contribute to the colors of foods, such as the deep purple of eggplant, the yellow of peppers, the red of wine.

Flavonoids and polyphenols have been associated with numerous health benefits. Until recently, it was a mystery how these compounds could provide benefit because about 90 percent or more are passed out in bowel movements and less than 10 percent are absorbed. It has now become clear that many of the benefits of such food compounds are due to their effects on bowel flora; flavonoids and polyphenols act much like prebiotic fibers. A special relationship appears to exist between flavonoids, polyphenols, and our friend *Akkermansia* because vigorous intake of foods containing flavonoids and polyphenols, such as with olive oil and prebiotic fibers, causes these species to bloom.[13] This effect may be most pronounced with the class of polyphenols called proanthocyanidins provided by grapes, pomegranate, cranberries, and other berries.

The polyphenols in green tea, epigallocatechin and epigallocatechin gallate, are especially important for intestinal health. They promote the proliferation of bacterial species that produce butyrate, which yields so many health benefits, including protection against colon cancer and reduced blood sugar and blood pressure.[14] Given their poor absorption—a feature that we desire because it keeps them in the gut instead of being metabolized and absorbed—green tea polyphenols exert their effects along the full length of the GI tract. Green tea catechins also cross-link the mucin proteins in mucus, strengthening semiliquid mucus into a stronger gel that forms a more effective barrier against microbes and inflammation.[15] For an especially potent mixture of factors that help heal the intestinal mucus barrier, try the Clove Green Tea recipe in Part IV that combines the mucin-cross-linking effect of green tea catechins with the mucus-thickening effect of clove eugenol and *Akkermansia*-stimulating fructooligosaccharide (FOS) fiber, a triple punch for healing the GI tract. Likewise, any weight loss effect of green tea is likely attributable to its ability to reduce endotoxemia by strengthening the mucus barrier. With green tea, it's all about the bowels and mucus.

Because of the wonderful health benefits of flavonoids and polyphenols, you will find them used generously in the Super Gut Recipes.

VOICES IN YOUR HEAD

Unlike lions, dogs, and fish, which largely respond to sensory input, most of us humans have an added dimension to our experience: some form of internal monologue going on in our heads. While much of it may be triggered by external people and events, you also carry on a monologue with yourself that is a series of images, emotions, words, or what University of Nevada psychologist Russell Hulberg calls "unsymbolized thinking," thinking without words or symbols.

It is becoming clear that, although no bacteria can think for you, microbes do influence your thinking and emotions. One of the most vivid illustrations of this appeared in the series of human experiments I described in Chapter 1 in which researchers injected normal, nondepressed volunteers with bacterial LPS endotoxin, which promptly triggered in these people all the feelings associated with depression along with its hallmark signs in the brain, as visualized by MRI. As you embark on your efforts to eradicate your Frankenbelly and kill off unhelpful bacteria and fungi, you may experience a flood of LPS endotoxin that brings on feelings of anxiety, anger, or depression. All of this influences your internal conversation—someone experiencing depression is going to have a different inner monologue than someone who is not depressed—and microbes in your GI tract can influence the content and tone of these conversations. People who are depressed are more likely to rehash thoughts about personal weaknesses and failures, feelings of inferiority, and an impulse to give up.

Conversely, one of the yogurts I will show you how to make includes strains of the bacterial species *Lactobacillus helveticus* and *Bifidobacterium longum*, which have been shown to reduce feelings of depression and anger. *Lactobacillus reuteri* yogurt yields feelings of empathy and closeness to other people—you are less likely to be suspicious or wary of another person, more likely to be trusting and friendly. You can imagine that a person's internal monologue can be dramatically changed when depression and anger are lifted, or if they are more inclined to like and trust people.

Just how far can we go in influencing our internal conversations? Can eradicating SIBO, for instance, thereby reducing the flow of endotoxins into the bloodstream, provide relief from depression or perhaps even subdue or abolish thoughts of suicide? Can the right mix of restored microbes bring a family closer or bring down the temperature in political discourse?

I believe that all of this is possible. You can get your start right here.

oregano
cloves
rosemary
ginger

cinnamon
peppermint
cumin

Bowel Power

167

HERBS AND SPICES

Herbs and spices such as oregano, cloves, rosemary, ginger, cinnamon, peppermint, and cumin contain polyphenols that stimulate the proliferation of _Lactobacillus_ and _Bifidobacterium_ species.[16] They thereby reduce likelihood of SIBO and SIFO and recurrences of these conditions because of their prebiotic fiber–like effects on beneficial species and their modest antibacterial effects on Enterobacteriaceae and other pathogenic SIBO species. Obviously, the effects of herbs and spices are modest, else all the people enjoying an Italian dish or pumpkin pie would not have SIBO or SIFO, which is, of course, far from true. But used liberally in the context of an otherwise microbiome-supportive lifestyle, they stack the odds further in your favor and should be part of your long-term culinary habits. Accordingly, I provide recipes that make generous use of these helpful herbs and spices.

Oregano, cinnamon, and cloves stand out for their antifungal properties, effective against numerous harmful species. Whereas the most potent effects come through their essential oils (components of our SIBO and SIFO management program), liberal use of these herbs and spices, fresh or dried, can help prevent fungal overgrowth.[17]

Cloves stand out further for their potential to heal the GI tract by increasing intestinal mucus. The essential oil pressed from cloves is composed mostly of a compound called eugenol that has been demonstrated to dramatically increase the thickness of the mucus lining of the GI tract. It yields this effect by encouraging proliferation of several healthy species of the class Clostridia. (Clostridia species are an example of how related species can be extremely different: in this case, beneficial Clostridia are responsible for stimulating mucus production, unlike _Clostridium difficile_, which is responsible for severe inflammation.[18])

Clove oil is potent and should not be consumed directly (we dilute essential oils in edible oils in our SIBO/SIFO-managing efforts, as described in Chapter 8). However, ground cloves are easy to include in many dishes such as the recipes I provide for Orange Clove Scones and Gingerbread Coffee. I also provide a simple recipe for Clove Green Tea that contains a potent combination of ingredients that helps heal the intestinal mucus lining for anyone with any form of intestinal inflammation; the recipe can be found in Part IV.

CAPSAICIN

Capsaicin is the ingredient found in hot chili peppers that makes you run for a cold drink. This phenomenon led to research that identified a unique thermal-sensing receptor in the human body that can be fooled by capsaicin. (Your mouth may feel like it's burning but, of course, it really is not.)

Because of this characteristic, capsaicin has been employed for a variety of purposes, such as in pepper spray and as a topical pain reliever for post-herpetic neuralgia. But it also exerts some interesting and useful microbiome effects.

Capsaicin has been found to confer the following benefits:[19]

- Reduces the species of SIBO. Although it is not powerful enough to be used as a treatment for SIBO, capsaicin can be useful over the long term to help prevent SIBO or recurrences after eradication.
- Promotes proliferation of several Clostridia species. You may recall that Clostridia species can serve as "gatekeepers" of the intestinal mucus barrier.
- More than doubles the population of the keystone species *Faecalibacterium prausnitzii*, which is the most vigorous producer of intestinal butyrate, which in turn provides beneficial effects such as reduced endotoxemia, blood sugar, and blood pressure.
- Reduces appetite. This effect is mediated via the glucagon-like peptide-I, which has proven to be effective in weight loss.

Obtain capsaicin by making a habit of topping fried eggs, stir-fries, Hot Chili Fries (recipe provided later), and other dishes with hot pepper sauces. The most recent evidence suggests that 10 milligrams of capsaicin per day yields these positive health effects. Capsaicin content in hot chili sauces varies with the species of pepper used, such as habanero or cayenne, and can be anywhere from 1.0 to 7.5 milligrams per tablespoon of liquid sauce. In general, the hotter the pepper (the higher the Scoville heat unit), the greater the capsaicin content.[20]

CURCUMIN

As previously discussed, curcumin is the active polyphenol in the spice turmeric. It is unique among popular herbs and spices in that it acts more like
an antibacterial and antifungal than a prebiotic fiber. Curcumin has also
been shown to be effective in reducing arthritic knee pain and the blood
markers of inflammation, yet, like most other polyphenols, it is very poorly
absorbed, if absorbed at all. As we've discussed, curcumin does *not* need to
be absorbed to exert its beneficial effects in the gut, where it (1) acts against
harmful bacterial and fungal species in the GI tract, and (2) helps rebuild
the intestinal barrier.

Among curcumin's properties:

• Increases alkaline phosphatase that deactivates bacterial LPS
• Increases strength of the intestinal mucus lining
• Decreases penetrability of intestinal cells
• Increases production of antimicrobial peptides

This combination of benefits also results in lower blood levels of LPS—
reduced endotoxemia—a critically important observation that explains why
curcumin reduces inflammation throughout the body.[21]

Curcumin's unique properties provide advantages when used as part of
your efforts to eradicate SIBO and SIFO and heal the intestinal barrier. But
there is one unsettled issue: Despite all its benefits, is it safe to supplement
with curcumin long term beyond efforts to eradicate SIBO and SIFO? No
one yet has an answer to this question, so we keep curcumin as part of our
SIBO/SIFO efforts and do not rely on it long term. After using it in the
Super Gut program, we resort to obtaining curcumin's intestinal mucus
barrier benefits by seasoning our food with a less-potent source, turmeric.

BERBERINE

The plant extract berberine, long used in traditional Chinese medicine,
has been shown to achieve a number of health benefits, including reduced
blood sugar and reduced measures of inflammation. But, like curcumin,
it is poorly absorbed, registering only minor rises in blood levels with

ingestion. In other words, berberine's negligible absorption suggests that it remains in the gut and exerts its outsized benefits on the bowel flora and intestinal mucus barrier. Also like curcumin, berberine's antibiotic and anti-fungal properties act against common SIBO species, including *Staphylococcus*, *Streptococcus*, *Salmonella*, *Klebsiella*, and *Pseudomonas* species, and SIFO species such as *Candida albicans*, while it also increases the population of *Akkermansia*, which helps improve intestinal barrier function, increase butyrate production, and reduce the level of bacterial endotoxemia.[22,23] Berberine is helpful in efforts to eradicate SIBO and SIFO and is a component of one of the herbal antibiotic regimens we use in the Super Gut program. It is unclear, however, given its antimicrobial effects, whether berberine is safe to consume outside a SIBO/SIFO-eradicating effort.

A MICROBIOME CALL TO ARMS

I won't kid you: Righting the wrongs of your intestinal microbiome can be physically and emotionally challenging. You will be wielding the microbial equivalent of a sword, hacking off heads and limbs, taking back several feet of territory that used to be yours but that are now unruly, chaotic, and serving another master.

I hope that you now understand that the monster within has profound effects on how you feel, your health, your state of mind, your internal monologue, and how you feel about other people—just about every aspect of human life. I hope that you also appreciate that many people turn to prescription drugs—antidepressants, anti-inflammatory drugs, pain-relieving drugs, drugs to reduce blood sugar, drugs to subdue behavioral outbursts in kids with ADHD, drugs to force digestive by-products to exit into the toilet—or to alcohol or other means to deal with the many struggles of being human in the twenty-first century . . . while overlooking the real cause of such struggles.

My hope is that, just as the bright sunlight of a new day dispels scary shadows and dark figures, so you and I will expose the dark corners of the microbiome to the light of day so that we can craft strategies that help undo this awful situation we've created. There's no need to grab a club or reject indoor plumbing, but we will nonetheless work to restore something as close to the early human's microbiome as possible. We won't necessarily restore the lost species carried now only by hunter-gatherers, but we will rebuild a microbiome that reverses conditions such as irritable bowel syndrome, fibromyalgia, and autoimmune diseases and that stacks the odds in favor of reversing type 2 diabetes, losing weight, smoothing the skin, and turning back the clock ten or twenty years.

The next part of the book details the how-tos of bringing back order and reason to this population of errant microbes.

PART IV

BUILD YOUR OWN SUPER GUT: A FOUR-WEEK PROGRAM

I'VE STRUCTURED THE SUPER GUT PROGRAM INTO FOUR WEEKS for good reason. Although you might like results to proceed over a shorter time period of, say, ten days, intestinal healing requires time for unhealthy microbes to die off (and not overwhelm you with die-off effects) and for healthy microbes to take "root." I also would like to see you get the program right and enjoy the extravagant health benefits that thousands of other people have enjoyed when they unwound a lifetime of microbiome-disruptive practices, and that takes time. It's also important that you proceed through the program in the order it is presented and not jump to the parts you find most interesting. Resist that temptation.

The first three weeks provide the foundation that helps reverse numerous health conditions. But we also want to achieve benefits beyond reversing health conditions—that's the part that comes in week 4, when I show you how to put gut microbes to work so you can enjoy healthier skin, accelerated healing, youthful muscle and strength, deeper restorative sleep—essentially turning back the clock ten or twenty years. By adopting these ideas, I truly believe that you can be forty for the next sixty years. (Of course, if you start the Super Gut program before age forty, at age thirty-six, say, can you remain that age for another sixty or more years? That is what we are aiming for.) In other words, by adopting the principles of the Super Gut program, I believe you can preserve the vigor, strength, energy, and appearance you had in your youth all through your middle and later years.

○ Strategies like eating fermented foods will be more effective in the context of your new and improved microbiome. Incorporating yogurt made by fermenting *Bacillus coagulans* to reduce pain from knee arthritis, for instance, will work better after you have already adopted the diet changes, nutritional supplements, and basic healthy microbiome strategies because these initial efforts reduce endotoxemia and inflammation dramatically— just consuming the yogurt without the other strategies will not yield the same results. You will enjoy bigger and better results by following the steps of the program in order.

So, without further delay, let's get down to the 1-2-3 of rebuilding your Super Gut, which will yield too-many-to-count health, weight loss, and age-reversing effects, all the wonderful benefits that emerge when you conquer your Frankenbelly.

Let's begin with week 1, when you prepare the soil for a garden of bowel flora.

PREPARE THE SOIL

SUMMARY

We begin by eliminating factors that disrupted bowel flora in the first place:

» Avoid sugars and sugar-containing foods. ✓
» Avoid the synthetic noncaloric sweeteners aspartame (and related acesulfame, neotame, and advantame), sucralose, and saccharine. ✓
» Avoid emulsifying agents such as polysorbate 80 and carboxymethylcellulose. ✓
» Choose organic foods whenever possible. ✓
» Avoid all wheat and grains and be prepared for the opioid withdrawal process that accompanies this dietary change.
» Avoid or minimize drugs, including stomach acid–blocking drugs, anti-inflammatory drugs, antibiotics, and statin cholesterol drugs. Of course, consult your doctor to do this or get a well-informed doctor to help you.
» Replace essential nutrients, lacking in modern diets, that impact the microbiome and intestinal barrier: vitamin D, omega-3 fatty acids from fish oil, iodine, and magnesium. ✓

» Drink Clove Green Tea, which rebuilds a healthy intestinal mucus barrier.
» Begin a four-week course of curcumin, 300–600 milligrams twice per day, to rebuild the intestinal barrier and address dysbiosis.

B ECAUSE I WANT THIS PROCESS TO BE MANAGEABLE FOR YOU AND not overwhelming, I've broken down the program into bite-sized pieces spread out over four weeks. This way, you can take seven days to get each part of the program right, building an effective and complete program over a total of four weeks.

In the first week, we address all the factors that have disrupted our bowel flora over our lifetimes, or at least the factors we are able to address at this point in our lives. As mentioned, we cannot undo certain factors, such as having been delivered by C-section instead of vaginally, but we can banish all synthetic sweeteners and emulsifiers and sources of glyphosate. Don't worry: this does not mean that we cannot enjoy safe, natural sweeteners or savor a bowl of chocolate mint ice cream—we simply must choose safer alternatives that will not negatively impact the microbiome.

In the second week, we tackle the issue of diet, eliminating factors that encourage unhealthy microbes and increase intestinal permeability. We also introduce nutritional supplements that further support the microbiome, strengthen the intestinal mucus barrier, and reduce endotoxemia. In week 3, we dive deeper into learning how and why it is crucial to feed the microbial universe in your abdomen so that the right microbes proliferate and maintain order on your behalf.

In the fourth week, we get to the really spectacular and fun business of restoring high quantities of specific microbes that yield numerous benefits. We go beyond the standard notions of taking a probiotic and getting more fiber. We supercharge microbiome strategies by using unique methods to grow microbes to high numbers that, when consumed, repopulate your gut and yield powerful and unexpected effects. If your experience is like mine and that of the many other people who have engaged these strategies, you will be asking, "Why didn't we know about these ideas earlier?" I have personally, for instance, lived with chronic insomnia for most of my adult life:

struggling to fall asleep, waking up several times during the night, finding myself awake at four a.m., eyes wide open, and failing to fall back to sleep for hours, all sleep habits that meant tomorrow would be another day of feeling crabby, hazy, and tired, and the process would repeat night after night. For many years, I relied on high doses of melatonin and other "crutches," not recognizing that microbiome management efforts held the key. With some of the yogurts that I show you how to make—it is NOT about yogurt; it is about obtaining high counts of specific microbial species and strains—I sleep nine hours every night, uninterrupted, and every night is filled with vivid, childlike dreams. And that's just the start. As tempting as it may be, resist the impulse to jump ahead to the Super Gut yogurt recipes that pack huge benefits because you will enjoy even bigger results when you consume those yogurts after implementing the important preliminary strategies.

In week 1, we start by addressing the factors that disrupted your bowel flora in the first place. We also make dramatic changes in dietary choices and add nutritional supplements to address the several nutrient deficiencies unique to modern people. In my analogy to a springtime garden, these are the steps we take to prepare the soil to rid it of weeds and rocks, changes so powerful that you may experience a detoxification or withdrawal process in these first seven days.

These are the steps you'll take to correct microbiome-disrupting factors:

- **Avoid sugar—in all its forms.** We avoid sucrose, dextrose, high-fructose corn syrup, coconut sugar, brown sugar, agave nectar, turbinado sugar, maltose, maltitol, maltodextrin, rice syrup, and the dozens of other code names for various forms of sugar—they're all sugar and they all cultivate unhealthy bacterial and fungal species even after just a few *days* of consumption.
- **Avoid synthetic, noncaloric sweeteners.** Avoid aspartame and related acesulfame, neotame, advantame, sucralose, saccharine, and all foods sweetened with them. This means that nearly all "diet" sodas are off the menu.
- **Banish emulsifying agents.** Especially avoid polysorbate 80 and carboxymethylcellulose but also carrageenan, sodium stearoyl lactylate, and lecithin.

NO GMO's
NO Bio-engineered

- **Choose organic.** Minimize exposure to herbicides, pesticides, antibiotics, and genetically modified foods that also contain glyphosate and the Bt toxin by choosing organically grown and raised foods.
- **Filter drinking water.** Filter tap water to avoid chlorine, chloramine, and fluoride. ✓
- **Avoid wheat and grains.** By eliminating wheat and grain foods from your diet, you avoid the protein gliadin, which increases intestinal permeability and slows intestinal peristalsis (the natural propulsive movement of the GI tract). You are also thereby reducing exposure to the antibiotic effects of the herbicide glyphosate and avoiding a major source of intestinal inflammation. This alone is a big step. (See below: Wheat and Grains: The Great Health Disrupters.)
- **Limit net carbs.** Keep the amount of carbohydrates you eat to no more than 15 grams per meal. (See box on page 179: The Blessings of Normal Blood Sugar.)

  Per meal, not, A Day

- **Hydrate.** Drink more than usual, and lightly salt food and water.
- **Go light on alcohol.** Have no more than one or two servings of alcohol per day. Be a teetotaler if you're trying to lose weight.
- **Get off microbiome-disrupting drugs.** Work with your health-care provider to eliminate or reduce the use of nonsteroidal anti-inflammatory drugs (NSAIDs like ibuprofen and acetaminophen), stomach acid–suppressing drugs, and statin cholesterol drugs.
- **Minimize exposure to antibiotics.** Accept a prescription only when it is truly necessary.

Opt for real, single-ingredient foods, preferably those that don't require a label. Avocados and eggs are safe, as are broccoli, salmon, and a handful of walnuts—no added sugar or synthetic sweeteners, no emulsifiers, no preservatives, no labels or nutritional panels required. When shopping, you will find yourself spending nearly all your time in the produce section, butcher/meat section, and dairy section, rarely needing to venture into the inner aisles, which are packed top to bottom with processed foods.

We also discard many other conventional ideas about a healthy diet. We never limit fats or oils, never limit calories, never push the plate away, reject "everything in moderation," common mistakes that lead to long-term weight gain, insulin resistance, and gallstones. If your doctor advises that these strategies will raise cholesterol and risk for heart disease, find a better-informed doctor who understands how heart disease is caused—there is no conclusive evidence, nor has any ever been generated, demonstrating that total fat intake or saturated fat intake causes heart disease.

Wheat and grain elimination can be among the most unsettling, confusing, but powerful strategies that begins the process of rebuilding healthy bowel flora. It means that, though you may be avoiding foods like breads, pizza, pasta, pretzels, and crackers, you will be unrestricted in including foods such as eggs, butter, vegetables, olive oil, beef, fish, poultry, and nuts—there are plenty of whole, unprocessed foods that are safe and healthy.

THE BLESSINGS OF NORMAL BLOOD SUGAR

Having normal blood sugar is a basic requirement for health and a healthy microbiome.

Having high blood sugar, as occurs in diabetes, prediabetes, and to a lesser degree with any amount of insulin resistance—conditions that now affect 75 percent of the US population—increases intestinal permeability. The effect can be so substantial that bacteria themselves, not just LPS or other by-products, move across the intestinal wall into the bloodstream and thereby travel to other organs. And it doesn't take much: the common hemoglobin A1c (HbA1c) test that reflects blood sugar fluctuations over the preceding ninety days shows that even levels of 5.0–5.6 percent, which are typically regarded as normal, are sufficient to allow intestinal permeability.[1]

One of the very important benefits of the Super Gut program is that it reverses insulin resistance. Insulin resistance occurs when the liver, muscles, brain, and other organs respond poorly to insulin, the pancreatic hormone that allows us to metabolize carbohydrates by taking blood sugar out of the blood to use as energy. This lack of response to insulin causes the pancreas to compensate by producing greater amounts of insulin in order to get organs to take up glucose from the blood. The (fasting) blood insulin level of a slender, healthy person without insulin resistance? Around 1–4 mIU/L (milli-international units per liter). But the insulin level of someone with prediabetes or someone who is overweight, with "love handles" around their waist, or who has high blood pressure, or who has any of the many other manifestations of insulin resistance? Many times greater at 30, 50, 80 mIU/L or more. This is the process that causes weight gain and drives numerous health conditions while also altering bowel flora, increasing intestinal permeability, increasing endotoxemia that, in turn, worsens insulin resistance, blocks weight loss, causes weight gain . . . around and around in a vicious cycle.

Reversing high levels of insulin in the blood also reverses sodium retention. This is why, during the first week of the Super Gut program, it is not uncommon for you to lose five or so pounds of body weight, nearly half of which is water. (Sodium accompanies water in urine.) Vigorous hydration is therefore key during the first week to maintain normal blood pressure while at the same time we no longer adhere to sodium restrictions. It actually helps if you lightly salt your food and even toss a dash of salt into drinking water.

To further augment the effects of wheat/grain elimination and restoration of nutrients that reverse high blood sugar and insulin resistance, it is also helpful to limit carbohydrate intake to no more than 15 grams net carbs per meal. You can calculate net carbs (as opposed to total carbs) using the information provided in a food's nutrition panel. On nutritional labels, fiber is included as a carbohydrate, even though humans are incapable of digesting fibers. We therefore subtract fiber from total carbs to yield "net" carbs. For example, a medium-sized ripe (not green) banana contains 27 grams of total carbs and 3 grams of fiber: 27 - 3 = 24 grams net carbs—far too much to eat in one meal. Anytime you exceed 15 grams net carbs in a meal, you raise blood sugar, raise insulin, contribute to insulin resistance, and gain weight. You can find the nutritional profiles of various whole foods that include values for total carbs and fiber in online resources (e.g., Nutrition Data), smartphone apps (e.g., Nutrition Lookup), and numerous handbooks.

The majority of people reading this book will be able to obtain ideal insulin levels (4.0 mIU/L or less), ideal blood sugar levels

Avoid, Correct, Address

(70–90 mg/dl), ideal HbA1c levels (5.0% or less) and break the vicious cycle and undo all the harmful effects high blood sugar levels cause. You achieve this by avoiding foods that raise blood sugar and insulin, correcting common nutrient deficiencies that exaggerate insulin resistance, and addressing the disrupted state of bowel flora and endotoxemia. For the occasional person who has incurred damage to their pancreas and is unable to achieve ideal blood sugar levels, you can at least minimize insulin and blood sugar and reliance on medication.

WHEAT AND GRAINS: THE GREAT HEALTH DISRUPTERS

Those of you familiar with my Wheat Belly series of books already know that, contrary to dietary guidelines, elimination of wheat and grains from the human diet is a spectacularly effective strategy for health and weight loss. This dietary strategy mimics dietary habits that humans adopted before the advent of agriculture, that is, it's similar to the eating habits of people who hunted and gathered their food. (People are often surprised to learn that humans have been consuming wheat and grains for less than one-half of 1 percent of our species' time on this planet.) Wheat and grain elimination removes an extravagant source of intestinal inflammation and begins the process of healing your GI tract. It means rejecting many modern notions of healthy eating such as reducing fat and saturated fat and centering your diet around "healthy whole grains."

There are numerous toxic components in the seeds of the grasses—grains—that humans mistakenly adopted as food twelve thousand years ago: the gliadin protein (within gluten) disrupts the intestinal barriers and initiates autoimmune diseases; gliadin-derived opioid peptides are potent appetite stimulants and impair intestinal peristalsis; the amylopectin A carbohydrate raises blood sugar higher than table sugar; and phytates bind essential minerals such as iron, zinc, calcium, and magnesium and cause them to be swept out of your system and into the toilet. Banishing all wheat and grains therefore begins a powerful journey back to health.

Can we argue in favor of removing wheat and grains to benefit gastrointestinal health and the microbiome too? We absolutely can. The following lists components of wheat and grains that impact GI health:

- **Gliadin:** Gliadin and gliadin-derived peptides (formed through partial digestive breakdown) are directly toxic to the intestinal wall. Removing gliadin thereby removes a potent bowel toxin.
- Gliadin also breaks down normal intestinal barriers, allowing foreign substances, including gliadin itself, entry into the bloodstream. This is the initiating process for many, perhaps most, autoimmune diseases while it also amplifies bacterial endotoxemia.[2] (You'd think that this fact alone—that the gliadin protein of wheat initiates autoimmune disease—would be a death sentence for grains in the diet.)
- **Gliadin-derived opioids:** Just as opioid drugs such as oxycodone and morphine cause constipation, so do gliadin-derived opioids slow intestinal peristalsis and cause constipation. (I have seen the worst kind of constipation in which people move their bowels only every few weeks, a condition labeled obstipation, reverse within days of banishing gliadin-derived opioids from the diet.) Slowed peristalsis is a major issue in many cases of SIBO, and it can be reversed in the majority with wheat and grain elimination.[3]
- **Wheat germ agglutinin (WGA):** WGA is a pest-resistant compound in wheat. Farmers and agricultural scientists have selected wheat strains for their greater WGA content to enhance the plant's resistance to molds and insects. But WGA is also a potent bowel toxin that damages intestinal villi (the hair-like projections on the intestinal wall that enhance nutrient absorption) as it passes through the GI tract. WGA also blocks the hormone cholecystokinin (see box on page 183: Lessons Learned from Gallstones) that provokes the gallbladder to release bile and the pancreas to release pancreatic enzymes to help digest food. WGA thereby impairs digestion, causing symptoms like heartburn, and adds to the risk for gallstones.[4]

Just by eliminating all wheat and grains, many people report complete relief or marked improvement of bowel urgency, acid reflux, heartburn, and constipation. Observations of the changes in bowel flora composition provoked by wheat/grain elimination are preliminary but suggest the potential for reversing an inflammatory microbiome with the eradication of inflammation-provoking species.[5,6]

Bottom line: removing wheat and grains yields substantial improvements in GI health that aid in your efforts to reverse dysbiosis, SIBO, and SIFO and regain overall health.

LESSONS LEARNED FROM GALLSTONES

When we study how gallstones develop, we can learn a lot about the microbiome and the effects of food choices and calorie counting.

Twenty million Americans, or about 15 percent of the adult population, have gallstones. Ask doctors why someone develops gallstones that eventually necessitate gallbladder removal (the number one most common abdominal surgery performed today), and they usually respond with the unhelpful answer that risk factors like obesity, being female, and getting older stack the odds in favor of developing stones.

An important insight has emerged from a series of simple studies that did nothing more than obtain ultrasound images of the gallbladder of people who had no gallstones at the start and who then initiated a diet of reduced calories, reduced fat, or reduced calories and fat.

The ages of participants, proportion of females to males, strictness of the diets, and other characteristics differed across these various gallbladder ultrasound studies, but one thing they had in common was that as many as 55–62 percent of participants engaging in such diets developed gallstones; many of them had to go on to surgery to have their gallbladder removed. In short, cutting calories, cutting fat, or—worst of all—cutting both calories and fat sets you up for gallstones within a few weeks.[11–14]

The concept is simple: Consume foods with fats, and the gallbladder is prompted by the hormone cholecystokinin (CCK) to squeeze out the bile required to digest dietary fats. Reduce calories, fat, or both, and the gallbladder is left idle, having no opportunity to squeeze out its stored bile. Over time, bile crystallizes (bile stasis), the process that leads to gallstone formation. It is therefore well established that cutting calories and/or fat leads to high likelihood of gallstone formation.

Let's go further. What if you cut calories and/or fat but continue to consume wheat and grains? One component of wheat and grains is wheat germ agglutinin. Besides being a potent bowel toxin, wheat germ agglutinin also blocks the action of the CCK hormone that causes gallbladder contraction. Just as cutting calories or fat does, wheat germ agglutinin prevents the gallbladder from squeezing out its contents.[15] Cut calories, cut fat, eat "healthy whole grains," and schedule your gallbladder surgery.

It gets worse. Examine gallstones removed from the gallbladder and you will find *E. coli*, *Salmonella*, *Klebsiella*, et cetera—stool organisms. How do stool organisms get into the gallbladder, which connects to the duodenum, twenty-some feet away from the colon where *E. coli* and friends originate? You're catching on: SIBO.

Yes, gallstones, like a good history teacher, can teach us many lessons. The lessons we take are to never cut calories, never cut fats, and eat no foods containing wheat germ agglutinin (i.e., wheat and grains) so as to push back those nasty stool microbes that have invited themselves into your upper GI tract and gallbladder.

WILL I LOSE WEIGHT?

Having had thousands of people engage in this program, I can tell you with confidence that weight loss is typically dramatic and effortless. Note that I did *not* say you will have to cut your calories, cut your fat intake, move more, and eat less, or any of the other advice you hear—which does not work or which works against you and can even cause gallstones.

The combination of strategies in the Super Gut lifestyle typically leads to extraordinary amounts of weight loss for the following reasons:

- **Eliminating wheat and grains eliminates gliadin-derived opioid peptides.** The gliadin protein of wheat and related proteins in other grains are poorly digested in the human digestive system. National Institutes of Health researchers determined a number of years ago that, rather than being digested into single amino acids, four- or five-amino-acid-long peptides result, and these cross into the brain and bind to opioid receptors that stimulate appetite: wheat and grains are potent appetite stimulants. Removing them thereby eliminates a powerful driver of appetite. This also explains the opioid withdrawal process that many people experience upon removal of all wheat and grains. Get through this process and you will find yourself wonderfully freed from appetite, content to not eat for extended periods, no longer driven by impulse or temptation.[3]
- **We reverse insulin resistance.** High levels of insulin drive weight gain. We reverse this situation by eliminating foods that provoke high insulin levels (wheat, grains, sugar), then address nutrient deficiencies that help reverse insulin resistance (vitamin D, omega-3s, magnesium). We then address disrupted bowel flora and the accompanying endotoxemia, which further reduces insulin resistance. The result: the weight you have been wanting to lose begins to fall off you effortlessly.
- **We correct iodine deficiency.** A substantial proportion of modern people can blame lack of iodine and associated hypothyroidism for their inability to control their weight, especially those who limit salt use. We therefore supplement this crucial trace mineral that everyone needs.

Once again: we *never* limit calories, we *never* limit fat, we *never* say things like "move more, eat less." Once they've experienced the weight loss that this approach facilitates, many people end up asking, "What if I don't want to lose any more weight?" Don't worry: Of the thousands of people following this program, no one has turned to a pile of dust or ended up emaciated. Weight loss naturally plateaus when your body achieves its ideal weight level.

PUT ON YOUR BEST LOINCLOTH

It's also time to introduce nutrients that are lacking in modern life—not because of the diet we follow but because of the modern lifestyle—that support your efforts to rebuild a healthy microbiome. These same nutrients also help reverse insulin resistance, reduce blood sugar, reduce blood pressure, reduce triglycerides, help reverse fatty liver, and facilitate weight loss. Because we live largely indoor lives and wear clothes that cover our skin, because we generally don't consume organ meats, because we filter our drinking water, we need to compensate for the nutrients lost as a result of such modern practices. We introduce these nutrients early in the Super Gut program because the changes in diet, especially removal of all wheat and grains, can be accompanied by withdrawal and detoxification phenomena. Introducing nutritional supplements is crucial to soften the process and helps to reduce transient unpleasant effects such as headache, leg cramps, and fatigue.

The following nutritional supplements are important for this early phase of your program.

Vitamin D

Recall that vitamin D plays an important role in sustaining a healthy microbiome and amplifying the intestinal immune response, as well as reversing insulin resistance, improving mental clarity and mood, and adding to heart health.

Choose oil-based gelcaps because they are the most effectively and consistently absorbed, unlike tablets and capsules, which are erratically absorbed or often not absorbed at all. Vitamin D drops are also useful, though dosing can be inconsistent. (Try to be as consistent as possible with your use of the dropper.) Most adults do fine taking a dose of 5,000–6,000 units per day, a dose that usually generates a 25-OH vitamin D blood level of 60–70 ng/ml, what I regard as the ideal level. (Should you track blood levels, recognize that it takes about three months for a "steady state" to be achieved, that is, a stable blood level, after starting vitamin D or with any dose change.) Because the occasional person requires much less or much more vitamin D to achieve this blood level, it is wise to check your blood level within six to twelve months after starting vitamin D supplementation or with any dose adjustment.

MUCUS-BUILDING TEA

Part of rebuilding a healthy microbiome is intestinal healing. And an important component of intestinal healing is restoring a vigorous, thick mucus lining of the intestines that acts as a barrier. Almost everyone starting the Super Gut program begins with a compromised mucus barrier. I've therefore developed a recipe for Clove Green Tea that strengthens the mucus lining while reducing intestinal and body-wide inflammation by reducing endotoxemia and helping soothe any residual intestinal discomfort you may have. This unique tea combines the following healing constituents:

1. The mucus-thickening power (via proliferation of Clostridia species) of the eugenol oil from cloves, which helps increase the thickness of the intestinal mucus lining[7]
2. The mucus protein cross-linking effect of green tea catechins that converts mucus from semiliquid to semisolid gel, thereby increasing its protective function[8]
3. The fructooligosaccharide (FOS) prebiotic that causes an *Akkermansia* bloom that further increases mucus production[9]

People who drink this tea have reported many interesting effects. Richard (not his real name) struggled with feelings of self-doubt for years, hearing an internal monologue that repeatedly told him that he was unqualified for the work he was doing, that he was a fake. Within forty-eight hours of consuming the tea, this painful internal conversation came to a stop. He was elated, noting that weeks passed without these thoughts. Holidays came, however, and he neglected making the tea, and the flood of self-doubt resumed. He restarted the tea, and the internal monologue stopped once again. Such on-again, off-again associations are good evidence of a genuine cause-effect relationship. But think about it: an internal and unremitting internal monologue turned off by the intestinal mucus–strengthening effect of Clove Green Tea.

Find the recipe for Clove Green Tea on page 247.

Omega-3 Fatty Acids

The only truly reliable source of the omega-3 fatty acids EPA and DHA, which are essential for preservation of intestinal health and reduction of endotoxemia, is fish oil. There are marketing claims made by alternatives, such as krill oil or algae-sourced omega-3 oil, but none provides the dose that you need to fully restore the intestinal mucus lining and the intestinal barrier. Once or twice per week, you should also include fish and shellfish in your diet, such as salmon, cod, mackerel, sardines, scallops, and oysters, because the amino acid taurine present in seafood but absent in fish oil increases the immune response within the colon, a potent effect.[10] Consuming fish more frequently, given the pollution levels in the world's oceans, can lead unfortunately to excessive exposure to mercury, which comes with a list of health concerns.

The ideal intake of EPA and DHA is higher than most people think: 3,000–3,600 milligrams per day of EPA + DHA (total)—this is the dose of EPA and DHA, *not* fish oil. Ideally, divide it into at least two doses, such as 1,500–1,800 milligrams in the morning and another 1,500–1,800 milligrams in the evening or with dinner.

Super Gut Success: Grace, 70, British Columbia

"I've been eating a half cup of *L. reuteri* daily for about a month and a half cup of the SIBO trio for about a week. Previous to this, I typically slept in one- to two-hour segments, often awake for hours between short periods of sleep during the night. For the past week, I have been able to go to bed earlier and sleep through the night, getting five to seven hours of uninterrupted sleep for the first time since my husband died four years ago. I feel so rested and energized.

"It also helps that I have much reduced inflammation with this way of eating so that my hip and shoulder joints are not waking me with pain. I'm almost reluctant to mention this next possible aspect because it sounds so unlikely, so take it with 'a grain of salt.' I play a certain set of songs from memory on the piano every day so that I don't forget what I've learned over the past six years. I started playing when I was sixty-three. It's hard work for me, and I'm not good at it. In the past week, I've been noticing that I am suddenly able to improvise as I play. It's as if my brain gained a level of creative confidence I did not previously possess.

"My thoughts toward other people have shifted. The best way I can describe it is that I am more accepting (empathetic?) of others' perspectives. Anger, annoyance, and feelings of negative judgment are no longer present. When I approach a discussion, my first impulse is a desire to bring positivity to the table. This is a terrific and welcome improvement in my ability to interact with people. I would call the benefit 'a higher form of sociability.'"

———

Iodine

We supplement iodine to provide your thyroid gland with the iodine it needs to manufacture thyroid hormones. Insufficient iodine intake leads to lower thyroid hormone levels, hypothyroidism, which slows intestinal activity and can lead to SIBO and SIFO. The Recommended Dietary Allowance of 150 micrograms per day advocated by conventional authorities is the quantity required to not have a goiter. We are, instead, aiming for *optimal* or *ideal* thyroid status, not just preventing a goiter. I advocate a daily intake of 350–500 micrograms per day from kelp tablets (dried seaweed) or potassium iodide drops. I prefer kelp tablets because they provide varied forms of iodine that, I believe, stack the odds in favor of supporting the function of not just the thyroid gland but also the salivary glands, intestinal lining, and breast tissue, all of which also require iodine.

"YOU MEAN I'LL NEVER HAVE PIZZA AGAIN?"

If reverting to preagricultural hunter-gatherer practices means no wheat or grains, then will you ever have a slice of sausage pizza, a wedge of strawberry cheesecake, or a few bites of birthday cake again?

You absolutely can. Simply replace problematic wheat and grain flours with benign flours and meals and replace sugar and synthetic sweeteners with natural non- or minimally caloric sweeteners that do not lead to endotoxemia, disrupt GI function, or raise blood sugar. This means that you can enjoy, for example, biscuits and gravy at Thanksgiving, a blueberry muffin spread with butter at breakfast, or a cinnamon scone with tea or coffee while not experiencing any of the health impairments of wheat, grains, and sugar.

Why not just stick to real, single-ingredient foods and not sweat trying to re-create such familiar wheat/grain-containing favorites? I learned long ago that, although you could indeed simply choose foods like eggs, meats, vegetables, and fruit, there are times when a slice of pizza or some blueberry muffins would be nice. Sometimes it is an advantage to be able to indulge in familiar foods re-created to be healthy, such as when you're entertaining friends, enjoying the holidays, or keeping the kids and grandkids happy. Without access to these healthier versions of comfort foods, I've watched many people return from Thanksgiving fourteen pounds heavier and in the midst of a metabolic disaster. Having safe and delicious alternatives could have prevented this from happening. And having the option of accompanying your coffee or tea with a muffin or enjoying a slice of cheese pizza really helps from time to time.

ALTERNATIVE FLOURS AND MEALS

Almond flour (from blanched almonds), almond meal (from whole almonds)

Walnut or pecan meal—best suited to making piecrusts
Coconut flour
Ground golden flaxseed
Sesame flour
Lupin flour
Ground psyllium seed

Combinations of flours and meals work best, for example, use 3 cups almond flour + ¼ cup ground golden flaxseed + 2 tablespoons ground psyllium seed. You can purchase flours and meals preground or you can grind them yourself in a food chopper, food processor, or coffee grinder. Flours and meals are best stored in the refrigerator and consumed within four to six weeks. You can find recipes for using these flours and meals in Part IV, including an easy and fragrant Herbed Focaccia Bread.

ALTERNATIVE NONCALORIC OR MINIMALLY CALORIC SWEETENERS

Stevia
Allulose
Monk fruit
Inulin
Erythritol
Xylitol

Alternative sweetener combinations are commercially available, such as Swerve (inulin + erythritol), Truvía (rebiana, an isolate of stevia + erythritol), Virtue (monk fruit + erythritol), and Lakanto (monk fruit + erythritol). Note that we avoid most sugar alcohols, such as maltitol, lactitol, and sorbitol, because they behave much like conventional sugar and can cause loose stools even with consumption of modest quantities.

Because different products provide different levels of sweetness, you'll find that you use different proportions of each sweetener to achieve the same level of sweetness. A table of sugar equivalents can be found in Appendix A.

Magnesium

We take advantage of magnesium's osmotic property, that is, it pulls water into the GI tract, thereby ensuring rapid transit that discourages proliferation of SIBO species. Wheat and grain elimination can unmask the presence of a magnesium deficiency, given the fact that the modern diet provides abnormally low intakes of magnesium. You may experience this as leg cramps, most common during the first week of wheat and grain elimination. Magnesium supplementation helps block or blunt cramps and provides many other health benefits.

We supplement magnesium early in the program. It is available in many different forms, including magnesium malate, glycerophosphate, glycinate, chelate, and citrate, all of which are among the best absorbed with the least potential for causing loose bowel movements. Purchase magnesium supplements that specify the amount of "elemental" magnesium contained, that is, the amount of magnesium by itself without the weight of the malate, glycinate, and so forth. The ideal intake of elemental magnesium is in the range of 450 to 500 milligrams per day for adults, divided into two or three doses. This level of intake contributes to reductions in blood pressure, blood sugar, and heart rhythm disorders, as well as adds to effortless episodes in the bathroom.

Curcumin

Unlike the previous four nutrients, there is no intrinsic human need for curcumin—nobody has a curcumin deficiency.

Instead, we supplement with this compound derived from the spice turmeric to help undo many adverse effects on the microbiome, intestinal mucus, and the intestinal barrier—curcumin is one of a few compounds that favorably addresses all three factors in intestinal health. It reduces the populations of several unhealthy bacterial species of the Enterobacteriaceae family as well as fungi, increases production of intestinal mucus, and improves the intestinal immune response. Curcumin is therefore front and center in our efforts to restore bowel health.

To minimize die-off effects, we start with a modest dose of 300 milligrams twice per day, and increase to 600 milligrams twice per day after several days. Recall that we avoid products with added ingredients such as piperine or bioperine that enhance absorption because we want the cur-cumin *not* to be absorbed and to stay within the GI tract.

What is not clear about curcumin is whether, given its antibacterial and antifungal properties, it is safe for long-term use. Just as it may not be safe to consume an antibiotic for a prolonged period, it is not clear whether exposure to the antimicrobial effects of curcumin is safe for an extended time. We therefore supplement with curcumin only for the four weeks of the Super Gut program. Should you temporarily divert from the four-week program in order to engage in SIBO/SIFO management, then you can take a longer course of curcumin; it is safe to use as part of a several-week- to several-month-long course of antifungal efforts.

During this first week, you've prepared the soil, so let's now go on to the second week of planting seeds.

RESEED YOUR GARDEN

SUMMARY

Now that we've prepared the soil, removing the microbiome equivalent of rocks and other debris, we next begin the process of "reseeding" your garden of bowel flora with healthy bacterial species, including keystone species.

» Begin a high-potency, multispecies probiotic from the list provided in Appendix A or make probiotic yogurt from the recipe provided.
» Include at least one fermented food, either purchased or homemade, in your diet every day.
» Start your own home fermentation efforts. (I'll show you how to get started fermenting at home.)

YOU'VE LAID DOWN THE FOUNDATION FOR A HEALTHIER MICRO-biome by preparing the soil during week 1. During week 2, we begin the work of planting our gardens by reseeding our GI tracts with healthy microbes. We delay the introduction of "water and fertilizer," that is, prebiotic fibers, polyphenols, and other nutrients that promote microbial growth, until we have had at least several days of these reseeding strategies. This sequence of steps is purposeful: Just as you wouldn't water your garden if you hadn't planted seeds yet, so we do not supply microbial nutrients until we have begun the reseeding process that shifts microbiome composition. Some people who begin the Super Gut program with substantial dysbiosis, for example, and who adopt prebiotic fiber intake too early, end up feeding the wrong bacterial species, an effect experienced as excessive gas, bloating, abdominal discomfort, and unpleasant emotional effects. Therefore, allow a week of reseeding to proceed first.

Rather than seeds for squash and watermelon, we're planting "seeds" in your garden of bowel flora with microbes from probiotics and fermented foods. Unfortunately, most commercial probiotic products do not deliver on promises to restore bowel health because they are nothing more than haphazard collections of bacteria with limited potential for benefit. Choose a probiotic at random and you might as well throw your retirement money at any stock or mutual fund available—you might make money, but it's little more than a crapshoot. Instead, choose a commercial probiotic from the list of preferred preparations included in Appendix A. Unlike most brands, these products specify the strains of bacterial species they contain—without knowing the strain, you cannot know whether the probiotic could actually achieve the health benefits you're after—or contain groups of microbes that have been proven to "collaborate" to form metabolic "guilds" or "consortia." Think about the power of the fecal transplant—get the microbial species and strains right, and wonderful things can happen.

The right probiotic provides the simple benefits you need at the start of the Super Gut program, such as increased mucus production and inhibited growth of undesirable species. But it should go further than that. A probiotic should, for instance, contain species that colonize the upper GI tract, not just the colon (e.g., *L. reuteri, L. gasseri*). It should contain species that produce bacteriocins, the natural peptide antibiotics that protect against the *Salmonellas* and *Klebsiellas* of the microbiome world. There should also be ample total numbers of species and strains included—you wouldn't go to battle against ten thousand soldiers with a band of twenty, would you? We're about to go to war against trillions of unhealthy bacterial species, so we must choose our microbes, species, strains, and live organism counts carefully.

Alternatively, you can create your own probiotic easily and inexpensively by making Super Gut yogurts. You start with a capsule of commercial probiotic or with a commercial kefir rich in bacterial species from the recipe I provide. And you can do both, of course, take a commercial probiotic and make your own—the actual numbers of bacteria we obtain with any of these options is relatively low and so doubling up to increase numbers may provide advantage.

Unfortunately, no commercial probiotic available on the market provides all the microbial species and strains that we need to reseed our GI tract, nor do we yet know all the species that are crucial to restore. Beyond failing to specify strains, most commercial probiotics lack keystone species, they do not factor in the "collaborative" effects among species in their formulations, nor do they provide microbes likely to take up residence for more than a few days or weeks before they are gone. This is why people who take probiotics obtain limited benefits that are usually transient. Probiotics in their current commercial form cannot serve as a standalone strategy to rebuild a healthy microbiome; they represent only a modestly helpful strategy with largely temporary benefits. Overreliance on commercial probiotics is a common mistake: People often take probiotics in the hopes that their efforts to restore or maintain a healthy microbiome can begin and end with taking a capsule. But, in their current form, commercial probiotics are among the *least* important strategies we employ.

Like the anonymous species and strains we obtain through most probiotic products, the microbes in kefir and fermented cucumbers, cabbage, and other foods are a haphazard collection of good microbes that provide modest effects. The microbes in the kimchi you bought at the specialty store or the sauerkraut you fermented on your kitchen counter do offer some health benefits such as promoting the production of intestinal mucus, muscling out pathogenic species, and producing needed metabolites—helpful effects, even if they do not yield the full panel of effects we are after. We plant the seeds of these beneficial species by including at least one serving of fermented food in our daily routine. As with commercial probiotics, the microbial species in fermented foods contain unspecified strains and do not take up permanent residence in our gut. But they are still helpful.

The fermentation projects we create later partially compensate for the inadequacies of most commercial probiotics and fermented foods. We choose each species and strain in a fermentation project for specific effects and then we amplify them using my unique method of fermentation, which increases bacterial counts into the hundreds of billions. Eat some commercial yogurt, and you'll experience virtually no health benefit. Consume kefir, and you'll experience modest health benefits. But make and consume daily portions of the Super Gut yogurts, and you can reverse fibromyalgia, experience smoother skin with fewer wrinkles, increase your bench press by fifty pounds, and develop greater fondness for your friends and neighbors. In other words, the strategies that we engage in seeding the garden of bowel flora make up for the inadequacies of commercial probiotic preparations and yield life-changing benefits.

If, however, you find that you are intolerant to either probiotics or fermented foods and experience symptoms such as excessive bloating or abdominal discomfort, diarrhea, mind fog, or anxiety, then it is time to divert from week 2 of the Super Gut program into SIBO and SIFO management efforts because these symptoms are nearly always due to bacterial and fungal overgrowth. (See Appendix B for the Super Gut SIBO and SIFO Protocols we follow.) There is no natural reason for a person to be intolerant to, say, naturally fermented onions or other food sources of microbial species that are perfectly compatible with human life. Any intolerance can therefore be blamed on SIBO or SIFO and the considerable health disruptions they cause. Once you address these two overgrowth conditions, lo and behold, such intolerances disappear. Go to Chapter 8 to find the rationale on why and how we manage these conditions, adopt the protocols in Appendix B, then, once SIBO and SIFO are under control, return right here to week 2 of the Super Gut program to resume where you left off.

MAKE YOUR OWN LOW-COST PROBIOTIC

You can use a number of methods to make your own low-cost probiotic: fermenting from a capsule of commercial probiotic, fermenting from a commercial kefir, and fermenting from a commercial starter culture. The first option is the best because it allows you to choose a probiotic with as many healthy species and strains as possible, including keystone species. The downside of fermenting from a commercial kefir or a starter culture, as with most commercial probiotics, is that you won't know the particular bacterial strains included and they may not contain keystone species. Choose to ferment starting with a capsule of commercial probiotic whenever possible.

When we make yogurt using one of these methods, we ferment for an extended period and add prebiotic fibers to the fermenting mix, all to obtain the greatest number of microbes in the end result. If you choose to use a starter culture, follow the same instructions for fermenting as for starting with a probiotic capsule. Using the unique fermentation method I advocate results in a ferment with very high bacterial counts in the hundreds of billions per half-cup serving.

MAKING YOGURT WITH A COMMERCIAL PROBIOTIC

As a starter, choose a probiotic with ten or more species but with no *Saccharomyces*, *Candida*, or *Kluyveromyces* fungal species (these will cause it to ferment into alcohol). Ideally, choose from the list of recommended probiotics in Appendix A. You will also find a list of recommended fermentation devices such as yogurt makers and sous vide devices in Appendix A, devices that maintain a temperature conducive to microbial reproduction (which differs for each species and which is specified in each recipe).

RECIPE

MAKES 1 QUART

Contents of one probiotic capsule
2 tablespoons prebiotic fiber (e.g., inulin, raw potato
    starch)
1 quart organic half-and-half

In a medium-sized bowl, combine the contents of the probiotic capsule (opened and emptied into the mix), the prebiotic fiber, and 2 tablespoons of organic half-and-half (or other fermentable liquid). Make a slurry to ensure the prebiotic fiber does not clump. Stir until well mixed. Stir in the remaining half-and-half (or other liquid). Cover lightly (e.g., with plastic wrap), place in your fermenting device, and ferment at 106°F for 36 hours. To make future batches, use 2 tablespoons of curds and/or whey from a prior batch.

MAKING YOGURT WITH KEFIR

Kefir is a fermented dairy product that typically contains a dozen or more bacterial species and several fungal species. Kefirs are some of the richest sources of probiotic microbes, providing more than the few bacterial species in most yogurts. You can put kefir to work to save yourself a lot of money by fermenting kefir microbes and creating your own edible probiotic.

Commercial manufacturers use the shortest possible fermentation time, a practice that yields minimal bacterial counts. This is why commercial yogurts offer almost no real health benefits. It's *not* about taste and texture; it's about bacterial counts.

Most commercial kefirs have likewise been fermented for as little time as possible. You can improve on this by simply leaving the container of commercial kefir out on the counter for another forty-eight hours or so, allowing further fermentation. But here is another little strategy you can exploit: referment the kefir. And, by doing so, you put the long list of bacterial species to work making a food you can use as a probiotic supplement.

Look for kefirs that do not contain fungi, such as various *Saccharomyces* species, because they ferment to alcohol. Some commercial kefirs have bacterial, but no fungal, species. (No strains are specified, of course, as is typical for fermented foods.)

The commercial Wallaby brand of kefir, for example, contains the following bacterial species:

- *Streptococcus thermophilus*
- *Lactobacillus bulgaricus*
- *Lactobacillus casei*
- *Lactobacillus acidophilus*

- *Bifidobacterium lactis*
- *Lactobacillus rhamnosus*
- *Lactococcus lactis*
- *Lactococcus cremoris*
- *Lactobacillus paracasei*
- *Lactococcus lactis* subspecies *lactis* biovar *diacetylactis*
- *Leuconostoc mesenteroides* subspecies *cremoris*
- *Lactobacillus delbrueckii* subspecies *lactis*

The Lifeway brand of kefir contains

- *Bifidobacterium breve*
- *Bifidobacterium lactis*
- *Bifidobacterium longum*
- *Lactobacillus acidophilus*
- *Lactobacillus casei*
- *Lactobacillus cremoris*
- *Lactobacillus lactis*
- *Lactobacillus plantarum*
- *Lactobacillus reuteri*
- *Lactobacillus rhamnosus*
- *Streptococcus diacetylactis*
- *Streptococcus florentinus*

Compare just these two brands, with an overlap of just four species, and you can appreciate that kefirs can be quite different in microbial species composition. The Wallaby product contains *L. paracasei*, which can suppress pathogens such as *Salmonella* and *H. pylori*, while the Lifeway product contains a strain of *Bifidobacterium longum* that may provide emotional health benefits. Ferment either of these kefirs and you will have amplified a broad collection of healthy microbes. You can even combine a little of each kefir and referment the combo to yield a yogurt with twenty different microbial species.

RECIPE

MAKES 1 QUART

2 tablespoons of kefir (or 2 tablespoons of each brand if using more than one)
2 tablespoons prebiotic fiber (e.g., inulin, raw potato starch)
1 quart organic half-and-half

In a medium-sized bowl, combine the kefir(s), prebiotic fiber, and 2 tablespoons of organic half-and-half or other fermentable liquid. Make a slurry to ensure the prebiotic fiber does not clump. Stir until well mixed. Stir in the remaining half-and-half or other liquid. Cover lightly (using plastic wrap or a lid fit on loosely), place in your fermenting device, and ferment at 106°F for 36 hours. To make future batches, use 2 tablespoons of curds and/or whey from a prior batch.

VEGETABLE FERMENTATION: A BASIC GUIDE

Before refrigeration, there was fermentation, one of the methods by which humans preserved food after harvest. This was one of the ways our great-grandparents harvested radishes, zucchini, asparagus, and other vegetables in summer, then consumed them throughout the fall and winter. They allowed foods to ferment, that is, to undergo degradation by bacteria and fungi. You're probably already familiar with fermented foods in the form of kefir and yogurt. Pickles and sauerkraut can also be fermented, but most store-bought products are not, instead being preserved in vinegar and brine and not allowed to ferment.

Fermentation preserves food when microbes consume the sugars and fibers present and produce lactate (responsible for the characteristic tartness) and other acids that inhibit growth of unsafe bacteria. Unlike yogurt and kefir, vegetable fermentation occurs in an anaerobic environment, that is, an environment without oxygen. Successful fermentation therefore requires keeping oxygen away from fermenting vegetables.

Many of the bacteria that ferment foods are among the healthiest strains for human bowel flora, such as *Lactobacillus plantarum*, *Lactobacillus brevis*, *Leuconostoc mesenteroides*, and *Bifidobacterium* species. Consuming fermented vegetables regularly, just as humans have done for thousands of years, inoculates your bowels with healthy bacterial strains.

Beyond the price of the food itself, fermenting foods is a virtually no-cost process. Fermentation also introduces unique flavors, as well as another opportunity to add herbs and spices with their own microbiome benefits.

You will need a jar or ceramic vessel and a means of keeping veggies submerged beneath the surface of the brine, away from oxygen. I use an old olive jar, and a heavy drinking glass that fits into the mouth of the jar keeps veggies below the surface of the liquid; others use a small plate weighted down with a stone. You can buy a fermentation kit, but it's really simple to assemble your own with items you likely already have on hand.

The basic ingredients are as follows:

- **Vegetables:** Raw onions, peppers, asparagus, cucumbers, radishes, garlic, carrots, cabbage, green beans, daikon radish, and others—any vegetable can be fermented. Chop the vegetables into bite-sized pieces. Combine vegetables to create unique flavors, for example, asparagus and onions, green beans and garlic.
- **Herbs and spices:** Peppercorns, dill, garlic cloves, coriander seeds, mustard seeds, caraway seeds, rosemary, oregano. Many people also add grape or berry leaves to increase crispiness.
- **Sea salt or other salt:** Use any salt, but not iodized salt (iodine kills microbes).
- **Water:** Use filtered water, spring water, or distilled water, that is, water without chlorine or fluoride.

Fermenting vegetables is, like baking or pottery making, an entire world to explore.

Basic Fermentation

Fill a jar or fermentation vessel with water, then add salt until the water tastes lightly to moderately salty, typically 1½ tablespoons per quart of water.

Add the vegetables and your choice of herbs or spices, such as peppercorns, dill, and coriander. Stir to mix the vegetables with the salt water and to release any trapped air bubbles.

Submerge the vegetables and cover them with a plate or other clean object to keep them below the surface, then cover the vessel to keep pests out. The system should not be airtight but only loosely covered because the process of fermentation produces gases that must be released.

Set the vessel aside for at least two days. The time required varies with the type of vegetables used and the temperature, but fermentation can go on for weeks. Once you obtain the flavor and degree of fermentation desired, refrigerate; this will slow further fermentation.

Optionally, after the vegetables have fermented, add a half cup of vinegar per quart of fermented mixture to enhance the flavor.

Should any white or other colored growth appear on the top, skim it off; this is mold. It does not harm the process, however, and your fermented foods will remain safe for consumption for at least four weeks in the refrigerator.

ADD WATER AND FERTILIZER

SUMMARY

In your third week of this health- and microbiome-rebuilding program, let's get comfortable with prebiotic fibers. They are the water and fertilizer for your garden of bowel flora, crucial for cultivating microbes and health. For maximum benefit, include a source of prebiotic fiber in *every* meal, a habit that will make this important strategy effortless over time. In the Super Gut program, we go beyond prebiotic fibers by using other strategies that also enable beneficial species to proliferate.

» Start with small quantities of prebiotic fiber–rich foods, such as 1 teaspoon of inulin or acacia fiber in coffee or yogurt, half a green unripe banana, or half a raw white potato coarsely chopped and blended into a smoothie or shake, or 1 to 2 tablespoons of a cooked legume. Most people tolerate up to 10 grams of prebiotic fibers during their first few days of week 3.
» Build up to 20 grams or more of prebiotic fibers per day from a variety of sources to help cultivate bacterial species diversity.

» If you prove intolerant to the initial level or to the increase in prebiotic fibers (excessive bloating, gas, or diarrhea), consider stopping them while continuing other Super Gut efforts (probiotics, fermented foods) for another four weeks, then try to reintroduce prebiotic fibers. If intolerance persists, move on to the SIBO and SIFO management program in Appendix B because prebiotic fiber intolerance is a reliable sign of a severely disrupted microbiome or SIBO.

Now that you have begun to shift bacterial species in your GI tract with probiotics and fermented foods, let's next get comfortable with introducing plenty of prebiotic fibers into your daily routine. While we try to consume at least one fermented food per day for its *probiotic* bacterial species, another good practice is to include at least one prebiotic fiber–containing food *in every meal*. This does not have to be complicated. It could be as simple as adding a couple tablespoons of black beans to a Spanish omelet, stir-frying with onions and garlic, dipping raw veggies into hummus, including leeks or dandelion greens in green salads, adding a teaspoon of inulin or acacia fiber to yogurt. The key is to include some source of prebiotic fibers every time you eat. Within just a few days of incorporating this practice, it will become second nature.

Obtaining plentiful prebiotic fibers in your daily routine is one of the most important steps you can take to rebuild both bowel and overall health, more important than even probiotics. Not only do prebiotic fibers feed healthy bacterial species, they also encourage bowel flora to produce metabolites that yield a range of health benefits, including weight loss; reduction of triglycerides, blood sugar, and blood pressure; reduction of inflammation and fatty liver; and better bowel habits.[16,17]

The average (unhealthy) American obtains between 3 and 8 grams of prebiotic fibers per day, about half of that from grains. Banishing all wheat and grains therefore means that we need to make up for the prebiotic fiber deficit. But with Super Gut we go even further for greater benefits.

Measurable health results begin at a prebiotic fiber intake of 8 grams per day, maximum benefits occur at an intake of 20 grams per day. We aim to obtain *20 grams or more each and every day*, which more than replaces the modest deficit caused by grain elimination, to stack the odds in favor of having a successful garden of bowel flora.[16–18] You therefore want to make a habit of including foods from the list that follows. You can also make a daily smoothie that includes one or more of the foods richest in prebiotic fibers, especially a raw white potato, unripe banana, or one or two teaspoons of acacia fiber, inulin/FOS, or a commercial prebiotic fiber mix. You will find recipes for a few variations below. Provided you tolerate prebiotic fibers at the beginning and with the increase to 20 grams per day, you cannot overdo them. (It is not uncommon for people in hunter-gatherer cultures to take in over 100 grams per day.)

Another key point: Vary your intake of prebiotic fiber. Don't just add inulin powder to coffee and call it a day, repeating the same habit over and over again while neglecting other prebiotic fiber sources. Not only does this fail to cultivate the wide bacterial species diversity you want, but it can even over-cultivate one or more bacterial species that can outgrow others and become unfriendly—essentially *creating* dysbiosis.

Some of our choices in prebiotic fibers may seem odd, such as raw white potatoes. But remember, we are trying to re-create the bountiful prebiotic fiber intake of hunter-gatherer populations, who dig for fiber-filled roots and tubers and enjoy variety in a diet that changes with season, terrain, and availability. You likely have no interest in uprooting your backyard or the forest to mimic such practices, so we turn to modern equivalents that are available and convenient. But it can mean making some unique choices unfamiliar to many people. Whereas early peoples naturally ate prebiotic fibers and had no need for gram counting, we must be purposeful and knowledgeable about it in our synthetic, prepackaged, marketing-filled world.

FOODS RICH IN PREBIOTIC FIBERS

The following foods offer lots of grams of prebiotic fiber to feed our friendly microbes.

Legumes: Kidney beans, black beans, white beans, other starchy beans, chickpeas, hummus, lentils, and peas are rich sources of galactooligosaccharide, or GOS, a form of prebiotic fiber. Keep servings small, for example, a quarter to half cup that

contains no more than 15 grams of net carbohydrates (total carbohydrates minus fiber) to minimize blood sugar consequences.
Hummus and chickpeas provide 8.0 grams of prebiotic fiber
per half cup (13.5 grams net carbohydrates). Lentils contain 2.5
grams of prebiotic fiber per half cup (11 grams net carbohydrates).
Most beans provide around 3.8 grams of prebiotic fiber per half-
cup serving. White beans are the richest source, with twice this
quantity (12 grams net carbohydrates per half cup).

Green bananas and plantains: And I mean *green*. Not
green-yellow, or a little green at one end, but green. If in doubt,
taste it: it should not have any sweetness at all. A medium, seven-
inch-long green banana contains 10.9 grams of prebiotic fibers
and 0 grams of net carbs in contrast to the high-sugar/high-carb,
low-fiber content of a ripe banana. A green banana is tough to
peel and virtually inedible, so slice it lengthwise and scoop out the
pulp, chop it coarsely, and use in one of the prebiotic smoothie
recipes below. Bananas generally stay green for four to five days
in the refrigerator, or you can peel, chop, and store them in the
freezer to use as needed.

Potatoes: Cooked potatoes (baked, fried, mashed) are high
in sugar and low in fiber. But when *raw*, they are rich in prebiotic fiber, with 10–12 grams per one-half medium-sized potato
(3½-inch diameter) and 0 grams of sugar/carbs. Some people
actually like eating raw white potatoes like an apple, others prefer to include potato in a prebiotic fiber smoothie or to slice
or dice it and toss it into a green salad. Avoid any raw potatoes
with green skin because this represents fungal growth. If en-
countered, peel off the skin. (Sweet potatoes and yams have
far less prebiotic fiber, even when raw. This means that, even
consumed raw, you chance excessive carbohydrate exposure.
Eat only small quantities, whether raw or cooked.)

Fruit: Because modern fruit has been bred for lower fiber
and higher sugar content, fruit as a source of prebiotic fiber is
accompanied by excessive sugars. So we navigate carefully. Fruit,
however, is an especially rich source of the important prebiotic
fiber pectin, which has unique properties that aid in cultivating healthy bacterial species, inhibiting pathogenic species, and

increasing intestinal butyrate and other fatty acids.[19] The richest fruit sources of pectin include avocados, blackberries, raspberries, pomegranates, and apples, each providing around 1–2 grams of pectin per serving, which is 1 cup of blackberries or raspberries or one medium apple. Avocados are the champions here, with the greatest quantity of pectin and only 4 net carbs per average avocado and plenty of healthy fat. You can also purchase pectin powders but use them sparingly because they typically contain sugar.

Chia seeds and flaxseed: Though not yet precisely quantified, chia seeds and flaxseed are two sources that provide a mixture of fibers, some prebiotic, as well as other compounds with beneficial effects on bowel flora. They are easily added to smoothies, yogurt, kefir, and baked dishes.

Nuts: Almonds, walnuts, pecans, hazelnuts, and pistachios are rich in polyphenol compounds with prebiotic fiber properties.[20] Meaningful prebiotic effects begin with around a half cup of nuts, and the skins should be included (meaning that almond flour made from blanched almonds does not provide the same benefits). With nuts, you are on pretty safe ground with carbohydrate exposure. A half-cup serving of almonds, for instance, yields 4.5 grams net carbs. Raw and dry roasted (with no added maltodextrin, sugar, or other unwanted ingredients) are your best choices.

Mushrooms: Mushrooms are an underappreciated source of polysaccharides with prebiotic fiber properties, compounds such as beta-glucan (distinct from the beta-glucan of fungi), mannan, galactans, as well as polyphenols, all of which nourish microbes. Of course, mushrooms are so easy to incorporate into dishes such as salads and stir-fries, to eat alongside meats, to puree into sauces and gravies, or to toss into soups. (See the recipe for a traditional, though improved, Cream of Mushroom Soup on page 255.)

Shirataki noodles: Shirataki noodles are made from glucomannan sourced from an Asian yam and are a rich source of prebiotic fiber. They are best used in Asian dishes such as stir-fries and ramen. Look for products without soy or oats. Eight ounces of noodles yields approximately 2 grams of prebiotic fibers. (See recipe for Yakisoba Noodles on page 269.)

Modest quantities of prebiotic fiber (generally around 1–3 grams per common serving size) can also be obtained from the following foods:

- Asparagus
- Jicama
- Turnips
- Parsnips
- Onions
- Garlic and shallots

- Carrots
- Leeks
- Dandelion greens
- Radishes
- Cabbage
- Brussels sprouts

Food should be your primary source of prebiotic fibers. For convenience, however, prebiotic fiber powders are available such as inulin powder, acacia fiber, glucomannan powder, and commercial sources that combine several forms of prebiotic fiber (listed in Appendix A). You can add a teaspoon or two of these prebiotic powders to coffee, tea, the fermented yogurts that we make, and other dishes, and they will provide approximately 3 grams of prebiotic fiber per teaspoon. Glucomannan powder can be used to thicken foods too. Raw potato starch and green banana flour can also be used as prebiotic fiber sources, but use them sparingly, for example, no more than 1 tablespoon at a time, because they are nearly 50 percent sugar, given the temperature used to dehydrate these foods into flours, which is high enough to degrade fiber into sugar.

At the start of this third week, limit prebiotic fibers to no more than 10 grams per day, for example, half a green banana or 2 teaspoons of acacia fiber. Increase your intake to 20 grams later in the week, but be sure to obtain the fiber from a mixture of sources. If all goes well and you have no reaction to the low starting quantity or the increase, this means it's safe to go on to the rest of the program.

However, if you prove intolerant to prebiotic fibers—you experience excessive bloating, gas, diarrhea, or emotional effects such as anxiety or dark thoughts—this can serve as a therapeutic test for SIBO. If you experience any of these symptoms within the first ninety minutes after ingestion, it is a highly reliable sign that bacterial overgrowth is present in the small intestine. In this case, opt for a more extended course of probiotics and fermented foods to prolong the "seeding" process. Try reintroducing prebiotic fibers after a further four weeks of probiotic seeding. If they still cause distress, then it's time to follow the Super Gut SIBO and SIFO Protocols detailed in Appendix B. Once you have dealt with those issues, return here to week 3 and start watering and fertilizing your microbiome again.

SOMEWHERE OVER THE RAINBOW

Violet, indigo, blue, green, yellow, orange, and red: We want to follow the colors of the rainbow not just in the sky but also in our diets.

For years, it was something of a mystery why the colorful compounds in vegetables and fruit—the purple of eggplant, the yellow of lemons, the green of kale—yielded beneficial health effects because very little of them is absorbed from the GI tract. In other words, we obtain health benefits by consuming cranberries, plums, and green tea that correlate with their content of colorful compounds called polyphenols, even though the bulk of such compounds never leave the confines of the ileum or colon.

It has become clear that indigestible polyphenols are metabolized by bacteria and the composition of bowel flora is, in turn, altered by polyphenol metabolites.[21] Similar to the effects of prebiotic fibers, polyphenols stack the odds in favor of maintaining healthy bacterial species. Liberal intake of polyphenols, for example, favors growth of healthy species such as *Akkermansia muciniphila*, which regulates blood sugar, and *Faecalibacterium prausnitzii*, which is a major producer of butyrate.[22] Other polyphenols, most notably the catechin in green tea, strengthen the intestinal mucus barrier by cross-linking mucus proteins, an effect that further encourages *Akkermansia* growth. (See the recipe for Clove Green Tea on page 247 for a powerful way to increase the strength of the intestinal mucus lining.) Yet other polyphenols, such as the quercetin found in onions, apples, and kale, exert potent antibacterial and antifungal properties, especially against the species that dominate in SIBO and SIFO. All these findings shed new light on the wisdom of including a variety of vegetables and fruits in our diet for the unexpected and broad health benefits.[23,24]

Differences in bowel flora composition between individuals also mean that polyphenols such as quercetin, curcumin, rutin, and epigallocatechin are metabolized differently by different people, and some are not metabolized at all. Until we make sense of this complexity, variety in polyphenol intake is key: cocoa flavonoids, green tea catechins, blueberry anthocyanins, citrus naringenin, flaxseed lignans, red wine resveratrol, apple rutin, and extra-virgin olive oil hydroxytyrosols and oleuropeins.

The key with prebiotic fibers is variety. Don't over-rely on just, say, inulin powder because of its convenience. Ingesting a variety of prebiotic fibers encourages species diversity in bowel flora, and that wide variety of bacterial species keeps unhealthy species at bay. Shaping the microbiome composition in your GI tract using prebiotic fibers is a project that will occupy you for many months, perhaps years. This third week of the program gets you off to a powerful start.

SUPER FERTILIZERS

You can add super fertilizers like rich compost or fish emulsions to your backyard garden that stack the odds in favor of yielding a rich bounty of peppers and zucchini. You can likewise add specific dietary ingredients that have outsized stimulating effects on certain species to build your Super Gut. This is a really exciting area of research that has only just gotten its start, so the list is short and we have no official label to assign to these effects yet, so I call them "super fertilizers" to convey the idea that these compounds cause certain bacterial species to bloom. In fact, this area of study is so exciting that I predict it is on the leading edge of a movement to create what I call "third-generation probiotics." First-generation probiotics are the less-than-ideal, haphazard preparations we currently have. Second-generation probiotics are those that provide keystone species.

Third-generation probiotics will provide keystone species as well as crucial microbe nutrients that cause a "bloom" in selected, often other keystone, species. Among these super-fertilizing nutrients are the following:

Eugenol: Eugenol is an oil extracted from cloves that is also present in lesser quantities in nutmeg and cinnamon. The essential oil of clove that we include in our SIFO efforts is mostly eugenol. This compound has antibacterial effects against pathogenic species such as *Salmonella*, but, perhaps more importantly, eugenol has a stimulatory effect on beneficial species of the Clostridia class that, in turn, dramatically stimulate intestinal mucus production.[24] For this reason, I include eugenol in my recipe for Clove Green Tea, a powerful and tasty way to strengthen the intestinal mucus barrier.

FOS and oleic acid: FOS is a prebiotic fiber related to inulin, just with a shorter chain structure, and oleic acid is the dominant fatty acid in mono-unsaturated oils such as olive oil. Both, via different means, stimulate a bloom in *Akkermansia*. The combination of the two is especially powerful. Recall that people who inadvertently take in too little prebiotic fiber, such as FOS, to adequately feed beneficial microorganisms cause *Akkermansia* to resort to its alternative source of nutrition, the human intestinal mucus lining. Providing FOS prevents this from happening.[25] Whereas root vegetables such as onions, garlic, leeks, and shallots contain FOS, adding a teaspoon of FOS powder to coffee, yogurt, or other foods is a way to ensure a healthy intake of this crucial fiber. And including olive oil in your diet in generous amounts, for example, adding it to eggs, salad dressings, Caprese salad and dipping Herbed Focaccia Bread (recipe on page 252) into extra-virgin olive oil with a little sea salt ensures vigorous stimulation of *Akkermansia*.

Capsaicin: You'll recall that capsaicin is the factor in hot peppers that gives them the hot sensation upon consumption. Including capsaicin in your daily routine, most convenient as hot sauces made from habanero, cayenne, tabiche, and others, provokes a bloom in the master butyrate-producing microbe *Faecalibacterium prausnitzii* that, in turn, yields metabolic benefits such as lower blood sugar and lower blood pressure and may make a modest contribution to weight loss. Capsaicin also encourages proliferation of the intestinal mucus "gatekeepers," *Clostridia* species.

The hotter the sauce, the greater the capsaicin content, so content varies depending on hotness. A tablespoon of habanero sauce, for instance, provides around 7 grams of capsaicin. Maximum benefits develop with intake of around 10 grams per day. You can find cayenne pepper as a nutritional supplement in capsules, but they provide relatively minor intakes of capsaicin.

GROW YOUR SUPER GUT MICROBE GARDEN

SUMMARY

Like choosing a meal off the menu at a nice restaurant, you can pick and choose the microbes that yield specific health effects. You can boost the benefits by increasing bacterial numbers by using modified Super Gut methods of microbial fermentation. Here is the menu of beneficial microbes:

» *L. reuteri* for skin smoothing and reduced wrinkle depth, restoration of youthful muscle and strength, deeper sleep, increased libido, appetite suppression, accelerated healing, increased empathy, reduced social anxiety, preservation of bone density
» *L. reuteri* and *L. casei* for deeper and longer sleep, reduced stress, and enhanced immune function
» *B. coagulans* for reduced inflammation and arthritis pain
» *L. helveticus* and *B. longum* for reduced anxiety, improved mood, and reduced depression
» *L. casei* for enhanced mental clarity and focus
» *L. reuteri* and *L. gasseri* for weight loss and reduced waist size
» *L. reuteri* and *B. coagulans* for increased strength and accelerated recovery in athletes

» *B. infantis* for mothers to pass on to their babies at birth
and breastfeeding to reduce the number of infant bowel
movements, reduce colic, and improve sleep and long-
term health
» *L. reuteri*, *L. gasseri*, and *B. coagulans* found in the Super
Gut SIBO Yogurt for eradication of SIBO

YOU'VE BEEN THROUGH THE TOUGHEST PART OF THE PROGRAM
these past three weeks, changing diet and learning how to restore
healthy species of the microbiome and strengthen the intestinal barrier.
All that sets the stage for a return to magnificent health by undoing the
harmful effects of conventional dietary guidelines, food indulgences, and
medical mismanagement. Let's now get to the really fun part.

We are going to put our garden to work to obtain benefits such as
smoother skin, greater strength, reduced inflammation and pain, and reduced anxiety, all the wonderful effects I've mentioned. (If you have diverted
to managing SIBO and SIFO, you can still undertake these fermentation
projects, though the benefits will not be as dramatic because your current
antimicrobial efforts can eradicate both good and bad species. For best
results, begin these fermentation projects once you are through with your
SIBO/SIFO efforts.)

People sometimes ask, "Can't I just eat store-bought yogurt or take a
probiotic to obtain the same benefits?" I hope that you now understand
that, no, you cannot—not even close. The magic in what we undertake in
week 4 comes from a number of factors:

- **We select bacterial species and strains to yield specific health
  benefits.** The "generic" species in commercial products like yogurt
  and probiotics do not provide such targeted benefits. You could consume gallons of commercial yogurt and still not experience the sorts
  of benefits we're discussing here.
- **We modify the fermentation process to exponentially increase
  bacterial counts.** In these fermentation projects, we typically obtain bacterial counts in the hundreds of billions compared to the
  millions or few billions of commercial products. "Millions" sounds

like a lot, but it's almost nothing when it comes to bacteria. We extend fermentation time to culture hundreds of billions of microorganisms. Whereas commercial yogurt is fermented for about four hours, we ferment ours for thirty-six hours, a time difference that makes a *thousand-fold* difference in benefit. Likewise, most commercial probiotics contain bacterial counts of only a few billion of each species and often the least costly strains rather than the most effective.

- **We add prebiotic fiber to the fermentation process.** Like adding fertilizer to your garden to grow bigger, more luscious tomatoes, adding prebiotic fibers that nourish microbes to a fermentation project helps push bacterial counts higher, and in yogurt, it increases the thickness and richness of the final product.

Not only can you obtain magnificent benefits from these fermentation projects, but you also get to enjoy delicious yogurts and other fermented foods that are nutritious and easy to fit into your daily routine.

If you are able to consume dairy products, great—dairy is the most effective and forgiving medium for bacterial fermentation. If not, don't panic: we can ferment coconut milk and other foods like hummus and fruit purees.

The Super Gut method of yogurt fermentation minimizes the potentially problematic tolerance issues with dairy. Prolonged fermentation reduces lactose (the milk sugar that people who are lactose-intolerant are troubled by) to negligible levels because it is maximally converted to lactic acid (the organic acid that is a helpful by-product of fermentation and that lends a tart flavor to some of the yogurts). The accumulation of lactic acid in the yogurt drops the pH to an acidic 3.5 (nearly tenfold more acidic than commercial yogurt), a level associated with denaturation, or the breakdown, of the casein protein, making it less likely to stimulate an immune response. These changes explain why these yogurts are better tolerated by many people than conventional dairy products.

Also included in our fermentation projects are mixed-culture yogurts (i.e., yogurts fermented with a mixture of bacterial species). We use these when high bacterial counts of a single species are not desired, such as for children.

I also introduce the idea of using a yogurt I call Super Gut SIBO Yogurt to push back the populations of hydrogen- and methane-producing microbes in SIBO. As you now know, conventional probiotics, because they are haphazardly assembled, have only modest effects on depopulating the gut of SIBO species. But what if we carefully choose probiotic species and strains for their specific characteristics that could provide advantages against SIBO, such as an ability to colonize the upper GI tract where SIBO occurs and to produce bacteriocins effective against SIBO species? The three-species Super Gut yogurt thereby has a better chance of reorganizing the microbiome and reducing or eliminating SIBO.

Super Gut Success: Anne, 60, Connecticut

"I USED TO WAKE UP AT LEAST FOUR TIMES EVERY NIGHT, AND take at least half an hour to get back to sleep, but since I have been eating the *L. reuteri/L. casei* combo, I generally wake up once a night and fall back to sleep within a few minutes. In the last two weeks, I have slept through the night three times, which I have never done. Prior to this, I was eating *L. reuteri* yogurt alone, and I noticed my nodular acne has improved tremendously, to a point where it is almost gone, where heavy-duty meds did nothing for it. I stopped eating it for two weeks to test for SIBO, and the acne returned. I also like the *L. casei* Shirota for the respiratory benefits because I have pulmonary fibrosis and am prone to respiratory infections.

"Today is my one-year anniversary of being grain and sugar free. Down forty-five pounds, down six prescription meds, reduced dose on two other meds. Cured my fatty liver, which the GI doctor said he rarely sees. Stopped the prediabetes. Arthritis greatly improved with a huge decrease in swelling and an increase in mobility—I can walk up the stairs like a normal person instead of like a toddler. I have a lot more energy and my outlook on life has improved tremendously. I'm healthier now at sixty than I was at fifty, or even forty.

"In my late fifties I developed cystic (nodular) acne. It's ugly, painful, long-lasting and leaves scars. They started in one area and spread to a large portion of my body. My back and shoulders were even worse. After about a year of various treatments that didn't work, I stopped going to the doctor and started searching for other answers. Eventually, I found Dr. Davis and the *L. reuteri* yogurt. I noticed an improvement right away after starting the yogurt, the new spots weren't as bad as before, then they started healing faster, then the number of new ones decreased. And I just realized I don't have as many scars as I did. Now I rarely get a new spot, and if I do, it's in a limited area. If I stop or decrease the *L. reuteri*, they come right back as bad as before, so I know it's due to the addition of the yogurt and the rest of the program.

"I am so excited to have gotten to this point in my life and know the best is yet to come. I forgot to add that this is the first time I have lost weight and gotten healthier instead of sicker. Thank you, Dr. Davis!"

———

WHAT'S ON YOUR MICROBIAL MENU?

I don't believe that I can exaggerate about what you and I are about to embark upon, a microbial journey in which you can essentially order a healthy body composition or emotional benefit just by choosing advantageous microbial species, cultivating them, then restoring them to your body. We do not have all lessons charted, but the list is growing faster than I can write them down. Imagine what you and I shall have after two, five, or ten more years of such experiences, with many of us fermenting microbes and learning and getting smarter and more effective every day.

In this section, I list the effects most people who consume these yogurts or other fermented foods experience. I also include optional strategies you can use to accelerate or amplify benefits. You can obtain some of these health effects by taking a probiotic that includes each species and strain, but making Super Gut yogurt amplifies the effects of probiotics because the unique fermentation process is like taking seeds from one green pepper and planting an entire garden of green peppers in generously fertilized soil: We markedly increase yield this way. And don't forget that bacterial strain is crucial; *Lactobacillus gasseri* BNR17 may cause you to lose an inch off your waist, but another strain of *Lactobacillus gasseri* may not necessarily re-create that effect.

For unclear reasons, not everyone experiences all these effects or intensity of effects. In a survey of my online audience, 60 percent of people consuming the *L. reuteri* yogurt experienced moderate to marked improvement in skin health, while 40 percent experienced only modest or no effect on skin health. Whereas some people can improve results by increasing the quantity of yogurt they consume (e.g., eating a half cup twice per day rather than once per day), others do not. Some effects may also require a longer time to manifest, such as three to six months. Differing results may result from different genetics, such as a genetically determined variant in the oxytocin receptor or a defect in the complex endocannabinoid system (which mediates oxytocin effects), or something else entirely. My team and I are actively exploring these issues so that we can develop strategies to improve benefits.

The recipes for all these fermented yogurts and other foods can be found in Super Gut Recipes, including the proper strains and where to source them.

Smoother Skin with Reduced Wrinkles, Accelerated Healing

L. reuteri yogurt, a half cup per day.

Consider mixing in collagen hydrolysates, 10 grams per day, to your yogurt.

Deeper Sleep with Extended REM

L. reuteri yogurt, a half cup per day. Can be combined with *L. casei* Shirota for greater effects. If these species are fermented separately, consume a half cup per day of each yogurt. If fermented together, consume half to one cup per day. If fermented together, ferment at 104°F–106°F.

Consider tracking your sleep with an actigraphic device such as an Apple Watch, Whoop, Oura Ring, or FitBit, and specifically track duration of sleep, deep sleep, and REM.

Reduced Inflammation and Arthritis Pain

Bacillus coagulans yogurt, a half cup per day.

Consider adding Clove Green Tea for its mucus barrier–strengthening effects that reduce endotoxemia.

Reduced Stress

L. casei yogurt, a half cup per day. The effect is increased by combining with *L. reuteri* yogurt. If fermented separately, consume a half cup per day of each yogurt. If fermented together, ferment at 104°F–106°F and consume half to one cup per day. Also consider *L. infantis* for added benefit.

Both species blunt the abnormal rise in morning cortisol that defines many stressful situations. (Prolonged stress that has reduced adrenal gland release of cortisol may not respond to this strategy and will need to be specifically addressed.)

Reduced Depression and Anxiety

Lactobacillus helveticus and *Bifidobacterium longum* yogurt, a half cup per day. Consider adding *L. casei* for more benefits (and then fermenting it at 104°F–106°F).

Enhanced Mental Clarity and Focus

L. casei yogurt, a half cup per day.

This effect is most marked when you first start consuming this microbe. For best effect, cycle on and cycle off every few days; the greatest boost in mental clarity and focus comes at the start or upon resumption of consumption.

PSYCHOBIOTICS: MATTER OVER MIND

Mood is like the background music playing while you are shopping in the grocery store: It's there, just below conscious awareness, but nonetheless registering somewhere in your brain, perhaps influencing your shopping behavior. Mood, likewise, colors your emotions, what you say to other people, how satisfied or dissatisfied you are with your day, what tasks you take on. We don't give enough credit to the impact of mood, perhaps because we feel that we are not in control over this phenomenon. If you are annoyed and irritable, will this influence how you interact with others? If you are upbeat or euphoric, will problems seem less formidable? It's dysphoria, unhappiness, dissatisfaction that drive us to take antidepressants, drink more beer, take more drugs, say things we should not say to the people close to us.

What if we instead change the music in the supermarket to tunes that make you feel energized, hopeful, confident, eager to make the acquaintance of the woman smelling the cantaloupe? A mundane, dull activity like grocery shopping might turn out to be an adventure.

How much of a role can silly microbes that find their way into the toilet every day really play in determining your outlook, your internal dialogues, the conversations you have with others, whether you view your day with dread and trepidation or with excitement and anticipation?

To illustrate, consider how different you would feel if I painted the walls of your living room black and covered all the windows. Compare this to a room with large windows that let in the sunlight, with views of grass, trees, birds, sky, and sun. Does it make a difference? Of course it does. You are the same person, dark or light, but the emotions you experience are quite different. That is the same sort of background mood and emotion that microbes play in your brain, influencing how light or dark you view life, your circumstances, the people around you.

Let's therefore consider what you and I are contemplating in our microbe-cultivating projects: *L. reuteri* restores empathy and desire for the company of other people.[26] *L. casei* enhances attentiveness—mindfulness?—and blunts the effects of stress.[27] *L. helveticus* and *B. longum* reduce anxiety and restore feelings of hope.[28] And these are just our starting lessons—many more are sure to come.

You are likely already aware of what an utter failure pharmaceutical "solutions" to depression, anxiety, and other disorders of mood and emotion have been. Antidepressants come with warnings about weight gain and suicide, antianxiety agents invite addiction, more potent agents can lead to irreversible neurological damage. You and I are instead talking about making yogurt with microbes that shift the mood from night to day, deepen sleep, make problems seem lighter, smooth out skin wrinkles—I get euphoric just thinking about it.

Weight Loss, Visceral Fat Loss

L. reuteri + *L. gasseri* yogurt—if fermented separately, consume a half cup per day of each yogurt. If fermented together, consume half to one cup per day (and ferment at 106°F).

The oxytocin boost generated by *L. reuteri* reduces appetite, often dramatically. Food still tastes great, but most people enjoy absolute control over appetite and temptation. (If you are wheat- and grain-free, the absence of gliadin-derived opioid peptide appetite stimulants also reduces appetite, and the added *L. reuteri* oxytocin effect confers even greater control over appetite.) *L. gasseri* reduces visceral fat and waist circumference.

Note that, to gauge fat loss, you need to track measures such as waist size and/or body fat percentage using a body composition scale because the oxytocin boost obtained with *L. reuteri* can also increase muscle. If you track only your weight, you might notice you actually *gain* net weight, that is, you gain muscle but lose fat. A scale that analyzes body fat can tell you this, as will tracking your waist circumference or just looking in the mirror. In other words, better than weight loss, you are improving *body composition*.

Increase Muscle and Strength

L. reuteri yogurt, a half cup per day. Consider adding collagen hydrolysates, 10 grams per day, and creatine at 2–5 grams per day.

This effect also includes halting the muscle loss and advancing frailty that accompany aging. For maximum benefit, combine the oxytocin-boosting effect of *L. reuteri* with strength training. The strength- and muscle-building benefits of strength training are magnified by the oxytocin boost.

Athletes: Increase Strength and Accelerate Recovery

Mixed culture of *L. reuteri* + *B. coagulans*.

The *L. reuteri* increases strength and muscle mass and the *B. coagulans* reduces muscle breakdown during strenuous training or competition, which in turn accelerates recovery.

We use a mixed culture to achieve lower numbers of *L. reuteri*; consume a half cup per day. Ferment the mixed culture at 106°F to accommodate the higher temperature needs of *B. coagulans*.

Pregnant Mothers: Pass Keystone Species Bifidobacterium infantis On to Your Baby

B. infantis yogurt, a half cup per day. Recall that *Bifidobacterium infantis* is a keystone species that allows your child to digest breast milk oligosaccharides, which, in turn, provide better nutrition for your baby while also cultivating other healthy bacterial species in your child's microbiome. The commercial probiotic Evivo with the EVC001 strain (see Appendix A) provides substantial benefits, including reducing bowel movements by 50 percent (thereby fewer diaper changes), reducing colic, reducing diaper rash, prolonging sleep, enabling longer naps, and reducing long-term potential for asthma and autoimmune conditions.

But why not restore *B. infantis* to *your* microbiome, which then allows you to pass it on to your child during vaginal birth and breastfeeding—the way it was supposed to happen all along? Once again, you can choose to make yogurt with *B. infantis* to generate higher bacterial counts instead of taking a commercial probiotic. (This yogurt is meant for *your* consumption, not the baby's. You can, of course, also provide *B. infantis* to your child by mixing the probiotic in breast milk.)

Enhanced Immunity

Mixed culture of *L. reuteri* + *L. casei* Shirota yogurt. Consume half to one cup per day. Ferment the combination at 104°F–106°F.

We all experience a progressive decline in immune response as we age, which explains why, for example, people in their seventies and onward are more likely to die from influenza or pneumococcal pneumonia or to develop cancer (failed immune surveillance). Selected microbes have huge potential to augment the immune response.

SUPER GUT SIBO YOGURT

I've discussed how conventional commercial probiotics are created haphazardly. The species included are not chosen because they provide a specific effect, such as effectiveness against SIBO species.

We instead choose species and strains with characteristics that provide advantage against the species of SIBO, characteristics such as taking up residence in the small bowel (where SIBO occurs) and production of bacteriocins, peptide antibiotics effective against the species of SIBO. We then increase the numbers of these microbes through fermentation and consume the resulting yogurt for several weeks.

Results are preliminary, but I have witnessed a number of people in my program reverse abnormal hydrogen gas in their breath as measured with the AIRE device by using this yogurt. Here is what many of us are doing:

We ferment *L. reuteri* DSM17938 + ATCC PTA 6475 + *L. gasseri* BNR17 + *Bacillus coagulans* GBI-30,6086 yogurt, and then eat a half cup per day.

This specific mixture combines the upper GI–colonizing effects of *L. reuteri* and *L. gasseri* with the bacteriocin-producing capacity of all three microbes. So far, most people have responded to this mix.

These three species and strains should be fermented in the same mixture with good results. See the recipe for Super Gut SIBO Yogurt in Super Gut Recipes.

THE LIBERATED BOWEL

I hope that you now recognize the enormous power you harbor just below your diaphragm. That thing that annoys you with its churning and gurgling after a meal is actually a factory that you can put to work to manufacture products that keep you young, help you sleep, shape your physical appearance, and brighten your outlook. It's like turning the light on in your garage and discovering that you have a shiny, brand-new automobile that can take you places you've never been before. Order up deep sleep: Make the right kind of yogurt. How about greater strength and libido? Have a half cup of yogurt. Help your newborn be healthier and sleep through the night: Eat some yogurt. You cannot buy it in the grocery, it will not come with high-fructose corn syrup or carrageenan, but you can still enjoy it topped with some raspberries and chia seeds.

You now have therapeutic tools to rebuild a healthy microbiome and reap the enormous health benefits that develop when you put the right species—and strains!—to work.

SUPER GUT RECIPES

YOU HAVE SURELY PERUSED MANY COOKBOOKS OVER THE YEARS and followed some of their recipes—but you've never seen recipes like these.

We are going to be growing various bacteria to obtain a whole range of wonderful health benefits, as well as enjoying delicious dishes that help support your efforts to beat back the monster that's taken over your GI tract.

The recipes provided here fall into four categories:

1. **Yogurt recipes:** These recipes yield large numbers of specific species and strains of bacteria and thereby substantial health benefits.
2. **Beverage and smoothie recipes:** A smoothie is an easy way to get a wallop of prebiotic fibers as a tasty snack or meal replacement.
3. **Side dishes, main dishes, and condiments:** Various dishes that make use of ingredients that aid your efforts to reprogram your intestinal microbiome, such as spices in a delicious tea that increase the thickness and protective capabilities of your intestinal mucus lining and rosemary in baking for its ability to discourage overgrowth of *Staphylococcus aureus* and *Candida albicans*.
4. **Desserts:** Dishes that illustrate how you can make your sugar- and grain-free life delicious and fun when entertaining friends or enjoying holidays and keep the children and grandchildren happy.

A three-day menu plan and shopping list to get you started falls at the end of this recipe section.

If you can consume dairy products, you will find that they are the most forgiving, least problematic vehicle for fermentation. We may call our various fermentation efforts "yogurt," but they are really not. FDA regulations stipulate that anything labeled "yogurt" must be fermented using not-very-exciting *Lactobacillus bulgaricus* and *Streptococcus thermophilus* species, which we are *not* using. (There's no harm in using these traditional microbes, but I believe that we can achieve more interesting results with other species and strains.) We may call it "yogurt," but our unique fermented foods provide health benefits more profound than the ho-hum effects of conventional yogurt, and in nutrition these foods are light-years ahead of the fancy-labeled products in the dairy section of your supermarket that are sweetened with high-fructose corn syrup and thickened with carrageenan, xanthan, and gellan gums to conceal their meager bacterial numbers and metabolites.

In addition to choosing specific microbes, we also super-power traditional yogurt-making methods by prolonging fermentation times and adding prebiotic fibers to nourish the hardworking bacteria. These additional efforts increase bacterial counts from the few millions in conventional yogurts to hundreds of billions, not uncommonly a *thousand-fold* increase. In general, the higher the bacterial count, the greater the biological effect. I have submitted a number of samples of our yogurts for bacterial counts to labs that use an automated method called flow cytometry. The most recently submitted batch of *L. reuteri* yogurt, for instance, had 262 billion microbes per half-cup serving—try getting those numbers in a commercial yogurt or probiotic supplement.

Dairy products are not without issues: lactose, casein beta A1, and whey protein being among the most potentially problematic components. Extended fermentation, however, serves to minimize potential adverse effects by maximally converting lactose to lactic acid (very little lactose remains in the yogurt, and the end result is tart from lactic acid). The accumulation of lactic acid reduces the pH to 3.5, a level that denatures, or breaks down, the casein protein, making it less immunogenic (i.e., reducing its potential to provoke immune responses). And you can minimize the effect of the whey protein that stimulates insulin release from the pancreas by pouring off the liquid whey or straining the yogurt through cheesecloth or a coffee filter for four to six hours to yield a thicker Greek-style yogurt. (Line a colander with cheesecloth or a coffee filter, place the colander in a large bowl or pot, then pour the yogurt into the colander and cover. The whey slowly drips out of the yogurt into the bowl, and you can toss it out or use it to begin your next batch of yogurt, as the whey contains plenty of microbes.) If you are intolerant of conventional dairy, you can use A2 dairy products made from cows that produce the less-immune-stimulating casein beta A2 protein, a form that is identical to that in human breast milk. You also have the option of using goat's or sheep's milk, both also A2. Or you can use non-dairy milks such as coconut milk. I also provide recipes to ferment various foods such as salsa and hummus.

Each yogurt recipe uses one quart of dairy liquid. If you choose to use dairy, I find that organic half-and-half (50 percent cream, 50 percent whole milk) yields the best result. (Yes: We choose high-fat and high-calorie sources because we *want* fat, and calories *do not matter*. Ironically, fat is the dairy component most frequently demonized, but it is the healthiest ingredient of all in dairy.) Whole milk also works well but yields a richer end result only after you strain out the whey. You can also begin with heavy cream, but in my experience, it yields a yogurt that is too thick, almost like cream cheese. Some people, however, seem to prefer this, so it's your choice. Whatever you choose to start with, just be sure it contains no additives like gellan or xanthan gum because these will encourage clumpy separation of the yogurt into curds (solids) and whey (liquid).

After we select the bacterial species that yield the specific, often extraordinary, effects we're after, we add prebiotic fiber to further increase bacterial counts. This step also increases the thickness and richness of the final product. You can ferment without adding a source of prebiotic fiber, but the end product is thinner, less rich, and might not produce the full effect you are looking for because of lower bacterial counts. Inulin powder and raw potato starch (e.g., Bob's Red Mill brand) work best, unless you are fermenting *Bifidobacterium* species, which seem to "prefer" sources of sugar such as raw potato starch (a chain of glucose molecules) or sucrose rather than inulin. Don't worry: I have included instructions on which source of prebiotic fiber to use with each fermentation project.

You need some means of maintaining your yogurt at the recommended temperature, which varies with bacterial species. *L. reuteri*, for example, grows best at human body temperature, 97°F–100°F (meaning that the rate of bacterial reproduction is maximized at these temperatures), while *Bacillus coagulans* "prefers" a higher temperature, between 115°F and 122°F. You are therefore best served by choosing a yogurt-making device that allows you to vary both temperature and fermentation time. Sous vide devices (basin or stick, ordinarily used to slow cook meat), some yogurt makers, and newer Instant Pots with lower temperature settings work well. (See Appendix A for a list of recommended devices.)

Don't be overwhelmed by these fermentation projects, and don't feel like you need to do all of them. When you are handed a menu at a restaurant, you don't feel like you have to order every appetizer, entrée, and dessert listed—you just order the dishes you want. Likewise, view these recipes as a menu and choose the bacterial species and strains for the effects you desire. Each yogurt begins with a different starter species or strain that you need to purchase only once because you can make subsequent batches of yogurt using a tablespoon or two of a prior batch. You can use the liquid whey, solid curd, or both to start the next batch.

Feel free to experiment. People following my program frequently report new and unique effects from these foods that we did not anticipate. Some have reported, for instance, increased mental clarity with *Lactobacillus casei* Shirota yogurt, increased strength with *Lactobacillus gasseri* BNR17 yogurt, and relief from compulsive behaviors with *Bifidobacterium longum* BB536 yogurt. Because your response to each fermentation product may vary, you might learn about new benefits simply by trying new yogurts.

Don't be discouraged if your first batch of each yogurt separates into curds (solid) and whey (watery liquid); this is typical with first batches. Subsequent batches tend to be richer and thicker. Once you obtain the thick and creamy end result, enjoy your delicious and filling yogurt with some strawberries, a bit of chia seed, and a squirt of benign noncaloric sweetener such as stevia.

SUPER GUT YOGURT RECIPES

With these unique recipes, you are going to be creating foods that have the power of miraculous drugs, but with none of the side effects. You will be creating foods that have age-reversing and mood-elevating effects, effects that can improve physical performance for an athlete or mental performance for a student or businessperson. Calling it "yogurt" is like calling a Rolls-Royce a go-kart: it's hardly a fair comparison. But it looks like yogurt, tastes like yogurt, even though it would not meet the FDA's definition of yogurt—you are going to eat in style with these recipes, enjoying benefits that you may have thought were long out of reach.

For greatest effect, make a monoculture yogurt (or other fermented food), that is, ferment the food using a single bacterial species or strain because this yields the highest bacterial numbers, in the hundreds of billions per half-cup serving. If you desire less-intense effects or, as with *L. reuteri* for children or young adults, we want the benefits of the bacterial species and strains but not at the intense levels of full-strength yogurt, make a *mixed-culture* yogurt; this is when you ferment a yogurt using several species and strains (example recipe provided). Think of it this way: If you have a garden and you plant only tomatoes, watering and fertilizing your garden will yield a huge bounty of tomatoes. But if you plant tomatoes with zucchini, cucumbers, squash, and eggplant, you will have fewer tomatoes. Bacteria behave the exact same way when they compete for available resources. Remember that my flow cytometry studies of our yogurts showed bacterial counts at over two hundred billion per half-cup serving, so we have plenty of leeway to combine two, three, perhaps four species—you will have fewer numbers of each species, but the overall count should still be quite high, for example, sixty to eighty billion per strain per half-cup serving.

The first batch of each yogurt ferments from the bacterial source, for example, crushed probiotic tablets for *L. reuteri* yogurt, then you make subsequent batches from 2 tablespoons that you have saved from a prior batch, curds (solids), whey (liquid), or both. You can re-inoculate subsequent batches using additional tablets or capsules of the starting microbe, but usually there is no need because the bacteria are wonderful at proliferating and do just fine even if you do not add more organisms.

If you want to limit your reliance on dairy products or just want a change of pace, see the list of alternative fermentation vehicles toward the end of this chapter.

LACTOBACILLUS REUTERI YOGURT

LACTOBACILLUS REUTERI YOGURT IS OUR STAR YOGURT THAT CAN YIELD SPECTACU-lar health effects such as smoother skin, increased skin moisture (more sebum), increased dermal collagen (fewer wrinkles), accelerated heal-ing, and restoration of youthful muscle that, in total, amount to an age-reversing effect.[1,2] Recall that the oxytocin boost you receive with this yogurt also increases feelings of empathy and that the colonizing effect in the upper GI tract also provides protection against SIBO or SIFO re-currences. If you are pregnant, I recommend not consuming this yogurt as a monoculture but making the *L. reuteri* mixed-culture yogurt from the recipe on page 238, which yields lower bacterial counts.

L. reuteri is the first probiotic species that I fermented. Interestingly, when I first discussed making *L. reuteri* yogurt with the producers of the Gastrus product that provides the original bacteria, they insisted that yogurt could *not* be made with it. When I told them that I had made dozens of batches (at the time; now hundreds) and that the end result was rich and thick, they were shocked. (The difference, of course, is that conventional yogurt making is typically a four-hour process that yields a watery result necessitating the addition of thickening agents, whereas I ferment for thirty-six hours and add prebiotic fiber to increase bacterial counts—no wonder they were surprised.) The Gastrus product contains the two *L. reuteri* strains, DSM 17938 and ATCC PTA 6475, we know are associated with the specific health effects I listed above. The same manufacturer also offers a product called Osfortis that contains only the 6475 strain, but at higher counts (5 billion CFUs per capsule). This sin-gle strain seems to provide most, perhaps all, of the benefits when the two strains are combined. If you use Osfortis as a starter, only one cap-sule is required to ferment to yogurt.

Because oxytocin receptors in the uterus of pregnant human females increase sharply in number in the days leading up to delivery, pregnant women should not consume the full-strength yogurt. A mixed-culture yogurt that restores this missing microbe is a safer way to obtain the ben-efits of *L. reuteri*, a microbe that all humans should have.

Note that, when *L. reuteri* is fermented alone, it prefers to ferment at human body temperature. When combined with other species that have higher temperature "preferences," such as 115°F–122°F of *B. coagulans*, we use a temperature of around 106°F—not the ideal temperature for *B. coagulans*, but below the temp that kills *L. reuteri*, which is 109°F–110°F and higher. After all, life can be about compromise.

10 Gastrus tablets, crushed (or the contents of one capsule of Osfortis)

2 tablespoons prebiotic fiber (inulin or raw potato starch)

1 quart half-and-half or other liquid

Pulverize 10 Gastrus tablets by placing them in a plastic bag and crushing them with a heavy jar, thick drinking glass, or rolling pin. If in capsule form, simply open the capsule and pour into a bowl.

In a medium to large bowl, combine the probiotic, prebiotic fiber, and 2 tablespoons of half-and-half. Make a slurry to ensure the prebiotic fiber does not clump. Stir until well mixed. Stir in the remaining half-and-half. Cover lightly (e.g., with plastic wrap), place in your fermenting device, and ferment at 100°F for 36 hours. To make future batches, use 2 tablespoons of curds or whey from a prior batch.

> *Bacterial source: BioGaia Gastrus tablets (L. reuteri strains DSM 17938, ATCC PTA 6475) or Osfortis capsules (ATCC PTA 6475 strain only). These products are available through Amazon (www .amazon.com) and the US distributor Everidis (www.everidis.com).*

BACILLUS COAGULANS YOGURT

THE GBI-30,6086 STRAIN CAN REDUCE INFLAMMATION, REDUCE ARTHRITIS pain, reduce symptoms associated with irritable bowel syndrome, and accelerate muscle recovery after strenuous exercise.[3,4] *B. coagulans* yields a delicious milder yogurt that is less tart than *L. reuteri* yogurt. In fact, many people who have made yogurt with this strain report that it makes the most delightful and tasty yogurt they have ever had.

1 capsule *Bacillus coagulans* GBI-30,6086
2 tablespoons prebiotic fiber (inulin or raw potato starch)
1 quart half-and-half or other liquid

In a medium to large bowl, combine the contents of one capsule of probiotic, prebiotic fiber, and 2 tablespoons of half-and-half. Make a slurry to ensure the prebiotic fiber does not clump. Stir until well mixed. Stir in the remaining half-and-half. Cover lightly (e.g., with plastic wrap), place in your fermenting device, and ferment at 115°F–122°F for 36 hours. To make future batches, use two tablespoons of curds or whey from a prior batch.

> Bacterial source: The Digestive Advantage product from Schiff is available in many major retail stores and pharmacies. Other sources of B. coagulans do not specify strain and we therefore avoid them.

LACTOBACILLUS GASSERI YOGURT

THE BNR17 STRAIN OF *L. GASSERI* CAN REDUCE WAIST SIZE BY ABOUT ONE INCH when consumed over ninety days even in the absence of any change in diet or exercise.[5] It can also reduce symptoms of irritable bowel syndrome, reduce blood and urinary levels of oxalate, which can lead to kidney stones, and can be instrumental in protecting against SIBO or SIFO recurrences because of its vigorous bacteriocin-producing properties.

1 capsule *L. gasseri* BNR17
2 tablespoons sugar (sucrose) or prebiotic fiber (raw potato starch)
1 quart half-and-half or other liquid

In a medium to large bowl, combine the contents of one capsule of probiotic, the sugar, and 2 tablespoons of half-and-half. Make a slurry to ensure the sugar dissolves and the prebiotic fiber does not clump. Stir until well mixed. Stir in the remaining half-and-half. Cover lightly (e.g., with plastic wrap), place in your fermenting device, and ferment at 109°F for 36 hours. To make future batches, use two tablespoons of curds or whey from a prior batch.

Bacterial source: L. gasseri BNR17 has just recently become available from a US source, Mercola Market: www.mercolamarket.com

Look for a product called "Biothin Probiotic" with 10 billion CFUs per capsule. Use a single capsule to start your yogurt.

LACTOBACILLUS CASEI SHIROTA YOGURT

THIS STRAIN OF THE SPECIES PROVIDES UNIQUE IMMUNE SYSTEM–BOOSTING EF-fects, particularly effective against viral respiratory illnesses.[6] Three human clinical trials demonstrate that intake of this microbe at 100 billion CFUs per day reduces the potential for viral illnesses by 50 percent and, should you develop a viral illness, abbreviates the illness by 50 percent. Because this effect appears to require high bacterial counts and the commercial source of the bacterial strain provides only 6.5 billion CFUs per bottle (sold as a product called Yakult), our prolonged fermentation with added prebiotic fibers provides the higher numbers for this effect. (The sugar and skim milk contents of the original product are lost with fermentation.)

1 2-ounce bottle Yakult
2 tablespoons prebiotic fiber (inulin or raw potato starch)
1 quart half-and-half or other liquid

In a medium to large bowl, combine the Yakult, prebiotic fiber, and 2 tablespoons of half-and-half. Make a slurry to ensure the prebiotic fiber does not clump. Stir until well mixed. Stir in the remaining half-and-half. Cover lightly (e.g., with plastic wrap), place in your fermenting device, and ferment at 109°F for 36 hours.

Bacterial source: Yakult

You can find the Yakult product at Walmart, at Meijer, in Asian grocery stores, and at several other major retailers in the refrigerated dairy section next to the yogurts and kefirs. The manufacturer provides a store locator on its website: www.yakultusa.com.

BIFIDOBACTERIUM INFANTIS YOGURT

B. INFANTIS IS A SPECIES THAT HAS BEEN LOST BY MANY MOTHERS, WHO THEREBY cannot pass it on to their newborn babies, which puts infants at a disadvantage for growth and long-term health. When this species is restored in infants as a probiotic, they have fewer bowel movements (fewer diaper changes), less colic, less eczema, less diaper rash, better sleep, and less risk for asthma, type 1 diabetes, and other autoimmune disorders later in childhood.[7]

However, instead of dosing an infant with a probiotic, I advocate a better strategy: Make yogurt with the EVC001 strain of this species that *the pregnant mother can consume* and thereby pass *B. infantis* on to the newborn with passage through the birth canal or through breastfeeding. This may provide advantage in that moms can deliver this species in the context of a broader microbiome made more diverse by restoration of *B. infantis* prior to delivery. It also saves money because the yogurt can be propagated over and over again starting with a single sachet. (The Evivo product source of this microbe comes in a sachet rather than a capsule.) The probiotic can also be given to the baby, of course, to ensure that the microbe is present.

Because this microbe is somewhat slow growing, we extend fermentation time to between 36 and 40 hours. Also, *B. infantis* is unable to metabolize inulin and will not ferment as vigorously when inulin is used as the prebiotic fiber, so choose raw potato starch or sucrose as your microbe feed.

> 1 envelope Evivo *B. infantis* EVC001 (8 billion CFUs)
> 2 tablespoons sugar (sucrose) or prebiotic fiber (raw potato starch)
> 1 quart half-and-half or other liquid
>
> In a medium to large bowl, combine the contents of one envelope of Evivo, the sugar, and 2 tablespoons of half-and-half. Make a slurry to ensure the sugar dissolves or the prebiotic fiber does not clump. Stir until well mixed. Stir in the remaining half-and-half. Cover lightly (e.g., with plastic wrap), place in your fermenting device, and

ferment at 100°F for 36–40 hours. To make future batches, use 2 tablespoons of curds or whey from a prior batch.

Bacterial source: Evivo

Obtain from the manufacturer: evivo.com

LACTOBACILLUS HELVETICUS AND *BIFIDOBACTERIUM LONGUM* YOGURT

THIS COMBINATION OF SPECIES HAS BEEN SHOWN TO REDUCE ANXIETY AND LIFT mood, contributing to a reversal of depression.[8] Once again, we put our microbes to work with prolonged fermentation and prebiotic fibers to ob-tain greater bacterial numbers for bigger and faster effects. This combina-tion may propagate a little more slowly than other species, so we ferment at 100°F for 36 to 40 hours. Not everyone experiences the lift in mood, but those who do can experience marked effects.

1 capsule Mood Probiotic
2 tablespoons sugar (sucrose) or prebiotic fiber (raw potato
    starch)
1 quart half-and-half or other liquid

In a medium to large bowl, empty the contents of one capsule; add the sugar and 2 tablespoons of half-and-half. Make a slurry to ensure the sugar dissolves or the prebiotic fiber does not clump. Stir until well mixed. Stir in the remaining half-and-half. Cover lightly (e.g., with plastic wrap), place in your fermenting device, and ferment at 100°F for 36–40 hours. To make future batches, use 2 tablespoons of curds or whey from a prior batch.

Bacterial source: InnovixLabs Mood Probiotic or Life Extension Florassist Mood Improve

Obtain from the manufacturer: InnovixLabs.com

Also available from Life Extension: www.lifeextension.com

MIXED-CULTURE *L. REUTERI* YOGURT

THIS IS HOW TO MAKE YOGURT FOR CHILDREN OR PREGNANT MOTHERS IN WHOM we don't want to boost oxytocin to high levels. We ferment *L. reuteri* with other species. Everyone should enjoy the health benefits of *L. reuteri* intestinal colonization, and we should have received it at birth from our mothers, but if that did not happen, a mixed-culture yogurt like this one can restore this species in a gentler way for children and pregnant women. This keystone species has the ability to colonize the upper GI tract and enhances healing and boosts oxytocin levels so that we can enjoy feelings of greater empathy.

We start with either 2 tablespoons of *L. reuteri* yogurt from a prior batch or 10 crushed tablets of *L. reuteri* probiotic. We then combine that with 2 tablespoons of any store-bought yogurt that contains live cultures or a starting culture you purchased. The Oui brand of yogurt is the simplest, containing only *Lactobacillus bulgaricus* and *Streptococcus thermophilus*. Culturing these two species with *L. reuteri* yields an absolutely delicious, nontart end result that even kids will enjoy. Other yogurt brands include additional strains. Different bacterial mixtures can yield subtle differences in flavor. Alternatively, you can make a mixed-culture yogurt by ferment-ing *L. reuteri* in combination with 2 tablespoons of one or more of the other yogurts you have fermented or their starter preparation (e.g., one capsule of *B. coagulans* or *B. infantis*).

> 2 tablespoons *L. reuteri* yogurt or 10 crushed Gastrus tablets
> 2 tablespoons live-culture store-bought yogurt or 2 tablespoons
>   of each of your other yogurts or 1 capsule of each starting
>   microbe
> 2 tablespoons prebiotic fiber (inulin or raw potato starch)
> 1 quart half-and-half or other liquid

In a medium to large bowl, combine 2 tablespoons of a prior batch of *L. reuteri* yogurt, 2 tablespoons each of other live-culture yo-gurts (or capsules), prebiotic fiber, and 2 tablespoons of half-and-half. Make a slurry to ensure the prebiotic fiber does not clump. Stir until well mixed. Stir in the remaining half-and-half. Cover lightly (e.g., with plastic wrap), place in your fermenting device, and ferment at 106°F for 36 hours. To make future batches, use 2 tablespoons of curds or whey from a prior batch.

HIGH-POTENCY PROBIOTIC YOGURT

THIS IS HOW TO CREATE A HIGH-POTENCY PROBIOTIC YOGURT STARTING WITH either a commercial probiotic or a commercial kefir that saves you money while providing super-duper-high bacterial counts with all the benefits of commercially produced high-potency probiotics. I paid around $4 for each of the commercial kefirs I used. A couple tablespoons of store-bought kefir can yield months and months of probiotic, saving you a lot of money on costly commercial probiotics.

Start with either a capsule of probiotic with at least 2 billion CFUs of one or more species or 2 tablespoons of a commercial kefir, which typically contain ten or more species. You can also combine different brands of kefir that include different bacterial species to increase the number of fermenting species.

1 capsule probiotic or 2 tablespoons of kefir (if combining kefirs,
     use 2 tablespoons of each product)
2 tablespoons sugar (sucrose) or prebiotic fiber (inulin or raw
     potato starch)
1 quart half-and-half or other liquid

In a medium-sized bowl, combine the contents of the probiotic capsule with the sugar and 2 tablespoons of organic half-and-half. Make a slurry to ensure the sugar dissolves or the prebiotic fiber does not clump. Stir until well mixed. Stir in the remaining half-and-half. Cover lightly (e.g., with plastic wrap), place in your fermenting device, and ferment at 106°F for 36 hours. To make future batches, use 2 tablespoons of curds or whey from a prior batch.

The end result will be thicker than the original kefir, given the prolonged fermentation time, more like yogurt in consistency and no longer the thin, drinkable liquid of regular kefir.

SUPER GUT SIBO YOGURT

MY TEAM AND I ARE EXPLORING WHETHER A CAREFULLY CURATED COLLECTION of probiotic species and strains, chosen for their positive effects against pathogenic species (H_2- and possibly methane-producing varieties), can be used to push back SIBO. Choosing species and strains capable of colonizing the upper GI tract and producing bacteriocins, for instance, make these species more likely to be successful in thwarting SIBO species. And we can now track success or failure by monitoring breath gases after the prebiotic fiber challenge. Even though our experience with curated yogurts is preliminary, I share this benign strategy with you in case you are nervous about making the leap to using herbal or conventional antibiotics against your SIBO-related symptoms because a growing number of people have had success with this route.

Rather than fermenting three different species separately, for Super Gut SIBO Yogurt we ferment all three together to generate our potentially anti-SIBO mix of probiotic species. This process limits the resulting microbial counts of *L. gasseri*, which preliminary experience suggests is quite potent, so that we do not induce an excessive die-off reaction too quickly.

To start this ferment, you can use the raw probiotic products or 1–2 tablespoons of yogurt made with each individual species or a couple of tablespoons that you saved from a prior batch of this mixed yogurt.

> 10 BioGaia Gastrus tablets, crushed (total 2 billion CFUs), or 2
>   tablespoons of *L. reuteri* yogurt (curds and/or whey)
> 1 capsule *Lactobacillus gasseri* BNR17 (10 billion CFUs), or
>   2 tablespoons of *L. gasseri* yogurt (curds and/or whey)
> 1 capsule *Bacillus coagulans* GBI-30,6086 (2 billion CFUs), or 2
>   tablespoons of *B. coagulans* yogurt (curds and/or whey)
> 2 tablespoons prebiotic fiber (inulin or raw potato starch)
> 1 quart half-and-half or other liquid
>
> In a medium-sized bowl, combine the starting probiotics, prebiotic fiber, and 2 tablespoons of organic half-and-half. Make a slurry to ensure the prebiotic fiber does not clump. Stir until well mixed.

Stir in the remaining half-and-half. Cover lightly (e.g., with plastic wrap), place in your fermenting device, and ferment at 106°F for 36 hours. To make future batches, use 2 tablespoons of curds or whey from a prior batch.

WHAT CAN WE FERMENT BESIDES DAIRY?

The extended fermentation method we use for our yogurts minimizes the problematic components of dairy products, reducing, for instance, lactose to lactic acid and denaturing casein in the resulting low-pH product. Even so, many people are interested in either minimizing or avoiding dairy products altogether. Thankfully, a number of other foods are suitable for fermentation.

Some starting foods are rich in sugar, such as mangos and bananas, but bacteria consume sugar in the process of fermentation, especially during the prolonged fermentation times of 48–72 hours that I suggest (longer than for dairy). Long fermentation times not only reduce sugar content dramatically but also increase bacterial populations exponentially.

You can purchase many of the starting products prepared or you can make them yourself. Fermenting salsa, for instance, can begin with either store-bought salsa or a salsa you made yourself in your food processor or food chopper. If you choose to start with store-bought products, be sure to choose products that contain no preservatives, emulsifiers, or other undesirable ingredients because these additives not only are not good for you but also can block or alter the fermentation process.

As with dairy fermentation, choose which bacterial species to use depending on the effect you desire, e.g., *Bacillus coagulans* probiotic capsules or some whey from a prior batch of yogurt to start the process.

COCONUT MILK

CHOOSE A CANNED COCONUT MILK (NEVER THE THINNER PRODUCTS IN CARtons) that contains nothing but coconut and water, with no thickeners or mixing agents such as xanthan gum or gellan gum—guar gum is okay, however—because these additives provoke separation upon fermentation. Because coconut milk (sometimes called coconut cream) has the tendency to separate into water and oil, several additional steps are required to obtain a uniform end result. Unlike dairy, which we do not preheat (if it's already pasteurized or ultra-pasteurized), we do preheat coconut milk. The key is to use the prebiotic fiber and the thickener guar gum to keep the milk from separating. Don't let the use of sugar in this recipe alarm you—the microbes consume the sugar and there should be little to none left after fermentation.

Following is the recipe for making coconut milk yogurt with *L. reuteri* as an illustration of the process; if you choose another species or a mixed culture, use the same temperature settings as specified in the dairy-based yogurt recipes for the included strains. Also, be sure to ferment coconut milk yogurt for 48 hours to obtain a thicker, richer end result.

Note that the blending step *precedes* addition of the bacteria because the blending process can kill microbes. We therefore add microbes as the last step before fermentation.

MAKES 2 SERVINGS

1 (13.5-ounce) can coconut milk
¾ teaspoon guar gum
2 tablespoons sugar
1 tablespoon raw potato starch
1–2 tablespoons *L. reuteri* yogurt, curds and/or whey, or
    10 Gastrus tablets, crushed

In a small or medium-sized saucepan, heat coconut milk over medium heat to 180°F or until it just begins to boil; remove from heat. Allow to cool 5 minutes.

Add guar gum, sugar, and potato starch to the cooled coconut milk and blend with a stick blender or pour these ingredients into a blender; blend for a minimum of 1 minute or until the mixture thickens to the approximate thickness of heavy cream.

Allow the mixture to cool to 100°F (or room temperature), then mix in the *L. reuteri* yogurt. Ferment for 48 hours at 100°F.

HUMMUS

CHICKPEAS WITH TAHINI (FROM SESAME SEEDS) PUREED INTO HUMMUS MAKES A wonderful vehicle for fermentation. The end result tastes a bit different from the original unfermented hummus, with a cheesy scent and flavor. It therefore makes a tasty spread for sandwiches or a dip for jicama and other vegetables.

> I find it necessary to dilute hummus by half with water before fermentation: add a half cup of water for every cup of hummus. Ferment for 48 hours. Follow the same temperature settings used in the dairy-based recipes, which vary with the microbe you choose.

SALSA

SALSA DEVELOPS A LIGHT EFFERVESCENCE WHEN FERMENTED. SALSA VERDE also ferments nicely. Ferment for 48–72 hours. Follow the same temperature settings used in the dairy-based recipes, which vary with the microbe you choose.

PUREED FRUITS, SWEET POTATOES

STRAWBERRIES, BLUEBERRIES, RASPBERRIES, BLACKBERRIES, BANANAS, MANgoes, and peaches are among the fruits that you can puree and put to work fermenting with chosen microbial species. You can also purchase fruits that are already pureed, but choose products without added sugar because the naturally occurring sugar in fruit is more than enough to support fermentation.

Ferment purees for at least 72 hours to maximally reduce sugar. You can also ferment baby foods such as pureed carrots, an excellent vehicle for fermenting with the *Bifidobacterium infantis* EVC001 strain, which provides so many benefits to babies, as discussed in the yogurt recipe for this microbe. Pureed sweet potatoes are also an especially fermentation-friendly food. Follow the same temperature settings used in the dairy-based recipes, which vary with the microbe you choose.

BEVERAGES AND SMOOTHIES

STRAWBERRY, CARROT, AND
DANDELION GREENS PREBIOTIC SMOOTHIE

THE BANANA, DANDELION GREENS, AND CARROT IN THIS TASTY SMOOTHIE ADD to your daily intake of prebiotic fiber. You can, of course, obtain even more prebiotic fiber by adding a teaspoon of inulin or acacia fiber.

MAKES 1 SMOOTHIE

1 medium green banana or 1 medium raw peeled white potato
1 cup fresh dandelion greens
1 medium carrot, coarsely sliced
½ cup strawberries, fresh or frozen
1 cup water
Sweetener equivalent to 1 tablespoon sugar
1 teaspoon of powdered inulin or acacia fiber (optional)

If using green banana, skin and chop it coarsely. It is easy to use a knife to cut the skin lengthwise, then scoop out the pulp. If using potato, chop it coarsely. Place the banana in a blender followed by the dandelion greens, carrot, strawberries, water, sweetener, and optional prebiotic fiber. Blend until well mixed and the banana has been liquefied. Serve immediately.

MATCHA STRAWBERRY KEY LIME SMOOTHIE

MATCHA GREEN TEA IS NOT THE USUAL TEA MADE BY STEEPING GREEN TEA LEAVES in water but is the leaves themselves, finely ground, which dissolve into the water. Since you consume the actual leaves, matcha is therefore a highly concentrated source of green tea polyphenols, which cross-link the proteins in the intestinal mucus barrier, especially helpful for anyone who has been diagnosed with any intestinal inflammatory disorder. You don't have to have ulcerative colitis, of course, to enjoy this smoothie, which provides other health benefits from green tea catechins, such as modest weight loss. And, of course, don't sweat the carbs from the banana because a green, unripe banana has zero carbs but plenty of prebiotic fiber.

MAKES 1 SERVING

1 cup water
2 tablespoons key lime juice (bottled or fresh-squeezed)
1 green, unripe banana, coarsely chopped
Sweetener equivalent to 1 tablespoon sugar
3–4 strawberries, fresh or frozen
1 teaspoon matcha green tea powder
1 teaspoon of powdered inulin or acacia fiber (optional)

In a blender, combine water, key lime juice, banana, sweetener, strawberries, matcha powder, and optional prebiotic fiber and blend until well mixed. Serve as is or on ice.

GINGER SNAP SMOOTHIE

HERE IS AN OPTION FOR OBTAINING THE ESSENTIAL OILS WE USE TO REDUCE intestinal fungal populations disguised as a Ginger Snap Smoothie. Recall that when you are just starting out using essential oils, you start with minimal quantities of the cinnamon and clove oils, no more than 1–2 drops of each. You can increase to a maximum of 5–6 drops over several weeks.

1 cup water
1 teaspoon ground cinnamon

½ teaspoon ground ginger
1–2 drops cinnamon bark essential oil
1–2 drops clove essential oil
½ teaspoon ground nutmeg
1 green, unripe banana, coarsely chopped
Sweetener equivalent to 1 tablespoon sugar
1 teaspoon of powdered inulin or acacia fiber (optional)

In a blender, combine water, cinnamon, ginger, cinnamon bark and clove oils, nutmeg, banana, sweetener, and optional additional prebiotic fiber and blend until well mixed.

CLOVE GREEN TEA

HERE'S A MUCUS-BUILDING POWERHOUSE OF A RECIPE, SO SIMPLE YET PACKING several intestinal health advantages into a simple cup of tea. Use this tea to help repair, rebuild, or maintain your intestinal mucus barrier and as part of your dysbiosis/SIBO/SIFO management program because it may make the journey smoother. This tea combines the mucus-increasing effect of eugenol oil from cloves, the mucus protein cross-linking effect of green tea catechins, and the *Akkermansia* growth-stimulating effects of fructooligosaccharides (FOS).

Whole cloves, rather than ground cloves, work best in this tea. Ground cloves include too many solids that cannot be separated from the eugenol, so if you filter the tea, you are removing much of the beneficial eugenol.

Whole cloves, on the other hand, retain their ingredients well, so I have found that you can reuse whole cloves three or four times without sacrificing quality.

Choose a green tea, preferably organic, that is high in green tea catechin content for maximum benefit. Matcha teas are high, as is tea brewed from Trader Joe's Organic Green Tea, Pique Tea Crystals, Newman's Own Organic Green Tea, and Numi Organic Gunpowder Green Tea.

Optionally, you can sweeten the tea with allulose, which has the properties of prebiotic fiber. (FOS and allulose both readily dissolve in tea, unlike some other powdered prebiotics.)

For added flavor, add a cinnamon stick to the tea upon serving.

MAKES 2 SERVINGS

2 cups water
1 tablespoon whole cloves
1 teabag green tea
1 teaspoon FOS powder
2 teaspoons allulose (optional)
Additional sweetener to taste
1 cinnamon stick (optional)

In a small saucepan, combine the water and cloves and bring to a boil. Reduce the heat and cover to maintain a low simmer for 10 minutes.

Add the teabag in the last 1–2 minutes of simmering, then remove from heat. Discard teabag.

Stir in the FOS, optional allulose, other sweetener, and optional cinnamon stick, and serve or sip throughout the day.

MATCHA, MINT, AND BLUEBERRY FROZEN SMOOTHIE

HERE'S ANOTHER WAY TO PUT YOUR YOGURTS TO WORK WHILE YOU OBTAIN THE mucus-strengthening effect of green tea catechins, especially potent in matcha green tea. Blueberry flavonoids add further to the benefits of this smoothie by boosting *Akkermansia*. We achieve all this while enjoying a drinkable frozen smoothie that, of course, does not rely on emulsifiers that wreak havoc on intestinal health.

In this recipe, we minimize the use of a mechanical blender because forceful agitation kills probiotic microbes. Once you have added the yogurt to the mix, pulse the blender as little as possible, just enough to mix the ingredients.

Choose the yogurt that provides the effects you desire, for example, *L. helveticus* and *B. longum* to boost mood or reduce anxiety, or *L. reuteri* to increase empathy and smooth skin. Whereas probiotic species are killed by excessive heat, they survive just fine in the freezer.

MAKES 2 SERVINGS

1 teaspoon matcha tea powder
7–8 mint leaves, coarsely chopped, or ½ teaspoon mint extract
1 cup fresh or frozen blueberries
½ cup cold water
Sweetener equivalent to 1½ tablespoons sugar
1 teaspoon inulin/FOS, acacia powder, or other prebiotic
    powder (optional)
1½ cups your choice of yogurt

In a blender, combine matcha tea, mint, blueberries, water, sweetener, and optional prebiotic fiber and blend until mixed. Use a spatula or spoon to release any frozen material from the sides of the blender.

Add yogurt and pulse briefly, just enough to mix all ingredients. If the smoothie is too thin, allow it to set in the freezer for 20–30 minutes before serving.

MOCHA MINT KEFIR

You'll love this Mocha Mint Kefir—it's almost like drinking melted ice cream. Kefirs are among the richest sources of microbial species. Despite the lack of information on which strains are included, adding kefir with its multiple species can still be a helpful part of your microbiome-building program.

Use either commercial kefir or a kefir you made yourself using a commercial kefir or kefir starter.

MAKES 2 SERVINGS

2 cups kefir
1 teaspoon instant coffee granules
1 tablespoon unsweetened cocoa powder
½ teaspoon mint extract
Sweetener equivalent to 1 tablespoon sugar

In a shaker, combine kefir, coffee, cocoa, mint, and sweetener and shake vigorously until well mixed. Serve cold or at room temperature.

GINGERBREAD COFFEE

HERE IS A WAY TO ENJOY COFFEE THAT WARMS YOUR INSIDES ON AN AUTUMN or winter morning while providing the potent mucus-increasing effects of cloves and the modest positive microbiome effects of cinnamon and ginger. If you are embarking on a SIFO-eradicating effort, this is a good opportunity to add 1–2 drops of cinnamon bark oil and/or a drop of clove oil.

MAKES 2 SERVINGS

1 teaspoon ground cinnamon
½ teaspoon ground cloves
Dash ground nutmeg
½ teaspoon ground ginger
1 teaspoon instant coffee granules
Sweetener equivalent to 1 tablespoon sugar or to taste
16 ounces boiling water

In a small to medium-sized saucepan, combine cinnamon, cloves, nutmeg, ginger, coffee, sweetener, and water. Bring to boil, then divide into two coffee mugs.

You may need to stir occasionally during consumption to keep the nondissolvable components suspended.

RASPBERRY LIME YOGURT
SMOOTHIE FOR SMOOTHER SKIN

HERE'S A WAY TO PUT YOUR *L. REUTERI* YOGURT COMBINED WITH COLLAGEN hydrolysates to work for smoother skin.

MAKES 1 SERVING

1 cup raspberries
7–8 mint leaves, coarsely chopped, or ½ teaspoon mint extract

1 tablespoon collagen hydrolysates
½ cup water
Sweetener equivalent to 1 tablespoon sugar
1 cup *L. reuteri* yogurt

In a blender, combine raspberries, mint, collagen, water, and sweetener and blend until pureed. Add the yogurt and pulse very briefly, just enough to mix, or use a spoon to mix in the yogurt. Serve immediately.

SMALL DISHES, SIDE DISHES, AND CONDIMENTS

SUPER GUT TZATZIKI

THIS TRADITIONAL GREEK AND MIDDLE EASTERN DISH CAN BE USED AS A SAUCE or a dip or to liven up lamb, kabobs, roasted veggies, or souvlaki for an authentic Greek experience.

Our version of tzatziki comes with added benefits, depending on which yogurt you include. If you choose to make this recipe with *L. gasseri* yogurt, for instance, you may enjoy reduced stress and a reduction in waist size while also increasing healthy *Akkermansia* populations with the olive oil and garlic. Tzatziki is best consumed within 72 hours.

MAKES ABOUT 3½ CUPS

1 medium cucumber
2 cups homemade yogurt (your choice of variety)
4 tablespoons extra-virgin olive oil
3 cloves garlic, minced or crushed
2 tablespoons lemon juice, freshly squeezed or bottled
2 tablespoons dill or mint, chopped
½ teaspoon sea salt

Grate or chop the cucumber into a colander that is set in a large bowl. Allow to sit for 30 minutes, stirring occasionally, to release water.

Meanwhile, in a medium bowl, combine yogurt, olive oil, garlic, lemon juice, dill, and salt. After the cucumber is drained, stir it in and mix thoroughly.

MOROCCAN ROASTED VEGETABLES

HERE'S A FRAGRANT MIX OF VEGETABLES AND SPICES THAT CAN SERVE AS A MAIN dish or side dish.

The onion, turnip, and garlic add a few grams of prebiotic fiber while the mushrooms provide prebiotic-like polysaccharides. Turmeric benefits the intestinal lining, and eggplant and cumin contribute polyphenols.

MAKES 6 SERVINGS

1 eggplant, sliced and quartered
1 large onion (yellow, white, or red), halved and sliced
1 turnip, sliced
8 ounces white button mushrooms, halved
½ cup extra-virgin olive oil
2 tablespoons garlic paste
1 teaspoon ground turmeric
1 teaspoon ground cumin
1 teaspoon ground cinnamon
1 teaspoon onion powder
Sea salt to taste

Preheat oven to 375°F.

On a large baking sheet, combine the eggplant, onion, turnip, and mushrooms. Drizzle olive oil over the vegetables, then mix in the garlic paste. Sprinkle on turmeric, cumin, cinnamon, onion powder, and salt. Toss the mixture to mix the ingredients well.

Roast for 30 minutes.

HERBED FOCACCIA BREAD

Here's an old favorite among readers of my Wheat Belly books and cookbooks, a fragrant, delicious, and virtually foolproof focaccia-style flatbread that we make with almond flour. I've tweaked the recipe to include a greater quantity of herbs for their bowel flora benefits.

You can use this flatbread as a sandwich bread, but my favorite way to eat it is to simply dip it into a high-quality extra-virgin olive oil seasoned with coarse salt.

MAKES 6 FLATBREADS

1 cup shredded mozzarella or other cheese
3 cups almond meal/flour
¼ cup ground psyllium seed
1½ teaspoons sea salt or kosher salt, divided
1 teaspoon onion powder
1 tablespoon garlic paste or 5 cloves garlic, minced
1 tablespoon rosemary, chopped, or 1½ teaspoons dried rosemary
1 tablespoon oregano, chopped (stems removed), or 1½ teaspoons
    dried oregano
½ cup black or kalamata olives, diced
¼ cup sun-dried tomatoes (preferably in oil, or as dried and
    presoftened in hot water), diced
2 large eggs
½ cup extra-virgin olive oil, divided

Preheat oven to 375°F.

In medium bowl, combine cheese, almond meal/flour, psyllium, ½ teaspoon salt, onion powder, garlic, rosemary, oregano, olives, and sun-dried tomatoes and mix well. Set aside.

In a small bowl, whisk the eggs, then stir in all but 1 tablespoon of olive oil. Pour the egg mixture into the almond meal/flour mixture and mix thoroughly.

Grease an 11x17-inch shallow baking pan. Place the dough onto the pan and shape it into a large rectangle by hand or by covering with parchment paper and using a roller or other flat cylindrical object to achieve a ½-inch thickness. Dough may not fill the entire pan.

Bake for 12 minutes. Remove from the oven. Use the blunt handle of a spoon or other small rounded instrument to make small depressions in the surface of the dough every inch or so. Brush the surface with the remaining olive oil and sprinkle with sea salt or kosher salt. Return the pan to the oven for an additional 8–10 minutes until the flatbread is lightly browned.

Use a pizza cutter to slice the flatbread into six pieces. Remove slices from the pan carefully using a pancake flipper.

HOT CHILI FRIES

SOME PEOPLE MISS FRENCH FRIES. SLICED TURNIPS ACTUALLY MAKE A PRETTY good substitute.

Here's a way to combine prebiotic fiber–rich, low-carb turnips in a baked version of fries that you can spice up by dipping in a hot chili sauce for the microbiome-molding benefits of capsaicin. You can further boost capsaicin content by adding your choice of chili pepper to the dry mix. (I used ancho chili powder made from poblano peppers. If you're using a very hot pepper, such as cayenne, cut back to taste, for example, use only a ¼–½ teaspoon.)

MAKES 2 SERVINGS

FRIES:
    2 teaspoons sea salt
    1 tablespoon onion powder
    2 teaspoons dried chili pepper powder (e.g., ancho chili powder)
    2 tablespoons grated Parmesan cheese
    ¼ cup extra-virgin olive oil
    2 turnips, sliced into ¼- to ½-inch-thick pieces

SAUCE:
    2 tablespoons hot chili sauce
    1 tablespoon melted butter

Preheat oven to 425°F. Line a large baking sheet with parchment paper.

In a large bowl, combine salt, onion powder, chili pepper powder, and Parmesan cheese and mix together. Pour in olive oil and mix.

Add sliced turnips to the mixture and toss to coat thoroughly.

Spread the turnip slices one-layer deep on the lined baking sheet. Bake for 35–40 minutes or until fries are slightly crispy.

In a small bowl, combine chili sauce with butter and mix.

CURRIED CAULIFLOWER WITH PEAS

MANY PEOPLE WHO LIMIT THEIR CARBS AVOID PEAS, BUT PEAS ARE NOT TOO TER-ribly high in carbs, with 14 grams net carbs per cup, while they provide 3–5 grams of prebiotic fiber. The galactooligosaccharide and amylose prebiotic fibers in peas add to your daily intake, along with the modest contributions made by the cauliflower and onion. The turmeric in the curry powder provides intestinal healing effects.

MAKES 4 SERVINGS

3 tablespoons butter
1 medium onion, chopped
4 cups riced cauliflower
1 cup frozen peas
1 (13.5-ounce) can coconut milk
2 tablespoons curry powder
Sea salt and black pepper to taste
¼ cup cilantro, chopped (optional)

In a large skillet over medium-high heat, melt the butter, then add the onion, cauliflower, and peas, stirring frequently until the onion is translucent and the cauliflower is tender, for 5–7 minutes.

Stir in the coconut milk, curry powder, salt, and pepper. Simmer for another two minutes, then remove from heat. Serve topped with cilantro.

CREAM OF MUSHROOM SOUP

YOU'LL LOVE THE EARTHY MIX OF FLAVORS IN THIS VERSION OF AN OLD-TIME favorite, tweaked to offer more prebiotic fiber and microbiome-balancing benefit. For you cilantro fans, this soup is a perfect match for the herb, which has modest antifungal properties.

Choose portabella or cremini mushrooms rather than white buttons for a slightly deeper flavor.

MAKES 8 SERVINGS

¼ cup extra-virgin olive oil or butter
1 onion, chopped
1 leek, white stem, halved and sliced
4 cloves garlic, minced
16 ounces white button mushrooms (or portabella or cremini),
    sliced
1 teaspoon ground turmeric
1 teaspoon ground cumin
1 tablespoon fresh thyme, stems removed and finely chopped,
    or ½ tablespoon dried thyme
1 teaspoon sea salt or to taste
½ teaspoon ground black pepper
1 (13.5-ounce) can coconut milk
4 cups chicken or vegetable stock
¼ cup cilantro, chopped (optional)

In a large skillet over medium-high heat, cook oil, onion, leeks, and garlic until the onion is translucent, about 3 minutes.

Stir in the mushrooms, and stir occasionally until softened, about 5 minutes.

Stir in turmeric, cumin, thyme, salt, and pepper. Add coconut milk and stock. Bring to a slow boil, then reduce the heat, cover, and simmer for 3 minutes. Remove from heat.

Ladle the mixture into a blender and blend until smooth (in batches, if necessary). Serve with cilantro sprinkled over top (optional).

FERMENTED ROASTED PEPPERS

ROASTED PEPPERS ARE TASTY TO BEGIN WITH. HERE IS HOW TO INCREASE THEIR tastiness while using them as a vehicle for fermenting your choice of probiotic microbe. You could begin with store-bought roasted peppers, but beware of those that contain preservatives, which have antibacterial properties. For this reason, you will have better luck roasting the peppers yourself for this recipe.

You will find that peppers are among the easiest vegetables to ferment because, unlike many other veggies, peppers sink to the bottom of the brine, obviating the need for a weight to keep them submerged.

Choose your microbe for the effect you desire, such as *B. longum* for reduction of anxiety or *Bacillus coagulans* for accelerated recovery after strenuous exercise or *L. reuteri* for youthful skin and muscle tone. You can begin with the contents of a probiotic capsule or whey from a batch of homemade yogurt.

MAKES APPROXIMATELY 4 CUPS

4 bell peppers (any color)
1 quart filtered or distilled water
1 tablespoon noniodized salt
1 tablespoon peppercorns
1 tablespoon whole coriander seeds
1 bay leaf
¼ cup white wine vinegar
Microbe of your choice from a probiotic capsule or 1 tablespoon
    of whey from your choice of yogurt

Preheat oven to 400°F.

Place the whole peppers on a baking sheet and roast for 15 minutes. Turn peppers and roast for an additional 15 minutes. Remove the peppers from the oven and allow to cool. Remove the seeds and stems, gently rub off the charred skins, then slice the peppers into strips.

In a jar you use for fermentation, combine water, salt, peppercorns, coriander, and bay leaf. Add the peppers, ensuring they are covered by the liquid, and your choice of microbe, and ferment for a minimum of 72 hours in your fermentation device to maintain the temperature appropriate for the microbe included. If your fermentation vessel is too large for your fermentation device, you can divide into several smaller containers. (See the yogurt recipes earlier in this chapter for the temperature appropriate for each species.)

After fermentation, add ¼ cup vinegar, then refrigerate. Peppers will keep for at least 4 weeks in the refrigerator.

ROSEMARY TURNIPS

BEFORE YOU TURN YOUR NOSE UP AT THE THOUGHT OF EATING TURNIPS, GIVE this tasty and healthier modification of Rosemary Potatoes a try. Turnips are much lower in carbohydrates than potatoes, thereby not adding to your waistline like baked potatoes do. They're also a great vehicle for the microbiome benefits of rosemary and olive oil with a little onion thrown in.

MAKES 4 SERVINGS

2 pounds turnips, cut into ½-inch cubes
¼ cup extra-virgin olive oil
1 tablespoon fresh rosemary, finely chopped, or 1½ teaspoons
    dried rosemary
1 teaspoon sea salt
1 teaspoon onion powder
½ teaspoon ground black pepper

Preheat oven to 400°F.

In a large bowl, combine cubed turnips, olive oil, rosemary, salt, onion powder, and black pepper, and toss to mix thoroughly.

Spread the mixture on a baking sheet and roast for 40 minutes or until lightly browned.

DANDELION GREENS AND RAW POTATO SALAD WITH AVOCADO LIME DRESSING

THIS RECIPE PACKS A LOT OF HEALTH BENEFITS INTO A SIMPLE SALAD: PREBIOTIC fiber from dandelion greens, raw potato, onion, and garlic; polysaccharide prebiotics from mushrooms; pectin fiber from avocado; and the antibacterial effects of cilantro. The Avocado Lime Dressing is best consumed within 48 hours of preparation.

MAKES 4 SERVINGS AS MAIN DISH OR 6 AS A SIDE; MAKES APPROXIMATELY 2 CUPS

SALAD:

8 ounces dandelion greens
1 medium raw white potato, quartered and thinly sliced
1 red onion, halved and thinly sliced
4 ounces white button mushrooms, sliced
4 hard-boiled eggs, sliced
5–6 strips bacon, cooked, drained, and broken or chopped into pieces

In a large bowl, combine the dandelion greens, potato, onion, mushrooms, eggs, and bacon. Toss and top with dressing (below).

AVOCADO LIME DRESSING:

2 medium avocados, pitted, skin removed
½ cup extra-virgin olive oil
¼ cup white wine vinegar
¼ cup fresh cilantro, coarsely chopped
1 clove garlic, minced, or 1 teaspoon dried garlic powder
Juice of one small lime
½ teaspoon salt
Sweetener equivalent to 1 tablespoon sugar
¾ cup water

In a blender or food processor, combine the avocado, oil, vinegar, cilantro, garlic, lime juice, salt, sweetener, and water. Blend or process until uniformly mixed. Use immediately or store in an airtight container in the refrigerator.

SPICY GARLIC PICKLES

THIS SIMPLE PICKLE RECIPE ILLUSTRATES HOW TO FERMENT VEGETABLES. AL-though you can begin the fermentation process by adding a teaspoon of whey recovered from one of your yogurt recipes, in this recipe we put to work the microbes that naturally populate the outer surface of the veg-etable. The key is to keep the veggies submerged beneath the surface of the liquid, out of the air.

These pickles require two or more weeks for full fermentation. You can judge when they are done by tasting: fully fermented pickles should be modestly tart.

6 cloves garlic, sliced in half
2 green onions, sliced
2 teaspoons whole mustard seed
1 tablespoon whole peppercorns
1 tablespoon whole coriander seed
1 sprig fresh oregano
4 cups filtered or distilled water
1 tablespoon sea salt or other noniodized salt
1 pound small pickling cucumbers
¼ cup white wine vinegar or apple cider vinegar

In a large jar or other glass or ceramic container, combine garlic, onions, mustard seed, peppercorns, coriander, oregano, water, and salt and stir. Add the cucumbers, then cover with a plate or other object that keeps the contents submerged below the surface of the brine. (Some of the spices will rise to the top, but that's okay.)

Ferment for about 2 weeks or until tart. Add vinegar, cover, and refrigerate. Pickles can keep for several weeks in the refrigerator.

MAIN DISHES

SPIRALIZED ZUCCHINI PASTA
WITH OREGANO PESTO

IN THIS DELICIOUS RE-CREATION OF PASTA SERVED WITH PESTO, WE TAKE AD-
vantage of the antibacterial and antifungal properties of oregano
(though the leaves used here are not as potent as the purified essential
oil), the *Akkermansia*-stimulating properties of oleic acid in olive oil, and
the modest quantity of inulin prebiotic fiber in garlic. This oregano pesto
serves as a delicious salad dressing too.

A spiral cutter, widely available in most department and cooking stores,
is used to shape the "noodles." You can now also save yourself a little work
by buying precut spiral noodles, found in the frozen food or refrigerated
section of the supermarket. To reduce moisture in the spiralized zucchini
(which can water down the sauce), some people like to wrap the noodles
in paper towels and press out excess water prior to cooking.

MAKES 2 SERVINGS

½ cup raw pine nuts
3 cloves garlic
½ cup oregano leaves, coarsely chopped
2 tablespoons lemon juice, freshly squeezed or bottled
½ cup + 2 tablespoons extra-virgin olive oil, divided
¼ cup grated Parmesan cheese
¼ teaspoon sea salt
Ground black pepper to taste
1 pound zucchini, spiral-cut into noodles

In a blender, combine pine nuts, garlic, oregano, lemon juice, ½ cup
olive oil, Parmesan cheese, salt, and pepper and blend until pureed.
Set aside.

In a medium to large skillet, heat the remaining olive oil over medium-high heat, add the zucchini, and sauté until tender, about 3 minutes.

Serve the zucchini topped with the pesto.

GINGER CHICKEN

HERE IS THE PREBIOTIC FIBER–RICH VERSION OF A PERENNIAL CHINESE RESTAUrant favorite.

I specify chicken thighs because many meat producers and grocers remove the skin and bones from chicken breasts, but those are what provide the flavor and health benefits. The last thing you want to do is buy skinless, boneless chicken. We do not limit fat, of course. And you can save the bones to make soup.

Be careful in your choice of fish sauce because many brands contain unhealthy additives. (Thai Kitchen brand is a safe choice.)

MAKES 4 SERVINGS

3 pounds chicken thighs, bone-in with skin
2 tablespoons coconut oil
5 cloves garlic, minced
1 leek stalk, halved and sliced
4 ounces shiitake mushrooms, sliced
6 green onions, white portion thinly sliced, green portion sliced
    into 1-inch lengths
2½ tablespoons gluten-free soy sauce, tamari, or coconut aminos
2 tablespoons freshly grated ginger or 2 teaspoons dried ginger
2 tablespoons vinegar
1 tablespoon fish sauce

Preheat oven to 375°F.

Place chicken in baking pan and bake for 45 minutes.

During the last 10 minutes of baking, heat oil in a large skillet over medium-high heat, then combine garlic, leek, shiitake mushrooms, and the white portion of green onions and cook until softened, for 4–5 minutes. Stir in gluten-free soy sauce and ginger followed by vinegar and fish sauce. Add green portion of green onions.

Remove chicken from oven and transfer to skillet, including all drippings. Reduce the heat to low and allow to simmer for 5 minutes, basting chicken thighs occasionally.

ITALIAN SAUSAGE SOUP

HERE'S A SPICY SOUP PACKED WITH PREBIOTIC FIBERS FROM ONION, GARLIC, daikon radish, and lentils, accompanied by the *Akkermansia*-blooming oleic acid of olive oil and the antifungal effects of oregano.

Lentils provide the galactooligosaccharide variety of prebiotic fiber, which is among the healthiest fibers you can get. A mix of inulin prebiotics comes from the onion, garlic, and daikon radish, with a little capsaicin from the hot sauce thrown in for good measure (which you can, of course, adjust depending on how hot your sauce is and your tolerance for this effect).

MAKES 8 SERVINGS

¼ cup extra-virgin olive oil
1 medium yellow onion, chopped
4 cloves garlic, minced
12 ounces Italian sausage, sliced
6 cups chicken stock or water
3 cups spinach, fresh or frozen, coarsely chopped
1 daikon radish, sliced
2 celery stalks, sliced
1 cup lentils
1 (14.5-ounce) can diced tomatoes
2 tablespoons fresh oregano, chopped, or 1 tablespoon dried
    oregano
1 tablespoon hot sauce
Sea salt and ground black pepper to taste

In a large saucepan, heat the oil over medium-high heat, then add onion, garlic, and sausage. Cover, stirring frequently, until the sausage is cooked and onions are translucent, for 5–6 minutes.

Transfer the sausage mixture to a large stockpot or other large vessel. Over high heat, add chicken stock or water, spinach, daikon, celery, lentils, tomatoes, oregano, hot sauce, salt, and pepper to the pot. Bring the soup to a boil, then reduce the heat to low and simmer, covered, for 30 minutes or until lentils have softened.

SICILIAN PIZZA

WITH THE MODIFICATIONS I INTRODUCE TO PIZZA MAKING, I CANNOT REALLY call this an authentic Sicilian Pizza. But this recipe illustrates how to modify a familiar favorite food to put it to work rebuilding your intestinal microbiome instead of destroying it.

The flaxseed and psyllium in the crust and the onion, garlic, mushrooms, oregano, and basil in the toppings all make a contribution. For an extra microbiome boost, you can even add inulin or acacia fiber to the pizza sauce.

MAKES 4 SERVINGS

CRUST:
- 3 cups almond meal/flour
- ¼ cup ground golden flaxseed
- ¼ cup ground psyllium seed
- 2 eggs
- ½ teaspoon sea salt
- 4 ounces cream cheese
- 4 ounces mozzarella cheese, grated or sliced
- ½ cup water

TOPPINGS:
- 4 tablespoons extra-virgin olive oil, divided
- 1 yellow onion, chopped
- 3 cloves garlic, minced

4 ounces white button or portabella mushrooms, sliced

2 tablespoons fresh oregano, chopped, or 1 tablespoon dried oregano

¼ cup fresh basil, chopped, or 1½ tablespoons dried basil

2 teaspoons inulin powder or acacia fiber (optional)

6 ounces pizza sauce

6 ounces mozzarella cheese, grated or sliced

TO MAKE CRUST:

Preheat oven to 375°F.

In a large bowl, add almond meal/flour, flaxseed, and psyllium seed and mix. Add the eggs and mix well.

In a microwave-safe bowl, combine cream cheese, mozzarella cheese, and water and microwave for 45 seconds to soften. Pour this mixture into the almond meal/flour mixture and mix thoroughly.

Line a baking pan or pizza stone with parchment paper. Place the dough on the parchment paper and, using your hands or a large spoon, spread the dough out to achieve ½-inch thickness with a raised border at the edge. Dip your hands in water to help smooth dough.

Bake the crust for 18–20 minutes or until it just begins to turn golden brown. Remove from oven.

TOPPINGS:

In a medium skillet, heat 2 tablespoons olive oil over medium-high heat, then add the onions, garlic, and mushrooms, and cook until the onions are translucent and the mushrooms have softened. Stir in oregano and basil, then remove from heat.

Spread this mixture over the baked crust. If adding inulin powder or acacia fiber to the pizza sauce, stir it in, then pour the sauce evenly over the toppings. Distribute mozzarella cheese over top.

Return the pizza to the oven until the cheese has melted, for 15–18 minutes. Remove and cut into 8 slices.

SALMON WITH AVOCADO LIME SAUCE

DRESS UP YOUR SALMON WITH THIS UNIQUE SAUCE THAT OFFERS THE ANTIBACTE-rial and antifungal properties of ginger, and cilantro and coriander (the leaf and seed from the same plant), and the prebiotic fiber of avocado plus the *Akkermansia*-cultivating effect of the oleic acid in olive oil.

MAKES 2 SERVINGS

1 avocado, pulp removed
3 tablespoons extra-virgin olive oil
2 tablespoons lime juice (fresh or bottled)
2 tablespoons onion, minced
¼ cup fresh cilantro, chopped
1 teaspoon freshly ground ginger, or ½ teaspoon dried ginger
½ teaspoon ground coriander
3 tablespoons white wine vinegar
½ teaspoon salt
2 tablespoons extra-virgin olive oil or butter
2 8-ounce salmon filets

In a blender, combine the pulp of one avocado with 3 tablespoons of olive oil and lime juice, onion, cilantro, ginger, coriander, vinegar, and salt and blend until smooth. Set aside.

Season both sides of the salmon with salt and pepper to taste.

In a large skillet, heat 2 tablespoons of oil over medium-high heat. Place salmon filets, skin side up, in the oil and cook for 4–5 minutes. Flip the salmon and cook for an additional 4–5 minutes.

Serve the salmon topped with the avocado lime sauce.

BEEF SHAWARMA WITH SUPER GUT TZATZIKI

BEEF (OR LAMB, CHICKEN, OR PORK) SHAWARMA IS AN OPPORTUNITY TO OBTAIN the microbiome health benefits of cumin, coriander, cloves, and cinnamon in the spice mixture called garam masala.

This is also another way to put Super Gut Tzatziki (recipe on page 250) to work, which combines the prebiotic fiber of garlic and antimicrobial effects of mint with the probiotic species of choice from one of your homemade yogurts. You may like this Beef Shawarma wrapped in a Turmeric Flax-seed Wrap (recipe on page 267) or simply put atop some riced cauliflower. (Riced cauliflower is cauliflower that has been put into a food processor or grated to yield a riced texture, then steamed; alternatively, you can now purchase, then steam, pre-riced cauliflower, a big time-saver.)

You can make your own garam masala by roasting roughly equal portions of cinnamon stick, cardamom pods, cumin seeds, coriander seeds, cloves, and peppercorns in a skillet over medium heat until fragrant (3–5 minutes), then grinding in a coffee grinder.

MAKES 4 SERVINGS

1½ pounds beef, thinly sliced (rib eye, chuck eye, top blade—
    the fattier, the better)
½ cup extra-virgin olive oil
1 tablespoon white wine vinegar
Juice of 1 lemon
1 teaspoon sea salt
¼ teaspoon ground black pepper
1 tablespoon garam masala

In a large bowl, combine the beef, olive oil, vinegar, lemon juice, salt, and pepper and cover. Marinate for 2 hours (or longer), stirring occasionally.

In a large skillet over medium-high heat, pour in the beef mixture, spreading the slices of beef so that each contacts the skillet directly. Cook to desired level of doneness, approximately 3 minutes. Shake garam masala over the top and stir into the mixture.

Remove the beef from the heat and spread it over riced cauliflower or lay it onto a Turmeric Flaxseed Wrap, roll it into a cone, and top with a tablespoon of tzatziki.

TURMERIC FLAXSEED WRAP

WHEN THE NEED ARISES TO ENCLOSE SOME FOODS—MEATS, CUCUMBERS, TOMA-
toes, tzatziki, and so forth—try this easy and inexpensive wrap rather than
resort to the various high-cost grain-free wraps at the store. We throw a
little turmeric into this wrap for its antibacterial and antifungal properties.

MAKES 1 WRAP

¼ cup ground golden flaxseed
½ teaspoon onion powder
½ teaspoon ground turmeric
1 teaspoon extra-virgin olive oil
1 egg
1 tablespoon water
Dash sea salt

In a small bowl, combine flaxseed, onion powder, turmeric, olive oil,
egg, water, and salt and mix thoroughly.

Grease a 9-inch microwave-safe pie pan. Pour the flaxseed mixture into the pan, tilting to spread it evenly. Microwave on high for
2–3 minutes or until cooked. Allow to cool 5 minutes, then remove
with a spatula. Alternatively, bake in a greased oven-safe pie pan at
375°F for 10 minutes or until the center is cooked. Allow to cool
for 5 minutes, then remove with a spatula.

ASPARAGUS, LEEK, AND WHITE BEAN QUICHE

START YOUR DAY WITH A SLICE OF QUICHE RICH IN PREBIOTIC FIBER FROM ONION,
garlic, leeks, and white beans. This recipe also illustrates how to make a
tasty piecrust using nongrain meals or flours.

MAKES 8 SERVINGS

CRUST:
1½ cups almond meal/flour (or ground walnuts or pecans)
¼ cup ground golden flaxseed

¼ cup butter or coconut oil, melted
¼ cup water
½ teaspoon sea salt

FILLING:
2 tablespoons olive oil, butter, or coconut oil
1 yellow onion, diced
4 cloves garlic, minced
1 leek stem, halved and sliced
1 pound ground pork, beef, turkey, or chicken
½ cup cooked white beans
¼ cup broth
1 tablespoon dried oregano
1 tablespoon dried basil
2 cups fresh or frozen asparagus, coarsely chopped
8 eggs
1 teaspoon sea salt
Ground black pepper to taste

Preheat oven to 350°F. Grease a 10-inch pie plate.

To make the crust, in a medium to large bowl, combine almond meal/flour, flaxseed, butter, water, and salt and mix thoroughly. Transfer the mixture to a greased pie plate and spread it with a spoon or spatula. Wet it with water if needed to help smooth it out. Spread it at least 1 inch up the sides of the plate.

Place in the oven and bake for 15–18 minutes or until the crust just turns golden brown. Remove and cool.

Meanwhile, in a large skillet, heat the olive oil over medium-high heat, then add the onions and garlic and cook until the onions soften and are translucent, for 3–5 minutes. Add the leek and pork, breaking it up as it cooks. Add the beans, broth, oregano, and basil, then cover, stirring intermittently until the meat is cooked through. Remove the mixture from the heat, uncover, and allow to cool for 10 minutes.

In a large bowl, add asparagus, eggs, salt, and pepper and mix. Pour the pork mixture into the egg mixture and mix thoroughly. Then, pour the combination into the cooled piecrust and bake for 35 minutes or until the eggs set.

YAKISOBA NOODLES

IF YOU HAVE EVER HAD YAKISOBA NOODLES IN A JAPANESE RESTAURANT, YOU know that they can be the height of umami comfort foods. But because we don't want the problems associated with wheat or buckwheat noodles, we use shirataki noodles made from the konjac root, which provides the fabulous prebiotic fiber glucomannan. Shirataki noodles are an ultra-low carbohydrate (3 grams or less per 8-ounce package). Look for shirataki without added tofu to avoid soy. You can also use spiral-cut kohlrabi noodles or hearts of palm noodles.

Shirataki noodles absorb the flavors of the foods they accompany, having little to no taste of their own. So don't be turned off by their peculiar odor right out of the package because it disappears with a brief rinse.

Shirataki noodles work best in Asian dishes, though you can experiment with Italian and other cuisines. Be careful with your choice of oyster or fish sauce used in this recipe because many brands add undesirable ingredients or additives; the widely available Thai Kitchen brand is a safe choice.

MAKES 2 SERVINGS

¼ cup coconut oil
1 pound ground pork (or beef, chicken, turkey)
4 garlic cloves, minced or crushed
4 ounces fresh shiitake mushrooms, stems discarded, caps sliced
5 green onions, sliced, white and green parts separated
1 tablespoon grated fresh ginger, or 1 teaspoon ground ginger
1 tablespoon sesame seeds
½ teaspoon red pepper flakes
2 to 3 tablespoons gluten-free soy sauce, tamari, or coconut aminos
2 tablespoons toasted sesame oil
1½ tablespoons oyster or fish sauce
2 packages (8 ounces each) shirataki noodles

Heat the coconut oil in a wok or large skillet over medium-high heat. Add the meat, garlic, mushrooms, white portions of the onions, ginger, sesame seeds, and pepper flakes and cook until the meat is fully cooked. (Add a touch of water if the pan becomes too dry.)

Reduce heat to low and stir in the soy sauce, sesame oil, oyster sauce, and green portion of the onions, maintaining the mixture at low heat for 1–2 minutes.

Meanwhile, bring 4 cups of water to a boil in a large saucepan. Rinse the shirataki noodles in a colander under cold running water for about 15 seconds and drain. Pour the noodles into the boiling water and cook for 2–3 minutes. Drain the noodles and transfer to the wok/skillet with the pork mixture. Toss and serve.

DESSERTS

CHOCOLATE CHIP FROZEN YOGURT

TO MAKE FROZEN YOGURT, WE AVOID USING ICE CREAM MAKERS AND MINIMIZE the forceful mechanical agitation of blenders so that we don't kill the probiotic microbes provided by our yogurts. Choose the yogurt for the effect you desire.

MAKES 2 SERVINGS

1½ cups yogurt of your choice
1 tablespoon unsweetened cocoa powder
1½ tablespoons dark chocolate chips
Sweetener equivalent to 3 tablespoons sugar
Optional: 1 teaspoon inulin/FOS, acacia powder, or other
    prebiotic powder

In a bowl, combine the yogurt, cocoa powder, chocolate chips, sweetener, and optional prebiotic fiber and mix thoroughly. Allow the mixture to set at least 1 hour in the freezer.

ONE-MINUTE STRAWBERRY ICE CREAM

HERE IS A WAY TO MAKE YOUR OWN ICE CREAM THAT INVOLVES ALMOST NO effort. Note that, for this time-saving shortcut to work, the strawberries (or other berries or fruit) must be frozen. This is how you can enjoy a bowl of ice cream sans the intestinal mucus- and microbiome-disrupting effects of synthetic emulsifying agents.

MAKES 2 CUPS

8 ounces heavy whipping cream or canned coconut milk
1 cup frozen strawberries or other berries or fruit
1 green, unripe banana, scooped out of the peel and coarsely
    chopped
Sweetener equivalent to 1 tablespoon sugar
½ teaspoon vanilla extract

In a blender, combine whipping cream, berries, banana, sweetener, and vanilla. Blend until the mixture is smooth.

ORANGE CLOVE SCONES

THE EUGENOL OIL OF CLOVES IS AMONG THE MOST POTENT OF NATURALLY OC-curring oils that thickens the intestinal mucus barrier, an effect achieved via proliferation of mucus-stimulating bacterial species. Here is a tasty orange-flavored scone with the added scents, flavors, and health benefits of ground cloves. These scones also offer you the opportunity of adding 4 teaspoons of inulin or acacia fiber into the dry portion of the recipe, yielding around 2 grams prebiotic fiber in each scone.

MAKES 8 SCONES

SCONES:
3 cups almond flour
Zest of one medium orange
¼ cup ground golden flaxseed
2 tablespoons ground psyllium seeds
½ teaspoon ground cloves

2 teaspoons baking soda
Sweetener equivalent to 1 cup sugar
Dash sea salt
4 teaspoons inulin or acacia fiber (optional)
1 egg
1 cup heavy cream or canned coconut milk
½ stick (4 oz.) butter, melted

VANILLA GLAZE:
¼ cup xylitol
2 tablespoons heavy cream or canned coconut milk
1 tablespoon coconut oil
1 teaspoon vanilla extract

Preheat the oven to 350°F. Line a baking sheet with parchment paper.

In a large bowl, combine the almond flour, orange zest, flaxseed, psyllium, cloves, baking soda, sweetener, salt, and optional prebiotic fiber and mix thoroughly.

In a separate small bowl, whisk together the egg, 1 cup of cream, and butter. Pour the egg mixture into the dry mixture and combine thoroughly to a doughlike consistency.

Spread the dough on the baking sheet and form into approximately an 8-inch round, ¾-inch thick shape. Cut the round into 8 triangular pieces (like slicing a pizza) using a knife or spatula.

Bake the scones for 30 minutes or until a toothpick withdraws dry. Allow to cool.

To make the glaze, combine the xylitol, cream, coconut oil, and vanilla extract in a small saucepan over low heat, stirring until foam forms. Remove from the heat and allow to cool.

Drizzle vanilla glaze over the tops of the cooled scones.

RASPBERRY CREAM PIE

EVEN IF THE PEOPLE AROUND YOU—FAMILY, FRIENDS, OTHERS IN YOUR SOCIAL circle—are simply uninterested in the health adventure you have embarked on, you can still enjoy delicious ways to deliver added prebiotic fibers (pectin from raspberries, added FOS/inulin in the filling) to your diet. You can share this pie with them, and no one is likely to notice that they are enjoying an enormously healthy alternative to the grain- and sugar-based conventional counterpart.

MAKES 8 SERVINGS

CRUST:
1½ cups ground pecans, walnuts, or almonds (or almond flour)
4 tablespoons butter, melted
Dash sea salt

FILLING AND TOPPING:
2½ cups raspberries, fresh or frozen, divided
½ cup water
16 ounces cream cheese, room temperature
½ cup sour cream
2 teaspoons FOS/inulin powder
Sweetener equivalent to ½ cup sugar

Preheat the oven to 375°F. Grease a 9-inch pie pan.

TO MAKE THE CRUST:
In a medium bowl, combine the ground nuts, butter, and salt and mix well.

Transfer the nut mixture to the pie pan and spread it along the bottom and approximately ½ inch up the sides. Bake for 10 minutes or until lightly browned. Lower oven temperature to 325°F.

TO MAKE THE FILLING AND TOPPING:
In a small or medium-sized saucepan over medium heat, combine 1½ cups raspberries and water. Bring to a boil and lightly simmer

and stir for 1 minute, then remove from the heat. Puree the berries using a stick blender or vigorously crush the raspberries using a spoon.

Meanwhile, in a large bowl, combine the cream cheese, sour cream, FOS/inulin, and sweetener and mix well.

Transfer approximately half the raspberry mixture into the cream cheese mixture. Using a stick blender, blend the ingredients until well mixed. Pour this mixture into the piecrust and bake for 15 minutes. Remove pie from the oven and allow it to cool to room temperature.

Spread the remaining raspberry mixture over the top, then distribute the remaining whole raspberries over the pie.

SUPER GUT SAMPLE THREE-DAY
MENU PLAN AND SHOPPING LISTS

THIS SAMPLE MENU PLAN DRAWS FROM SUPER GUT RECIPES TO get you off to a confident start. Although the Super Gut lifestyle introduces some major changes in food choices, you will quickly recognize that there are plenty of healthy, delicious foods to choose from while you're rebuilding and empowering a healthy microbiome. You may find that three meals a day is too much now that you have banished the gliadin-derived opioid peptides found in wheat that used to stimulate your appetite, are not limiting fats or oils that are satiating, and may even have added *L. reuteri* yogurt, which further suppresses appetite via oxytocin. Many people who follow this lifestyle eat no more than two meals a day. Listen to your appetite signals for when to eat—don't eat because it's time to eat.

Feel free to substitute foods that you are already comfortable with and that still fit into the Super Gut lifestyle. You likely do not need a recipe to make a familiar breakfast of three fried eggs with some sliced ham, topped with a hot chili sauce (for its microbiome-modifying effects of capsaicin) and accompanied by a small serving of black beans for prebiotic fiber.

Remember to make a habit of including some source of prebiotic fiber in every meal. If you are having one of the yogurts or a smoothie, for example, stir in a teaspoon of inulin or acacia fiber. Add some beans, peas, or other legumes to omelets, salads, or as a side dish. Include asparagus, sliced leeks, sliced avocado, or dandelion greens in salads along with thinly sliced raw potato.

A shopping list follows this menu plan. Don't be intimidated by the number of items—you are restocking your kitchen with healthier replacements. Once you are comfortably on the Super Gut lifestyle, you won't have to buy so many new foods.

DAY 1

BREAKFAST

L. reuteri + *B. coagulans* yogurt with a ½ cup of blueberries and dash of liquid stevia
Clove Green Tea

LUNCH

Dandelion Greens and Raw Potato Salad with Avocado Lime Dressing
Hot Chili Fries dipped in Hot Chili Sauce

DINNER

Sicilian Pizza
One-Minute Strawberry Ice Cream

DAY 2

BREAKFAST

Asparagus, Leek, and White Bean Quiche
Clove Green Tea

LUNCH

Cream of Mushroom Soup
Orange Clove Scones

DINNER

Salmon with Avocado Lime Sauce
Mocha Mint Kefir

DAY 3

BREAKFAST

Matcha Strawberry Key Lime Smoothie
Clove Green Tea

LUNCH

Bacon, lettuce, and tomato (or your choice of meat and fixings) on
Herbed Focaccia Bread
Gingerbread Coffee

DINNER

Beef Shawarma with Super Gut Tzatziki
Fermented Roasted Peppers (will need to be fermented at least
72 hours beforehand)
Raspberry Cream Pie

SHOPPING LISTS

FREQUENTLY USED FOODS

These are foods that you will rely on frequently and are therefore worth
stocking up on. Don't sweat the up-front costs—you are likely restocking
your fridge and pantry with a lot of new items at first. Over time, you will
see that this lifestyle either costs no more than a conventional diet or even
saves you a modest amount because of the marked reduction in appetite we
experience when we eat this way.

The day-by-day lists do not include items on this Frequently Used
Foods list.

Acacia fiber
Almond flour or meal
Butter
Chili pepper sauces
Cloves, whole

Coconut milk, canned

Coconut oil

Extra-virgin olive oil

Fructooligosaccharide (FOS) powder

Garlic cloves

Green tea (bags or loose leaf)

Ground golden flaxseed

Ground psyllium seed

Half-and-half (or your choice of fermenting vehicle)

Herbs and spices—fresh and/or dried basil, oregano, rosemary, nutmeg, cinnamon, coriander seeds, cayenne or other hot peppers, turmeric, cumin, curry powder, garam masala, thyme, ginger

Inulin powder

Sweeteners (See list of safe sweeteners on page 300)

Here are the foods you'll need in addition to Frequently Used Foods to follow this menu plan:

DAY 1

Blueberries, fresh or frozen

Dandelion greens

Raw white potatoes

Red onion

White button mushrooms

Eggs

Bacon

Avocados

White wine vinegar

Fresh cilantro

Lime

Turnips

Onion powder

Grated Parmesan cheese

Hot chili sauce

Cream cheese
Mozzarella cheese
Pizza sauce
Cream
Frozen strawberries

DAY 2

Yellow onion
Leek
Ground pork, beef, turkey, or chicken
Cooked white beans
Chicken or beef broth
Asparagus, fresh or frozen
Eggs
Yellow onion
Leek
White button mushrooms (or portabella or cremini)
Coconut milk, canned
Chicken or vegetable stock
Cilantro, fresh
Baking soda
Choice of sweetener (See list of safe sweeteners on page 300)
Avocado
White wine vinegar
Salmon filets
Kefir
Instant coffee granules
Cocoa powder, unsweetened
Mint extract

DAY 3

Matcha tea powder
Mint leaves
Blueberries, fresh or frozen

Bacon
Lettuce
Tomato
Mozzarella cheese, shredded
Dried onion powder
Olives, black or kalamata
Sun-dried tomatoes
Eggs
Beef
Lemon
Cucumber
Lemon juice, freshly squeezed or bottled
Dill or mint, fresh
Bell peppers
Bay leaf
Ground pecans, walnuts, or almonds (or almond flour)
Raspberries, fresh or frozen
Cream cheese
Sour cream

AFTERWORD: SWEAT THE SMALL STUFF

CONTRARY TO THE POPULAR ADAGE, I BELIEVE THAT YOU *SHOULD* sweat the small stuff.

I certainly do not want you to lose sleep agonizing over the creepy-crawlies inhabiting your GI tract, just as you did when you learned that your bedsheets were crawling with bed mites. But, just as we must, given modern life, be mindful of the teenager or soccer mom who, texting while driving, crosses the dividing line head-on into your lane, so we must now be mindful of the microscopic creatures inhabiting our internal world after the utter destruction we have inflicted on this microcosm.

The absolutely crazy and disturbing thing about all of this is that trillions of creatures, none of whom collect a paycheck or pay income taxes, can exert a more profound effect on your life than your doctor, are more important than any nutritional supplement you take, and are closer to you than any love you've shared with another human. They play a deep and intimate role in your life. And yet, in recent human history, most of us have done nothing more than throw bombs into their midst.

As a result, for too many of us, they've gone rogue. You may label it ulcerative colitis, rosacea, panic attacks, or unexpected urgent bowel movements that strike at the most inopportune moments. But it's not you, it's not a lack of prescription medications, it's not bad luck—it's those microscopic creatures that, even now, are tracking your every movement, every bite, every thought you have, good or bad. They are, in so many ways, a cumulative reflection of all you have been through: bad dietary choices, a course of ciprofloxacin for a urinary tract infection in 1998, too many beers in college, the birth control pill you took for ten years before having children, the painful divorce you endured in 2005, the many bowls of strawberry ice cream rich in emulsifying agents you ate while crying into your bowl for two years afterward.

It is therefore hazardous *not* to sweat the small stuff. I don't mean that you should sweat the offhand comment from a rude colleague or the cut of your hair. I don't mean that you should lose sleep over your teenager's sloppy hygiene or social media activities. I mean that you should sweat the effects of the trillions of microbes who "talk" to you, experience and share your stressful moments, your successes accompanied by celebratory glasses of champagne, and succumb to the microbial disaster that results when a doctor, who, not mindful of microbiome consequences, hands you prescriptions for statins, antibiotics for a "just-in-case" bacterial infection, stomach acid–reducing drugs, or anti-inflammatory medication.

It all matters. But the solution cannot be found in a prescription bottle. A drug won't back off bowel urgency (without a lot of unwanted side effects), a surgery won't healthfully shrink the size of your stomach, an antidepressant drug won't naturally lift your mood, and antibiotics won't eradicate the microbes that have burst through the intestinal wall to create a diverticular abscess without decimating the good bugs that could heal the root cause of the diverticular process in the first place.

None of us have all the answers or know exactly how to undo all the harm we have inflicted on the modern human microbiome. But new insights are coming to us at an unprecedented rate. Just as technology advances at breakneck speed, yielding new tools and innovations faster than any one person can comprehend—how many smartphone apps can you juggle?—so do answers unfold in the world of the microbiome. A day does not pass that some new lesson—or ten—does not present itself, causing us to consider how this new information might shed light on our microbiome predicament.

Let's now entertain a question that goes beyond just correcting previous wrongs: Can we not just undo all the mistakes we've made over our lifetimes but do *better*, taking health, well-being, body weight and body composition, feelings of optimism and success *above* what we can accomplish if we simply accept the limited benefits of, say, eating healthy and taking a probiotic supplement?

I believe we can.

As revolutionary and enlightening as some of the concepts in *Super Gut* are, I liken where we are at now with our understanding of the human microbiome to the early efforts of Henry Ford, who, when asked about his revolutionary Model-T automobiles, declared, "Any customer can have a car painted any color that he wants so long as it's black." From that humble start, we now have Teslas, self-driving cars, manned space flight, and other transportation innovations that Ford likely never imagined. I believe that we are in a similar situation, the microbiome equivalent of a 1908 Model-T, crank-started and belching smoke. These health concepts are evolving rapidly, likely to yield powerful and effective health solutions in coming months and years. Whereas it required more than a century to progress from a black $400 Model-T to the modern multicolored, computerized electric automobiles of today, I predict that progress in the world of the human microbiome will take just a few years before we have the equivalent of a self-driving car guiding microbiome health.

Nonetheless, it is clear that we are already capable of truly impressive feats with our microbiome management efforts. Just a few years ago, who would have thought that we could obtain smoother skin, restore youthful strength and muscle tone, preserve bone density, cultivate empathy, shrink our waist, and reduce anxiety simply by restoring a single microbe to our inner ecosystem? Or reduce blood sugar and blood pressure and realize other metabolic benefits—health corrections that most of the world still believes are the province of prescription drugs?

Soon we will witness a flood of fascinating new ideas, products, and practices that will help us better manage the microbial universe contained within us, such as the following:

- Second-generation probiotics that include keystone species and strains, which thereby increase their effectiveness, rapidly phasing out current minimally effective probiotic products. It is conceivable that we could take a probiotic for, say, a few weeks that then populates our GI tract for a lifetime. An increasing number of probiotics will also incorporate guild or consortium effects, that is, put "collaborations" among microbes to work to yield synergistic metabolic benefits for both bacteria and their hosts.

- Production of what I call "third-generation probiotics" that combine keystone microbes with nonmicrobial factors to exert potent microbiome-shaping effects.

- Targeted probiotics that eradicate SIBO and SIFO without the need for antibiotics or antifungals. These approaches will harvest the "Power of Normal." I believe that my Super Gut SIBO Yogurt may be a step in that direction. ✔

- Microbiome management becoming the method of choice to manage numerous health conditions, from type 2 diabetes to rheumatoid arthritis and Parkinson's disease(Imagine the potential of managing a condition like depression or anxiety through healing the microbiome)–it is conceivable that some serious mental and mood conditions will be readily and more effectively managed with efforts targeting the microbiome, eliminating the need for numerous ineffective, toxic, costly prescription drugs.

- A reduced need for many supplemental vitamins and disappearance of their related deficiencies as we learn how to cultivate bacterial species that produce vitamins, such as vitamins B_1, B_2, B_3, B_6, B_9 (folate), B_{12}, and K_2. In the foreseeable future, women of childbearing age who reduce non-nutrient-producing Enterobacteriaceae species and increase nutrient-producing *Lactobacillus* and *Bifidobacterium* species may no longer need to rely on grain products for folate supplementation, for instance(but can instead rely on bacterial species to provide it for them.)

- Food intolerances and allergies becoming a thing of the past as we learn how to manage the microbes that allowed such reactions to develop.

- Health conditions that involve the accumulation of some potentially harmful metabolite, such as uric acid in gout or oxalates in kidney stones, being managed by specific manipulations of the microbiome. ☑

Consider this: Can we go even further and *improve* on "normal" human health and behavior? In other words, with an eye toward indigenous populations like the Hadza and Yanomamo, who have a leg up on us in many aspects of health because of their microbiome-friendly lifestyles, can we find ways to improve on even their version of the human microbiome to achieve advances in health and function that traditional cultures have not yet achieved? Can we craft microbiome strategies, for instance, that improve memory, increase energy, or heighten physical performance? I believe that we are just a few steps—or yogurt batches—away from such insights.

Given the pace of innovation, you and I may see the emergence of microbiome management techniques that help us achieve a Bradley Cooper–like acceleration of mental capacity, as in the film *Limitless*, or that eliminate fatigue and depression—are you beginning to appreciate the incredible magnitude of change that may be possible?

But before we can realize any of these astounding benefits, first we must conquer the monster we harbor within, restructuring, rebuilding, and then improving upon this strange but magnificent thing we carry around just south of our diaphragm, responsible for all the gurgling and other unsettling noises and whose work product you witness every day (hopefully) in the bowl of your toilet.

CAN YOU BE FORTY YEARS OLD . . .
FOR THE NEXT SIXTY YEARS?

No one has yet cracked the code on living an additional twenty, fifty, or hundred years. Sure, claims are made, but real evidence? Outside of worms and mice, there is no evidence that shows humans can live longer by adopting this or that strategy. And does living longer mean hobbling around with a cane or walker, living with a deteriorating memory that keeps you from recognizing family and friends, and being so frail that you need to rely on others to accomplish the most basic activities of life? The achievable goal here is not to extend life span but improve life quality so you feel like you can still run, jump, dance, make love, and do the things that make humans human for as long as possible. And we hope to achieve this by understanding and applying the wisdom of the trillions of microbes we carry, not through some macabre Frankenstein-like experiment involving stitched-together body parts and lightning.

What if we instead could arrest aging at, say, age forty, and go on to celebrate birthday after birthday still capable of doing fifty pushups, with no deepening wrinkles, no osteoporotic fractures, no lost interest in social interaction? What if we could still laugh and attend social events at age ninety-eight after biking twenty miles or dancing the samba? What if we could still look lustily at our partner and plan the next holiday trip? With Super Gut strategies, I think that we take several steps closer to such a reality.

Many still think of microbes as "germs" that need to be eradicated. But what if we choose advantageous microbes and then provide the nutrients they need and an environment suitable to their proliferative success? Will they prop up our health, undo our health impairments, and reverse aspects of aging and deterioration? It is not eradication we are after, but *collaboration*. We may have to kill off the nasties that glyphosate, statin drugs, cheap chocolate ice cream, and diet soda have cultivated in our Frankenbelly of monstrous microbes. But what if we cultivate and support the proliferation of the microbial species that, after all, depend on us for survival? Can we then unlock the many secrets for our health that they hold?

I predict that we can. And we are closer to such enormous insights than we thought. Now go toss some chia seeds into that homemade *L. reuteri* yogurt and have a cup of Clove Green Tea to get started on age reversal and your return to youthfulness.

ACKNOWLEDGMENTS

I T IS 2022, BUT IF THIS WERE THE AUTOMOTIVE INDUSTRY, IT would be the equivalent of 1908. If it were the emergence of a nascent computing industry, it would be 1982 and you'd have a Commodore computer, complete with green screen and Pong. In other words, in the world of the intestinal microbiome, we are just getting started.

It is shocking, breathtaking, and exciting all at once to know that we are yet again witnessing the birth of an industry that has potential to change the world, all by concentrating on restoring and rebuilding this ecosystem that you and I may have thought was responsible for little more than indigestion or loose bowels after a course of antibiotics.

Most leaps in knowledge are incremental, building on prior knowledge and the work of many people. In *Super Gut*, that is precisely what I have done: I have built upon the impressive body of work assembled by thousands of researchers, microbiologists, and other scientists. I practiced cardiology for many years, a discipline that seems as far away from the intestinal microbiome as quantum physics is from Bingo. But great wisdom can be gained by anyone and any process that works to bridge divides among unconnected disciplines, combining the collective wisdom across different perspectives, coming to new and unique conclusions.

But there is a growing and powerful force that is accelerating the pace of growth in knowledge: crowdsourced knowledge and experience. If we combine the wisdom and experience of schoolteachers, businesspeople, engineers, scientists, hairdressers, production line workers, phone center operators, mothers, fathers, grandparents, and so forth, all devoting themselves to answering the same questions in health—you know what? We eventually find answers, answers to questions that have even stumped doctors for years.

I tell my readers and online audiences that if you do not ask the question, you will never receive the answer. So, ask the question. The answers may not come tomorrow, the next day, even the next year. But once the question is posed, your mind is tuned in to stumbling upon anything that brings you closer and closer to the answer.

My biggest thanks, therefore, goes to the countless number of people all seeking better answers, who took the time and trouble out of their busy lives to make a contribution to this huge, chaotic, but wonderful process called "crowdsourced wisdom." One person may not have the answer, neither may ten nor even one hundred. But combine the wisdom and experience of thousands of people and wonderful things happen. Obviously, it means that there are far too many people whom I would like to thank: the mother from California who discovered how her daughter's health, eating habits, and food intolerances were essentially cured by simply addressing her child's lost microbes. And the woman in Florida who experienced reduced skin wrinkles that were making her feel like retirement years were closer than anticipated, all reversed to 1990s-like youthfulness just by fermenting microbes as a thick, delicious yogurt that contained a species that boosted oxytocin and reduced inflammation.

But I do indeed have specific individuals to thank who have played crucial roles in producing this collection of insights that are purposefully *prescriptive*—I am not content just to jabber on and describe but must show you a path to newly rediscovered health, slenderness, and youthfulness that, I am confident, will genuinely change the course of your life. I am truly grateful for all the people who came to my aid in gathering together my thoughts collectively labeled as *Super Gut*. Among those to whom I am grateful for contributing are the following:

Chris Kliesmet, my longtime friend and muse, with whom I have spent many—too many—nights debating, countering, but navigating this disaster called the American health-care system and seeking out better solutions than the current awful status quo. I have thanked Chris previously in other books, but let me thank you again.

My agent, Rick Broadhead, who has endured my ups and downs as I publicly and vocally voiced my views and findings that run contrary to conventional wisdom. I am sure that Rick has spent a number of sleepless nights wondering what seemingly crazy ideas he has tied his fortunes to. But, given the success that Rick and I have seen with the Wheat Belly books, I am thankful he has stuck with these projects.

Although not directly tied to the content and ideas in *Super Gut*, here are people who played roles in shaping my thinking, helped develop the funding to support the research needed to evolve these ideas, and whom I regard as long-term friends and colleagues:

Mark Nottoli—rarely does someone in business also show a deep interest in applying science to derive benefit. Although I have known Mark for over fifteen years, I did not appreciate his brilliance to bridge disciplines until the last couple of years. Thank you.

Roy Bingham—Englishman, gentle and wise businessman, reaffirmed to me that there are bigger goals in the world and that, with grace and dignity, we can accomplish them. Roy recently moved back to the American Midwest, and I can only hope that this brings even greater synergy and collaboration.

Of course, I owe my editors at Hachette, Lauren Marino, Cisca Schreefel, Mollie Weisenfeld, and Christina Palaia, a deep and grateful thank-you for taking on a project that must have felt like wading through a swamp packed with alligators lurking under every lily pad: cold, slow, waiting for your leg to be bitten off, as they helped me craft a message that, as powerful as it is, is a bit complicated and that might struggle to resonate with people who have busy lives to conduct.

Lastly, I wish to thank friends, family, neighbors, and others who provided me feedback, knowingly or not, on this grand human experiment, who told me, for instance, how they had far fewer facial wrinkles with the *L. reuteri* yogurt, could perform almost superhuman physical feats with the *B. coagulans* yogurt, and are helping all of us chart a course to new and unique insights into how these microscopic creatures, unseen and generally unthanked, can make the difference between a life endured and a life fully lived.

RESOURCES

AIRE DEVICE FOR BREATH H_2, METHANE, AND H_2S TESTING

Because the AIRE device was originally conceived as a means to detect H_2 gas in people with irritable bowel syndrome when they are exposed to FODMAPs-containing foods, the instructions included with the device do not lay out the entire story on how to use this device for detecting SIBO. Until the company updates instructions, follow the instructions I provided in Chapter 8 to detect H_2 gas and methane in your breath to help identify SIBO and understand any food intolerances you may experience. (The AIRE device also detects hydrogen sulfide gas, but the science behind this application is preliminary. Please follow our online conversations at www.DrDavisInfiniteHealth.com to understand how to apply this measure.)

The device is available from the manufacturer, FoodMarble: www .foodmarble.com.

H_2 BREATH TESTING

These are the tests for breath H_2 and methane that can be performed at home or under the supervision of your doctor. At home, you consume either the sugar glucose or lactulose, then submit multiple breath samples by mail to a lab, and the results are then mailed back to you. Because glucose is not a satisfactory sugar for assessment of SIBO, I recommend only using lactulose, which is usually available only through a doctor. However, the Life Extension Foundation makes lactulose available directly and can provide results for both H_2 and methane breath testing for around $250:

Lactulose H2 and methane breath testing: www.lifeextension .com/lab-testing/itemlc100063/sibo-home-breath-kit-lactulose

A new service called trio-smart breath testing, developed in part by SIBO expert Dr. Mark Pimentel, is now available to test for hydrogen (H_2), methane, and hydrogen sulfide (H_2S). The cost for one round of testing is just under $300 and the company says that many health-care insurance policies and Medicare cover most or all of the cost.

Trio-smart H2, methane, and H2S breath testing: www.triosmart breath.com

STOOL TESTING

A number of methods may be used to assess the composition of bowel flora. Older methods that relied on growing microbes in a petri dish have proven unreliable because many bowel species do not grow in those conditions. Instead, "culture-independent" methods have uncovered far greater species diversity than we previously suspected. The following testing services rely on culture-independent assessment methods, such as DNA analysis by polymerase chain reaction, or PCR. (Despite the progression of technology, some testing services still use the older outdated methods; I advise against using this sort of testing unless you are unable to access the services listed below.)

Unfortunately, stool tests can only be ordered by a health-care practitioner. You should ask your doctor (who may not be familiar with them) for these tests, and he or she will have to register and create an account with the test company if they are not already associated. If your doctor refuses, find a health-care practitioner who is willing to work with you to assess this aspect of your health. Customer service representatives at each testing company can also identify practitioners in your area who use their service.

Costs are in the range of $200 to $300, except for Vibrant Wellness Gut Zoomer, the most comprehensive test, which is priced around $700, and Thryve, the least costly at around $100.

Vibrant Wellness Gut Zoomer

The oddly named Gut Zoomer is the most comprehensive stool test, reporting the following markers:

- Identification and quantification of bacterial species with strain designations
- Identification of Archaea
- Identification of fungi
- Identification of parasites
- Identification of some viruses
- Identification of physiological markers such as pancreatic elastase, calprotectin, bile acids, and fatty acids

www.vibrant-wellness.com/tests/gut-zoomer/

Diagnostic Solutions Laboratory GI-Map

This microbial assay relies on quantitative PCR testing to identify stool species.

www.diagnosticsolutionslab.com

Genova GI Effects Comprehensive Profile

Opt for the Comprehensive Profile for the most complete analysis. The GI-Map and GI Effects stool profiles are good services that yield plenty of helpful information but have major drawbacks, namely, the inability to identify species and strains. These tests therefore provide only broad insights into bowel bacterial composition. They do identify Archaea, fungi, and parasites, as well as a number of important physiological markers.

www.gdx.net

Thryve Gut Health Test

Thryve testing is comprehensive, able to identify bacteria down to species and strain and to quantify each. The test, however, does not identify

Archaea, fungi, or viruses. The company also steers you toward its brand of probiotics on the basis of test results, and I find that not a very helpful strategy. The upside is that Thryve is among the most affordable of tests, often priced lower than $100.

    www.thryveinside.com/products/thryves-gut-health-test

Viome Gut Intelligence

I find the Viome service to be the least helpful. Although comprehensive in identifying microbial species and strains, it provides no quantification. In other words, if an undesirable species such as a *Klebsiella* species or *Clostridium difficile* is identified, without quantification there is no way to know whether it is a problematic finding or not. The dietary advice prompted by results is also, in my view, not helpful.

    beta.viome.com/products#tests

HERBAL ANTIBIOTICS

CandiBactin-AR + CandiBactin-BR

These two products are available from Amazon, but health-care practitioners can obtain them from the manufacturer, Metagenics:

    metagenics.com

FC-Cidal + Dysbiocide

These two products are available from Amazon:

    Amazon.com

PREFERRED PROBIOTICS

Synbiotic 365

This probiotic contains 20 billion CFUs of the following strains: *L. rhamnosus* GG, *L. reuteri* UALre-16 (also designated NCIMB 30242), *L. gasseri* BNR17, which are keystone species, and a number of other important strains. It also contains *Saccharomyces boulardii*, a yeast that provides an additional advantage in rebuilding a microbiome.

    Unitednaturals.com

Ther-Biotic Synbiotic

This product has 50 billion CFUs per capsule of seven strains, many of which are on our list of keystone microbes, such as *L. rhamnosus* GG and *L. reuteri* UALre-16 (also designated NCIMB 30242). It is available from Klaire Labs or through selected health-care practitioners. You can make yogurt with this product.

Klaire.com

Vital Flora

Vital Flora from Vital Planet takes a different approach: include as many species and strains as possible at high counts. Vital Flora accordingly contains 60 billion CFUs of 60 strains, consistent with cofounder Brenda Watson's (cofounder of Renew Life, also) philosophy of cultivating species diversity.

VitalPlanet.com

Sugar Shift

Noted microbiologist Dr. Raul Cano developed this collection of unusual species on the basis of his research into synergistic "guilds" of species that yield greater-than-expected levels of various metabolites. Preliminary experience suggests this collection provides important benefits that include reduction of blood sugar. Strains are, unfortunately, not specified on the label, but the application of the guild effect puts this preparation at the forefront of the science. You can make yogurt with this product.

Biotiquest.com

Jarro-Dophilus EPS Digestive Probiotic

The mix of species and strains in this product, including some potentially keystone strains, may make it especially helpful for managing mood and emotional health. Each capsule provides only 5 billion CFUs, so you can make a tasty yogurt with this product to increase bacterial counts.

Jarrow.com

DS-01 Daily Synbiotic

This is an interesting probiotic in that there is a lot of science behind the preparation of over twenty species/strains with a total count of 53.6 billion.

Seed Health has created a capsule that survives passage through the small bowel and purportedly releases into the colon, but that, in my view, is a downside because for our SIBO-eradication purposes we want release into the small intestine. Should you take this probiotic, I would remove the external capsule and take only the internal capsule. Also, only some strain designations are recognizable, and many are proprietary. Nonetheless, Seed is an interesting addition to the mix of choices.

Seed.com

Pendulum Glucose Control

Pendulum has launched the world's first probiotic to deliver a strain of *Akkermansia* along with four other butyrate-producing species. The Glucose Control product is targeted to help manage blood sugar in people with type 2 diabetes, but it can also be taken by nondiabetics for other purposes, such as reintroducing *Akkermansia* in people who lack this species.

I advocate that only those of us who completely lack *Akkermansia* by stool analysis take the Pendulum product. If you have *Akkermansia* as identified via stool testing, then I would suggest you instead follow strategies that cause *Akkermansia* populations to bloom rather than supplementing with this very costly product, which is priced around $160–$200 per one-month supply. (See Chapter 5 for the discussion on how to bloom *Akkermansia*.) You cannot make yogurt with this probiotic because the *Akkermansia* dies upon exposure to air (although some of the other species included in the Pendulum product will indeed ferment to yogurt).

Pendulum Glucose Control provides
- *Akkermansia muciniphila* WB-STR-0001
- *Clostridium beijerinckii* WB-STR-0005
- *Clostridium butyricum* WB-STR-0006
- *Eubacterium hallii* WB-STR-0008
- *Bifidobacterium infantis* 100

Obtain Pendulum from the manufacturer:
Pendulumlife.com

Evivo

Bifidobacterium infantis EVC001 is the keystone strain of *Bifidobacterium infantis* that, with breastfeeding, has been demonstrated to cultivate a healthy microbiome in newborns and infants when taken during the first few months of life. (It is not yet clear whether similar benefits develop in babies who are formula fed and therefore not receiving oligosaccharides from breast milk, though there is certainly no harm in supplementing formula-fed babies with this probiotic.) However, I suggest that pregnant moms make yogurt with this strain for their own consumption, which will then allow t 1⅓ hem to pass this microbe on to their child during delivery and breastfeeding. The resulting yogurt is thick, rich, and delicious.

Obtain Evivo from the manufacturer:

Evivo.com

Florastor

Recall that *Saccharomyces boulardii* is a beneficial fungal species that is especially helpful for recovering from diarrhea after a course of antibiotics. Because it is a fungus, it is not a microbe you can make yogurt with, but it can still be a helpful component of your probiotic efforts to rebuild a healthy microbiome.

It is also unclear which strain is preferred, so we stick to the strain that is among the best studied, *Saccharomyces boulardii lyo* CNCM I-745. (The relative efficacy of various *S. boulardii* strains has not been well mapped out.)

This strain of *Saccharomyces boulardii* is available as the commercial product Florastor from major pharmacies and other major retailers, including Walmart, Meijer, and Amazon.

Sources of Specific Microbial Species/Strains for Fermentation

Lactobacillus reuteri DSM 17938, ATCC PTA 6475

The BioGaia Gastrus tablets are available through Amazon as well as BioGaia's US distributor Everidis. Likewise, Osfortis capsules with the 6475 strain alone are available through the same routes.

Everidis.com

Another source of *L. reuteri*, the NCIMB 30242 strain, also likely a keystone strain, is available from Life Extension as their Florassist Heart Health product, with 2.5 billion CFUs per capsule. However, do not use this strain to make the Super Gut SIBO Yogurt because it lacks a bacteriocin.

Lifeextension.com

Lactobacillus reuteri SD 5865

Here's another option: a yogurt-making kit using a different strain of L. reuteri that, in preliminary experience, yields many of the same effects, called "LR Superfood Starter."

www.cuttingedgecultures

Lactobacillus gasseri BNR17

While we previously could only source this microbe from the South Korean company that commercialized it, Dr. Joseph Mercola has finally made it directly available in the US on his Mercola Market. You only need to purchase it once to obtain a single capsule that you can ferment into yogurt or other fermented food (from the 10 billion CFUs per capsule). Many of my followers will purchase a product like this, then share with others (via my Facebook pages) for a modest price to reduce costs. Also stay tuned to updates for availability on my website, www.DrDavisInfiniteHealth.com.

https://www.mercolamarket.com

Bacillus coagulans GBI-30,6086

B. coagulans is available as the Digestive Advantage Daily Probiotic product from Schiff that is widely sold by many major retailers and online sources, including Meijer and Walmart.

Lactobacillus helveticus R0052 and *Bifidobacterium longum* R0175

This combination of species, which lifts mood and reduces anxiety, is available from the manufacturer, Innovix Labs, as well as Life Extension, Amazon, and other major retailers:

Innovixlabs.com
Lifeextension.com

Lactobacillus casei Shirota

This strain, which helps increase immunity against viral illnesses, increases mental clarity, and provides deep sleep for some people (especially in combination with *L. reuteri*), is available as a commercial drinkable product called Yakult. We ferment Yakult to increase the number of bacteria and to make a yogurt that no longer contains the skim milk or sugar in the original source product.

Retailers such as Walmart, Meijer, and Asian specialty stores carry Yakult. The manufacturer also has a store locator on its website:

Yakult.com

Lactobacillus rhamnosus GG

L. rhamnosus GG strain has proven, time and again, superior to other strains of *L. rhamnosus* for such effects as recovery from diarrhea after a course of antibiotics or for antifungal effects.

L. rhamnosus GG is commercially available as the Culturelle product, with 20 billion CFUs per capsule, at major retailers such as Walmart, Meijer, Target, and Walgreens. As always, you can amplify the health effects using our Super Gut "bacterial count amplification system," aka yogurt making, which achieves hundreds of billions of CFUs.

A growing number of products are making this strain available, including SuperSmart (www.supersmart.com) and Pure Encapsulations (www.pureencapsulations.com).

Lactobacillus plantarum 299v

L. plantarum is another interesting probiotic species that has been shown to reduce the symptoms of bloating, abdominal discomfort, and bowel frequency in people with irritable bowel syndrome (and likely SIBO). Although its disadvantage is that it does not colonize the upper GI tract, only the colon, it does exert substantial antibacterial and mucus-stimulating effects. And, of course, it makes a tasty yogurt.

Jarrow Formulas has a product with 10 billion CFUs per capsule that can serve as a starter for fermentation. You can obtain it through major nutritional supplement retailers such as iHerb or through Jarrow directly:

Jarrowonline.com

Starter Cultures for Fermentation

Cutting Edge Cultures provides products that are useful to accelerate fermentation of vegetables and other foods, not just relying on the microbes present on the surface of the food. They provide a starter culture for fermenting vegetables as well as a kefir starter.

cuttingedgecultures.com

Cultures For Health offers starters for yogurt, kefir, kombucha, and cheeses in an astounding choice of varieties.

culturesforhealth.com

COMMERCIAL PREBIOTIC FIBERS

In addition to inulin, acacia fiber, glucomannan, and galactooligosaccharide powders, the following are several excellent commercial sources of prebiotic fibers that are obtainable through major nutrition retailers such as Vitacost, iHerb, and Amazon and health food stores:

Garden of Life Organic Fiber
Swanson Ultra Inulin
NOW Inulin Prebiotic Pure Powder
Jarrow Formulas Prebiotic Inulin–FOS
Cutting Edge Cultures Prebio Plus
Micro Ingredients Organic Inulin Powder
NOW Certified Organic Acacia Fiber
Hyperbiotics Organic Prebiotic Fiber Blend
Please add:

FERMENTED MEATS

In addition to salamis, pepperonis, sopressatas, and other fermented meats that are mostly from Italy and found in the refrigerated section of the grocery or specialty shop, one online retailer makes fermented grass-fed beef sticks available: Paleovalley. They provide five varieties that are delicious.

www.paleovalley.com

NON-ABSORBED CURCUMIN

Despite all the commercial hullaballoo about adding this or that ingredient to enhance the absorption of curcumin, *we do not want absorption*—we want it to stay within the GI tract so as to exert its antifungal and intestinal barrier–fortifying effects there. I therefore advise that you avoid brands that have added ingredients such as bioperine, piperine, or other formulations. The following products are straight curcumin, which has notoriously low bioavailability, meaning it will stay in your gut:

NOW Curcumin Softgels

Jarrow Formula Curcumin 95

Life Extension Curcumin Elite Turmeric Extract

Solaray Curcumin

SAFE SWEETENERS

To replace sugar (sucrose) in recipes, here is a conversion chart that lists the equivalents of safe noncaloric or minimally caloric sweeteners to 1 cup sugar. Although monk fruit and inulin are safe sweeteners, they are rarely if ever used alone.

EQUIVALENT TO 1 CUP OF SUGAR:

Stevia, powder or liquid—Variable depending on brand; consult label

Allulose—1⅓ cups

Erythritol—1⅓ cups

Xylitol—1 cup

(Inulin)

(Monk fruit)

COMBINATION SWEETENERS:

Truvía (erythritol + rebiana, an isolate of stevia): 1¼ cups

Pyure (erythritol + stevia): ½ cup

Virtue (erythritol + monk fruit): ¼ cup

Swerve (erythritol + inulin): 1 cup

Lakanto (erythritol + monk fruit): 1 cup

RECOMMENDED FERMENTATION DEVICES

Actually, any means of maintaining the temperature "preferred" by the bacterial species you are fermenting can get the job done and yield a delicious, healthy "yogurt" with health effects far beyond the stuff available in grocery stores. I made my first thirty batches of *L. reuteri* yogurt, for instance, by putting the bowl in the oven and turning the oven on to any temperature (e.g., 300°F) for one to two minutes, just enough to make the oven tropical or desert warm, every four to six hours. But sharing this method confused readers, who thought I was baking the yogurt, or occasionally plagued those who would forget to turn off the oven and killed all their microbes. Therefore, the simplest approach involves using a device that you can turn on, place your fermenting mixture into, then walk away.

Note that many yogurt makers and older Instant Pots have preset temperatures, which work with only some bacterial species. *L. reuteri*, for example, does best at human body temperature, around 97°F–100°F, but dies at 108°F–114°F, the temperature range preset in most such devices. Ideally, you will use a device that allows you to vary the temperature within the range of 97°F to 125°F to accommodate different species. By saying that bacterial species "prefer" a temperature range, I mean this is the temperature range in which a species proliferates at maximum rate and remains viable. *L. reuteri*, for example, proliferates rapidly at 100°F but dies at a temperature of 122°F, an ideal temperature for *Bacillus coagulans*.

If you struggle to obtain a thick, rich, pleasant-scented end result, put a thermometer into your device, either into the water bath or the yogurt itself, to assess the accuracy of the set temperature. Unfortunately, it is not uncommon for some devices to display inaccurate temperatures that impair fermentation. (One popular yogurt-making device that I tested, for instance, showed a temperature of 116°F despite being set to 106°F, an inaccuracy that yielded soured milk rather than yogurt.)

Sous Vide

Sous vide devices are simply temperature-controlled water baths designed for slow-cooking meats and other foods. However, we can redirect use of these handy devices for our fermentation projects.

I began the entire yogurt-fermenting process with a basin sous vide from Gourmia that I paid $79 for at Bed, Bath, and Beyond. Unfortunately, I started talking about the device on my social media sites, and that triggered a surge in demand, and the price jumped up to over $400. Prices on many other sous vide devices likewise went up. This has put basic sous vides into unreasonable price ranges for some brands, so I do not include those brands in the short list below. Thankfully, there are still some brands within a reasonable price range, around $100.

Sous vide devices come as either a basin style or a "stick" that attaches to a basin of your choosing. If you choose a stick-style sous vide device, you will therefore need a basin to attach the sous vide; a large pan or other large vessel can work, or you can purchase inexpensive plastic basins (offered in the "People who buy this also buy this . . ." function on Amazon).

Dash Chef Series Sous Vide (basin style)

This basin sous vide has a variable temperature range of 104°F to 194°F, just low enough for our low-temperature fermenting species like *L. reuteri*. Unlike some other retailers who raised their prices skyward with the attention my yogurt-making conversations have prompted, this device is still reasonably priced under $120 on the Dash Amazon store.

Instant Accu Slim

This stick sous vide from the same company that makes Instant Pots has a wide temperature range of 68°F to 203°F and adjustable timing control. It is priced around $80.

Instantpot.com

Anova Culinary Sous Vide Precision Cooker Nano

This stick sous vide is the least expensive of the several Anova sous vide devices because of its low wattage. But, for yogurt-making purposes, this low-wattage device works fine. Temperature range is 32°F to 197°F, with an impressive 0.1°F accuracy. The device also connects to your smartphone via Bluetooth.

Anovaculinary.com

Yogurt Makers

Many yogurt makers are preset to maintain a temperature range of 108°F to 114°F. Whereas this is great for conventional yogurt making, it kills some of the microbes that we are interested in, such as *L. reuteri*. If you have a conventional temperature preset yogurt maker, run the device for a couple of hours with a thermometer inserted to assess the actual temperature. If too hot, you will need to obtain another device.

Here are some good choices among yogurt makers, with variable temperature and timing controls:

MV Power

This low-cost (around $33) option is a favorite, with variable temperature (68°F–131°F) and timing (up to 48 hours) controls. Amazon has been the most popular source for this device.

Luvelle

The Luvelle yogurt maker is another popular brand for making yogurts at various temperatures. Downside: Three temperature choices are preset: 97°F, 100.4°F, and 104°F, meaning the occasional microbe (e.g., *Bacillus coagulans*) cannot be fermented at its ideal temperature. The device also has to be reset after running for 24 hours.

Luvele.com.au

Suteck

The Suteck yogurt maker is available for modest cost and is programmable for up to 48 hours of fermentation with a variable temperature range of 68°F to 131°F. Walmart (and Walmart.com) and Amazon are among the sources for this device.

Instant Pots

Many people have had success using their Instant Pots if a yogurt setting is available. (Contrary to the instructions included with these devices, we do not preheat pasteurized dairy because we are using higher-fat half-and-half and similar starting liquids that do not improve with preheating, unlike skim or low-fat milks.) The only difficulty is that the yogurt temperature setting is preset on most older models. If you have a preset yogurt temperature, run the device with some water and a thermometer to assess the actual temperature achieved.

Newer devices allow you to vary the temperature, but, once again, verify with a thermometer before committing.

Other

Brod & Taylor has an oddly named device called a "Folding Proofer and Slow Cooker." Don't be scared away by its claim to be a "Breadmaker's dream machine" because it can be repurposed for yogurt making and other fermentation projects. This device has a wide temperature range of 70°F to 195°F. The device is more costly than others, at around $170, but it also serves as a slow-cooking device.

Brodandtaylor.com

ERADICATING YOUR FRANKENBELLY: SUPER GUT SIBO AND SIFO PROTOCOLS

O NCE YOU HAVE IDENTIFIED AND/OR CONFIRMED SIBO BY, FOR example, high H_2 readings on the AIRE device (see page 112 for instructions on how to use), you have the option of addressing overgrowth of the unhealthy bacterial species that have ascended in your gastrointestinal tract to where they don't belong.

For ideal results, we currently combine at least some antifungal efforts with SIBO efforts because fungal overgrowth accompanies SIBO in at least a third of cases and because reducing bacterial populations often invites fungal overgrowth. Recall that you also have the option of putting the Super Gut SIBO Yogurt to work in place of herbal antibiotics, based on its capability, in preliminary testing, to normalize breath H_2. (You should still consider adding antifungal efforts.)

SUPER GUT SIBO PROTOCOL

You have some choices to make in addressing SIBO:

1. **Herbal antibiotic regimen:** Choose between the CandiBactin-AR/ BR or the FC-Cidal + Dysbiocide regimen.

2. **Super Gut SIBO Yogurt:** You can choose this yogurt to manage your SIBO in place of herbal antibiotics.
3. **Antifungals:** We include curcumin regardless of whether you have SIFO. If you believe that you do indeed have SIFO, then you can add the additional strategies listed below for SIFO.

Herbal Antibiotics

Take an herbal antibiotic to purge pathogenic species from the upper GI tract. Two herbal antibiotic regimens have proven efficacy: CandiBactin-AR + CandiBactin-BR and FC-Cidal + Dysbiocide. Choose one of the two and follow the regimen for fourteen days or until prebiotic fiber challenge yields low values (less than 4) on AIRE device readings (low H_2 readings after consumption of prebiotic fiber).

> CandiBactin-AR: 1–2 capsules twice per day, and CandiBactin-BR: 2 capsules twice per day, for 14 days

Or

> FC-Cidal: 1 capsule twice per day, and Dysbiocide: 2 capsules twice per day, for 14 days

Super Gut SIBO Yogurt

Make and eat Super Gut SIBO Yogurt in place of herbal antibiotics. This is the yogurt you can choose to consume in place of herbal antibiotics that has, in preliminary experience, normalized breath H_2 readings, which means it purges the upper GI tract of problematic microorganisms. Because it is a probiotic preparation, not an antibiotic, people have had success by consuming this yogurt for four weeks rather than the two weeks of antibiotics. The three species in this yogurt should be co-fermented at 106°F. To hear the latest in our emerging experience with this SIBO-fighting yogurt strategy, join my conversations at www .DrDavisInfiniteHealth.com.

> **Super Gut SIBO Yogurt:** ½ cup per day

Here is a quick refresher on which specific strains to use in making Super Gut SIBO Yogurt. See the text in the Week 4 section for all the details of the yogurt-making process:

- *Lactobacillus reuteri* DSM 17938, ATCC PTA 6475
  The BioGaia Gastrus tablets are available through Amazon as well as BioGaia's US distributor Everidis.

  www.everidis.com

- *Lactobacillus gasseri* BNR17
  L. gasseri BNR17 is available from Mercola Market: www.mercolamarket.com. Look for a product called "Biothin Probiotic" with 10 billion CFUs per capsule.

- *Bacillus coagulans* GBI-30,6086
  B. coagulans is available as the Digestive Advantage product from Schiff that is widely sold by many major retailers and online sources such as Meijer and Walmart.

Add curcumin. Regardless of whether you choose either herbal antibiotic regimen or the Super Gut SIBO Yogurt, I believe that it is a good practice to add curcumin. Because of its antifungal and intestinal barrier–strengthening effects, add curcumin in a nonabsorbable form, 300 milligrams twice per day, building up to 600 milligrams twice per day over several days.

Curcumin: 300–600 milligrams twice per day, for 14 days

Super Gut SIFO Protocol

If you are pursuing an antifungal campaign without addressing SIBO, begin curcumin 300–600 milligrams twice per day and add one or two food-sourced essential oils (oregano, cinnamon, or clove) to your regimen. Remember: *Never* take the oils directly or undiluted. Start with one or two drops of essential oil diluted in 1 tablespoon of olive, avocado, or coconut oil (melted) twice per day, and build up gradually to five or six drops per tablespoon of food oil for a minimum of four weeks or until signs of fungal overgrowth have receded.

If you began with an herbal antibiotic regimen, or if you consumed the Super Gut SIBO Yogurt for SIBO: Continue curcumin: 300–600 milligrams twice per day, and add one or two essential oils of oregano, cinnamon, and/or clove diluted in 1 tablespoon of food oil for at least 4 weeks. Start with one or two drops of essential oil diluted in 1 tablespoon of olive, avocado, or coconut oil (melted) twice per day, and build up gradually to five or six drops per tablespoon of food oil for a minimum of four weeks or until signs of fungal overgrowth have receded.

You can enhance the likelihood of a successful response to your SIBO efforts by considering the following two additional strategies:

1. **Biofilm disruption: Add N-acetyl cysteine for its biofilm-disrupting capabilities.** Adding an agent that disrupts the biofilm that bacteria create can increase the efficacy of the herbal antibiotics. Biofilms provide a hiding place for microbes and make them less susceptible to antibiotics. Our biofilm disrupter of choice, given its long and proven track record, is N-acetyl cysteine (NAC).

   Efforts to disrupt biofilm with NAC are not required during antifungal efforts because the essential oils of oregano, cinnamon, and clove provide biofilm disruption.

   N-acetyl cysteine: 600–1,200 milligrams twice per day with herbal antibiotic, for 14 days

2. **Prevent sporulation: Add back prebiotic fiber to your diet.** Some bacteria can enter a spore-forming stage during their life cycle and thereby become impervious to antibiotics. Providing prebiotic fibers may help prevent bacteria from entering this mode, making them more susceptible to the antibiotics. After several days of antibiotics, you will likely be able to add back prebiotic fibers to which you may previously have been intolerant. Increase prebiotic fiber intake, as tolerated, up to a long-term target intake of 20 or more grams

per day. Sources such as legumes, garlic, asparagus, leeks, dandelion greens, jicama, raw white potato, unripe banana, inulin powder, pectin, and acacia fiber are good sources of prebiotic fibers.

Prebiotic fiber: 20 grams or more per day; eat some prebiotic fiber at each meal

PREVENT SIBO RECURRENCE

Continue eating prebiotic fibers, add a multispecies probiotic supplement, and add fermented foods to your diet to prevent recurrences of bacterial and fungal overgrowth. SIBO and SIFO commonly recur. It is not entirely clear why recurrences happen, but the most likely explanations involve continued exposure to an unhealthy diet (i.e., a diet containing grains and sugars), intestinal wall inflammation, a defective mucus barrier, or failure to sufficiently reduce undesirable species. To reduce the potential for future recurrences, once you complete the course of herbal antibiotics or Super Gut SIBO Yogurt, continue to include prebiotic fibers every day. Add a high-potency, multispecies probiotic (see the list of preferred products in Appendix A); include fermented foods such as kombucha, fermented sauerkraut, kefir, and fermented vegetables; and add *L. reuteri* yogurt (see below). If the AIRE device is available, monitor for and assess recurrences by taking an H_2 reading after prebiotic fiber challenge. Note that you must stop eating *L. reuteri* yogurt two weeks prior to any AIRE testing to avoid false positives.

ROLE OF *L. REUTERI* YOGURT IN PREVENTING SIBO/SIFO RECURRENCES

Recall that *L. reuteri* is unique among probiotic microbes in that it naturally colonizes the upper GI tract and produces bacteriocins, both of which provide advantage in preventing SIBO and SIFO. *L. reuteri* yogurt is therefore included in our efforts to prevent recurrences of SIBO and SIFO after these conditions have been managed initially.

However, there is a complication. Whereas *L. reuteri* yogurt likely helps eradicate or prevent recurrences of SIBO, it also generates positive H_2 readings on the AIRE device, making it impossible to distinguish SIBO from the H_2 generation by healthy *L. reuteri*. If you plan to use the AIRE device to track H_2 readings during or immediately following a course of herbal antibiotics, you should stop consuming *L. reuteri* yogurt for at least two weeks until negative H_2 readings are obtained, then resume enjoying this yogurt and all its benefits.

METHANOGENIC SIBO

For methanogenic SIBO, follow the same protocol as for H_2 SIBO using the CandiBactin-AR/BR regimen. Alternatively, the Super Gut SIBO Yogurt can be consumed for four weeks, since preliminary evidence suggests that *L. reuteri* reduces methanogens. You can assess your breath methane levels with a prebiotic fiber challenge after completing the herbal antibiotic or Super Gut SIBO Yogurt regimen.

H_2S SIBO

Stay tuned to our online discussions as we discuss and experiment with the evolving science around hydrogen sulfide gas measurement as related to the microbiome. We're likely to uncover a great number of cases of SIBO in people who test negative for H_2 and methane but positive for H_2S.

APPENDIX C
ERADICATING H. PYLORI

I F YOU HAVE TESTED POSITIVE FOR *HELICOBACTER PYLORI* (USING an *H. pylori* fingerstick antibody or stool antigen test), here are strategies to consider that have proved to contribute to eradication of this bacterium, which is associated with long-term health complications. Because of the increasing failure of conventional antibiotics to eradicate *H. pylori*, there is abundant evidence for the efficacy of such "alternative" therapies.

To document successful eradication, a stool antigen test (but not the antibody test, which remains positive even after eradication because you now have antibodies against this species) can be repeated after the course of treatment.

Probiotics: Probiotics alone have not been shown to eradicate *H. pylori* but have been demonstrated to modestly improve treatment efficacy when combined with conventional therapy, though the specific species responsible for these effects are not clear. The *Lactobacillus reuteri* strains that we use in our yogurt have also been shown to suppress (though not eradicate by themselves) *H. pylori* through production of antibacterial bacteriocins and hydrogen peroxide. *L. reuteri* is also resistant to stomach acid and can colonize the stomach, effects that allow it to protect against *H. pylori* overpopulation. *Lactobacillus rhamnosus* GG has also been shown to help suppress *H. pylori*.

Nigella sativa: The seeds of this plant have been used for thousands of years in southern Europe, the Middle East, and Asia to treat a variety of disorders, and they can be eaten as a food, used much like poppy seeds to top baked products. Nigella has come under study most recently as a source of antibacterial compounds. A recent small clinical trial demonstrated that 2 grams (approximately 1 level teaspoon) of ground nigella seed eradicated *H. pylori* in 67 percent of participants, making it nearly as effective as conventional triple therapy. *Nigella sativa* seeds are available from a number of online retailers. Add nigella to yogurt and smoothies, or sprinkle it on food.

Mastic gum: The oddly named mastic gum is a traditional food and folk treatment for stomach upset in Greece and the Mediterranean that dates back twenty-five hundred years. It is sourced from an evergreen shrub that grows in that region. There is evidence that even 1 milligram per day taken over two weeks can eradicate *H. pylori* and thereby heal peptic ulcers, though higher doses were typically used in the few small clinical trials. In one study, 350 milligrams three times per day and 1,050 milligrams three times per day over fourteen days eradicated *H. pylori* in one-third to one-half of participants.

Bismuth subsalicylate/subcitrate: Available over the counter as Pepto Bismol tablets and liquid, bismuth was the original treatment for *H. pylori* in combination with H_2 blocking agents. This antacid and antidiarrheal was, in the early history of *H. pylori* eradication efforts, nearly as effective as modern triple or quadruple therapy, but it has become less effective in recent years. However, it may still provide advantage when used in combination with other agents.

Vitamin C: Five hundred milligrams of vitamin C twice daily taken orally has, in several studies, demonstrated an *H. pylori*–reducing or eradicating effect, particularly when used along with other therapies. This may be due to vitamin C's ability to block the urease enzyme expressed by *H. pylori*.

N-acetyl cysteine (NAC): NAC is a biofilm disrupter, that is, it disrupts the layer of mucus that *H. pylori* produces for its own protection. When used in combination with other therapies, 600 milligrams of NAC twice per day has been shown to substantially improve treatment efficacy, including in people who have proven resistant to conventional treatment, presumably by making the organism more susceptible to antibiotics.

A combination of natural agents used in a small study of thirty-nine participants successfully eradicated *H. pylori* in twenty-nine people (74.3 percent), as confirmed by stool antigen testing. These results are on a par with conventional three- and four-drug treatments. The following regimen was used:

- Mastic gum (Jarrow Formulas): 500 milligrams, 1 capsule three times daily
- Emulsified oil of oregano as ADP (anti-dysbiosis product; Biotics Research Corporation): 50 milligrams, 1 tablet three times daily
- Pepto Bismol: 4 to 6 tablets daily in divided doses between meals

In addition, a probiotic containing 5 billion CFUs of ten species taken twice daily (Vital 10; Klaire Laboratories) and a prebiotic fiber supplement were included.

REFERENCES

CHAPTER 1

1. Carrera-Bastos P, Fontes-Villalba M, O'Keefe J, Lindeberg S, Cordain L. The Western diet and lifestyle and diseases of civilization. *Res Rep Clin Cardiol.* 9 March 2011;2:15–35.

2. Data and Statistics: Inflammatory Bowel Disease Prevalence (IBD) in the United States. Centers for Disease Control website. https://www.cdc.gov/ibd /data-statistics.htm. Reviewed August 11, 2020. Accessed May 25, 2021.

3. US Cancer Statistics Working Group. US Cancer Statistics Data Visualizations Tool, based on 2019 submission data (1999–2017). US Department of Health and Human Services, Centers for Disease Control and Prevention, and National Cancer Institute. https://gis.cdc.gov/Cancer/USCS/DataViz.html. Published June 2020. Accessed May 25, 2021.

4. Cani PD, Amar J, Iglesias MA, et al. Metabolic endotoxemia initiates obesity and insulin resistance. *Diabetes.* 2007;56(7):1761–1772.

5. Lasselin J, Lekander M, Benson S, et al. Sick for science: experimental endotoxemia as a translational tool to develop and test new therapies for inflammation-associated depression. *Mol Psych.* 2020. doi.org/10.1038/s41380 -020-00869-2.

6. Takakura W, Pimentel M. Small intestinal bacterial overgrowth and irritable bowel syndrome—an update. *Front Psych.* 2020;11:664.

7. Pimentel M, Wallace D, Hallequa D, et al. A link between irritable bowel syndrome and fibromyalgia may be related to findings on lactulose breath testing. *Ann Rheum Dis.* 2004;63(4):450–452.

8. Weinstock LB, Fern SE, Duntley SP, et al. Restless legs syndrome in patients with irritable bowel syndrome: response to small intestinal bacterial overgrowth therapy. *Dig Dis Sci.* 2008;53(5):1252–1256.

9. Mikolasevic I, Delija B, Mijic A, et al. Small intestinal bacterial overgrowth and non-alcoholic fatty liver disease diagnosed by transient elastography and liver biopsy. *Int J Clin Pract.* 2021;75(4):e13947.

10. Losurdo G, D'Abramo FS, Indellicati G, et al. The influence of small intestinal bacterial overgrowth in digestive and extra-intestinal disorders. *Int J Mol Sci.* 2020;21(10):3531.

11. Polkowska-Pruszynska B, Gerkowicz A, Szczepanik-Kulak P, et al. Small intestinal bacterial overgrowth in systemic sclerosis: a review of the literature. *Arch Dermatol Res.* 2019;311(1):1–8.

12. Yan LH, Mu B, Pan D. Association between small intestinal bacterial overgrowth and beta-cell function of type 2 diabetes. *J Int Med Res.* 2020;48(7):300060520937866.

13. Wijarnpreecha K, Werlang ME, Watthanasuntorn K, et al. Obesity and risk of small intestine bacterial overgrowth: a systematic review and meta-analysis. *Dig Dis Sci.* 2020;65(5):1414–1422.

14. Erdogan A, Rao SSC. Small intestinal fungal overgrowth. *Curr Gastroenterol Rep.* 2015;17(4):16.

15. Zhang W, Zhang K, Zhang P, et al. Research progress of pancreas-related microorganisms and pancreatic cancer. *Front Oncol.* 2021;10:604531.

16. Alonso R, Pisa D, Aguado R, Carrasco L. Identification of fungal species in brain tissue from Alzheimer's disease by next-generation sequencing. *J Alzheimers Dis.* 2017;58(1):55–67.

17. Nicoletti A, Ponziani FR, Nardella E, et al. Biliary tract microbiota: a new kid on the block of liver diseases? *Eur Rev Med Pharmacol Sci.* 2020;24(5):2750–2775.

CHAPTER 2

1. Global Health Observatory data repository: births by Cesarean section. World Health Organization website. https://apps.who.int/gho/data/node.main .BIRTHSBYCAESAREAN?lang=en. Updated April 9, 2018. Accessed May 25, 2021.

2. CDC releases 2018 breastfeeding report card [press release]. Centers for Disease Control and Prevention website. https://www.cdc.gov/media/releases

/2018/p0820-breastfeeding-report-card.html. Published August 20, 2018. Accessed May 25, 2021.

3. Goedert JJ, Hua X, Shi J. Diversity and composition of the adult fecal microbiome associated with history of Cesarean birth or appendectomy: analysis of the American Gut Project. *EBioMedicine*. 2014;1(2–3):167–172.

4. Lundgren SN, Madan JC, Emond JA, et al. Maternal diet during pregnancy is related with the infant stool microbiome in a delivery mode–dependent manner. *Microbiome*. 2018;6:109.

5. Vinturache AE, Gyamfi-Bannerman C, Hwand J, et al. Maternal microbiome—a pathway to preterm birth. *Seminars Fetal Neonat Med*. 2016;21(2): 94–99.

6. Torres J, Hu J, Seki A, et al. Infants born to mothers with IBD present with altered gut microbiome that transfers abnormalities of the adaptive immune system to germ-free mice. *Gut*. 2020;69(1):42–51.

7. Barcik W, Boutin RCT, Solokowska M, Finlay BB. The role of lung and gut microbiota in the pathology of asthma. *Immunity*. 2020;52(2):241–255.

8. Stewart CJ, Ajami NJ, O'Brien JL, et al. Temporal development of the gut microbiome in early childhood from the TEDDY Study. *Nature*. 2018;562(7728):583–588.

9. Robertson RC, Manges AR, Finlay BB, Prendergast AJ. The human microbiome and child growth—first 1000 days and beyond. *Trends Microbiol*. 2019;27(2):131–147.

10. Solomon S. The controversy over infant formula. *New York Times*, December 6, 1981. https://www.nytimes.com/1981/12/06/magazine/the-controversy-over-infant-formula.html?pagewanted=all.

11. Palmer C, Bik EM, Di Giulio DB, Relman DA, Brown PO. Development of the human infant intestinal microbiota. *PLoS Biol*. 2007;5:e177.

12. Ip S, Chung M, Raman G, et al. Breastfeeding and maternal and infant health outcomes in developed countries. *Evid Rep Technol Assess*. 2007; 153:1–186.

13. Frese SA, Hutton AA, Contreras LN, et al. Persistence of supplemented *Bifidobacterium longum* subsp. *infantis* EVC001 in breastfed infants. *mSphere*. 2017;2(6):e00501–e00517.

14. Vangay P, Ward T, Gerber JS, Knights D. Antibiotics, pediatric dysbiosis, and disease. *Cell Host Microbe*. 2015;17(5):553–564.

15. Hicks LA, Taylor TH, Hunkler RJ. U.S. outpatient antibiotic prescribing, 2010. *N Engl J Med*. 2013;368:1461–1462. doi:10.1056/NEJMc1212055.

16. Su T, Lai S, Lee A, et al. Meta-analysis: proton pump inhibitors moderately increase the risk of small intestinal bacterial overgrowth. *J Gastroenterol*. 2018;53(1):27–36.

17. Muraki M, Fujiwara Y, Machida H, et al. Role of small intestinal bacterial overgrowth in severe small intestinal damage in chronic non-steroidal anti-inflammatory drug users. *Scand J Gastroenterol.* 2014;49(3):267–273.

18. Saffouri GB, Shields-Cutler RR, Chen J, et al. Small intestinal microbial dysbiosis underlies symptoms associated with functional gastrointestinal disorders. *Nat Commun.* 2019;10:2012.

19. Mao Q, Manservisi F, Panzacchi S, et al. The Ramazzini Institute 13-week pilot study on glyphosate and Roundup administered at human-equivalent dose to Sprague Dawley rats: effects on the microbiome. *Environ Health.* 2018;17:50.

20. Claus SP, Guillou H, Ellero-Simatos S. The gut microbiota: a major player in the toxicity of environmental pollutants? *NPJ Biofilms Microbiomes.* 2016;2:16003.

21. Zhan J, Liang Y, Liu D, et al. Antibiotics may increase triazine herbicide exposure risk via disturbing gut microbiota. *Microbiome.* 2018;6:224.

22. Cho Y, Osgood RS, Bell LN, et al. Ozone-induced changes in the serum metabolome: role of the microbiome. *PLoS One.* 2019;14(8):e0221633.

CHAPTER 3

1. Appelt S, Drancourt M, Le Bailly M. Human coprolites as a source for paleomicrobiology. *Microbiology Spectrum.* 2016;4(4). doi:10.1128/microbiolspec.PoH-0002-2014.

2. Adler CJ, Dobney K, Weyrich LS, et al. Sequencing ancient calcified dental plaque shows changes in oral microbiota with dietary shifts of the Neolithic and Industrial revolutions. *Nat Genet.* 2013;45:450–455.

3. Tito RY, Knights D, Metcalf J, et al. Insights from characterizing extinct human gut microbiomes. *PLoS One.* 2012;7(12):e51146.

4. Pasolli E, Ascinar F, Manara S, et al. Extensive unexplored human microbiome diversity revealed by over 150,000 genomes from metagenomes spanning age, geography, and lifestyle. *Resource.* 2019;176(3):649–662.

5. Schnorr SL, Candela M, Rampelli S, et al. Gut microbiome of the Hadza hunter-gatherers. *Nat Commun.* 2014;5:3654.

6. Obregon-Tito A, Tito R, Metcalf J, et al. Subsistence strategies in traditional societies distinguish gut microbiomes. *Nat Commun.* 2015;6:6505.

7. Clemente JC, Pehrsson EC, Blaser MJ, et al. The microbiome of uncontacted Amerindians. *Sci Adv.* 2015;12(3):e1500183.

8. Abdel-Gadir A, Stephen-Victor E, Gerber GK, et al. Microbiota therapy acts via a regulatory T cell MyD88/RORγt pathway to suppress food allergy. *Nat Med.* 2019;25(7):1164–1174.

9. PeBenito A, Nazzal L, Wang C, et al. Comparative prevalence of *Oxalobacter formigenes* in three human populations. *Sci Rep.* 2019;9(1):574.

10. Dwyer ME, Krambeck AE, Bergstralh EJ, et al. Temporal trends in incidence of kidney stones among children: a 25-year population based study. *J Urol.* 2012;188:247.

11. Henrick BM, Hutton AA, Palumbo MC, et al. Elevated fecal pH indicates a profound change in the breastfed infant gut microbiome due to reduction of *Bifidobacterium* over the past century. *mSphere.* 2018;3(2):e00018–e00041.

12. Underwood MA, German JB, Lebrilla CB, Mills DA. *Bifidobacterium longum* subspecies Infantis: champion colonizer of the infant gut. *Pediatr Res.* 2015;77(1–2):229–235.

13. Frese SA, Hutton AA, Contreras LN, et al. Persistence of supplemented *Bifidobacterium longum* subsp. infantis EVC001 in breastfed infants. *mSphere.* Dec;2(6):e00501–e00517.

14. Del Giudice MM, Indolfi C, Capasso M, et al. *Bifidobacterium* mixture (*B longum* BB536, *B infantis* M-63, *B breve* M-16V) treatment in children with seasonal allergic rhinitis and intermittent asthma. *Ital J Pediatr.* 2017;43(1):25.

15. Giannetti E, Maglione M, Alessandrella A, et al. A mixture of 3 Bifidobacteria decreases abdominal pain and improves the quality of life in children with irritable bowel syndrome: a multi-center, randomized, double-blind, placebo-controlled, crossover trial. *J Clin Gastroenterol.* 2017;51(1):e5–e10.

16. Molin G, Jeppsson B, Johansson ML, et al. Numerical taxonomy of *Lactobacillus* spp. associated with healthy and diseased mucosa of the human intestines. *J App Bacteriol.* 1993;74(3):314–323.

17. Walter J, Britton RA, Roos S. Host-microbial symbiosis in the vertebrate gastrointestinal tract and the *Lactobacillus reuteri* paradigm. *Proc Nat Acad Sci.* 2001;108(suppl 1):4645–4652.

18. Erdman SE, Poutahidis T. Microbes and oxytocin: benefits for host physiology and behavior. *Int Rev Neurobiol.* 2016;131:91–126.

19. Poutahidis T, Kleinewietfeld M, Smillie C, et al. Microbial reprogramming inhibits Western diet–associated obesity. *PLoS One.* 2013;8(7):e68596.

20. Levkovich T, Poutahidis T, Smillie C, et al. Probiotic bacteria induce a "glow of health." *PLoS One.* 2013;8(1):e53867.

21. Varian BJ, Poutahidis T, DiBenedictis BT, et al. Microbial lysate upregulates host oxytocin. *Brain Behav Immun.* 2017;61:36–49.

22. Elabd C, Cousin W, Upadhyayula P, et al. Oxytocin is an age-specific circulating hormone that is necessary for muscle maintenance and regeneration. *Nat Commun.* 2014;5:4082.

23. Elabd S, Sabry I. Two birds with one stone: possible dual-role of oxytocin in the treatment of diabetes and osteoporosis. *Front Endocrinol* (Lausanne). 2015;6:121.

24. Nilsson AG, Sundh D, Backhed F, Lorentzon M. *Lactobacillus reuteri* reduces bone loss in older women with low bone mineral density: a randomized, placebo-controlled, double-blind, clinical trial. *J Intern Med.* 2018;284(3):307–317.

25. Faria C, Zakout R, Araujo M. *Helicobacter pylori* and autoimmune diseases. *Biomed Pharmacother.* 2013;67(4):347–349.

26. Mounika P. *Helicobacter pylori* infection and risk of lung cancer: a meta-analysis. *Lung Cancer Int.* 2013;2013:131869. doi:10.1155/2013/131869.

27. Kato M, Toda A, Yamamoto-Honda R, et al. Association between *Helicobacter pylori* infection, eradication and diabetes mellitus. *J Diabetes Investig.* 2019;10(5):1341–1346.

28. Dardiotis E, Tsouris Z, Mentis AFA, et al. *H. pylori* and Parkinson's disease: meta-analyses including clinical severity. *Clin Neurol Neurosurg.* 2018;175:16–24.

29. Bjarnason IT, Charlett A, Dobbs RJ, et al. Role of chronic infection and inflammation in the gastrointestinal tract in the etiology and pathogenesis of idiopathic parkinsonism. Part 2: response of facets of clinical idiopathic parkinsonism to *Helicobacter pylori* eradication. A randomized, double-blind, placebo-controlled efficacy study. *Helicobacter.* 2005;10:276–287.

30. Yang X. Relationship between *Helicobacter pylori* and rosacea: review and discussion. *BMC Infect Dis.* 2018;18(1):318.

31. Kato M, Toda A, Yamamoto-Honda R, et al. Association between *Helicobacter pylori* infection, eradication and diabetes mellitus. *J Diabetes Investig.* 2019;10(5):1341–1346.

32. Atherton JC, Blaser MJ. Coadaptation of *Helicobacter pylori* and humans: ancient history, modern implications. *J Clin Invest.* 2009;119:2475–2487.

33. Mao Q, Manservisi F, Panzacchi S, et al. The Ramazzini Institute 13-week pilot study on glyphosate and Roundup administered at human-equivalent dose to Sprague Dawley rats: effects on the microbiome. *Environ Health.* 2018;17:50.

34. Sonnenburg ED, Smits SA, Tikhonov M, et al. Diet-induced extinctions in the gut microbiota compound over generations. *Nature.* 2016;529:212–215.

35. Sonnenburg JL, Xu J, Leip DD, et al. Glycan foraging in vivo by an intestinal-adapted bacterial symbiont. *Science.* 2005;307(5717):1955–1959.

36. Olson CA, Vuong HE, Yano JM, et al. The gut microbiota mediates the anti-seizure effects of the ketogenic diet. *Cell.* 2018;173(7):1728–1741.

CHAPTER 4

1. Olsan EE, Byndloss MX, Faber F, et al. Colonization resistance: the deconvolution of a complex trait. *J Biol Chem.* 2017;292(21):8577–8581.

2. 2018 Update: Antibiotic Use in the United States: Progress and Opportunities. Centers for Disease Control and Prevention website. https://www.cdc

.gov/antibiotic-use/stewardship-report/pdf/stewardship-report-2018-508.pdf. Reviewed November 11, 2020. Accessed May 28, 2021.

3. Manyi-Loh C, Mamphweli S, Meyer E, Okoh A. Antibiotic use in agriculture and its consequential resistance in environmental sources: potential public health implications. *Molecules.* 2018;23(4):795.

4. Hensgens MPM, Keessen EC, Squire MM, et al. *Clostridium difficile* infection in the community: a zoonotic disease? *Clin Micro Infect.* 2012;18(7):635–645.

5. Severe *Clostridium difficile*–associated disease in populations previously at low risk—four states, 2005. *MMWR.* 2005;54(47):1201–1205.

6. Marlicz W, Loniewski I, Grimes DS, Quigley EM. Nonsteroidal anti-inflammatory drugs, proton pump inhibitors, and gastrointestinal injury: contrasting interactions in the stomach and small intestine. *Mayo Clin Proc.* 2014;89(12):1699–1709.

7. Sabate JM, Coupaye M, Ledoux S, et al. Consequences of small intestinal bacterial overgrowth in obese patients before and after bariatric surgery. *Obes Surg.* 2017;27(3):599–605.

8. Czepiel J, Drózdz M, Pituch H, et al. *Clostridium difficile* infection: review. *Eur J Clin Microbiol Infect Dis.* 2019;38(7):1211–1221.

9. Maziade PJ, Pereira P, Goldstein EJ. A decade of experience in primary prevention of *Clostridium difficile* infection at a community hospital using the probiotic combination *Lactobacillus acidophilus* CL1285, *Lactobacillus casei* LBC80R, and *Lactobacillus rhamnosus* CLR2 (Bio-K+). *Clin Infect Dis.* 2015;60(suppl 2):S144–S147.

10. Schubert AM, Rogers MAM, Ring C, et al. Microbiome data distinguish patients with *Clostridium difficile* infection and non-*C. difficile*–associated diarrhea from healthy controls. *MBio.* 2014;5:1–9.

11. Wu J, Peters BA, Dominianni C, et al. Cigarette smoking and the oral microbiome in a large study of American adults. *ISME J.* 2016;10(10):2435–2446.

12. Engen PA, Green SJ, Voigt RM, et al. The gastrointestinal microbiome: alcohol effects on the composition of intestinal microbiota. *Alcohol Res.* 2015;37(2):223–236.

13. Saffouri GB, Shields-Cutler RR, et al. Small intestinal microbial dysbiosis underlies symptoms associated with functional gastrointestinal disorders. *Nat Commun.* 2019;10(1):2012.

14. Suez J, Korem T, Zeevi D, et al. Artificial sweeteners induce glucose intolerance by altering the gut microbiota. *Nature.* 2014;514(7521):181–186.

15. Caparrós-Martín JA, Lareu RR, Ramsay JP, et al. Statin therapy causes gut dysbiosis in mice through a PXR-dependent mechanism. *Microbiome.* 2017;5(1):95.

16. Martinez KB, Leone V, Chang EB. Western diets, gut dysbiosis, and metabolic diseases: are they linked? *Gut Microbes.* 2017;8(2):130–142.

17. Schroeder BO, Birchenough GMH, Stahlman M, et al. Bifidobacteria or fiber protect against diet-induced microbiota-mediated colonic mucus deterioration. *Cell Host Microbe.* 2018;23(1):27–40.

18. Fuke N, Nagata N, Suganuma H, Ota T. Regulation of gut microbiota and metabolic endotoxemia with dietary factors. *Nutrients.* 2019;11(10):2277.

19. Everard A, Lazarevic V, Gaia N, et al. Microbiome of prebiotic-treated mice reveals novel targets involved in host response during obesity. *ISME J.* 2014;8(10):2116–2130.

20. Ghosh SS, Wang J, Yannie PJ, et al. Dietary supplementation with galactooligosaccharides attenuates high fat, high cholesterol diet–induced disruption of colonic mucin layer and improves glucose intolerance in C57BL/6 mice and reduces atherosclerosis in Ldlr-/- mice. *J Nutr.* 2020;150(2):285–293.

21. Yildiz H., Speciner L, Ozdemir C, Cohen D, Carrier R. Food-associated stimuli enhance barrier properties of gastrointestinal mucus. *Biomaterials.* 2015;54:1–8.

22. Kaliannan K, Wang B, Li X-Y, et al. A host-microbiome interaction mediates the opposing effects of omega-6 and omega-3 fatty acids on metabolic endotoxemia. *Sci Rep.* 2015;5:11276.

23. Bresciani L, Dall'Asta M, Favari C, et al. An in vitro exploratory study of dietary strategies based on polyphenol-rich beverages, fruit juices and oils to control trimethylamine production in the colon. *Food Funct.* 2018;9:6470–6483.

24. Samsel A, Seneff S. Glyphosate, pathways to modern diseases II: celiac sprue and gluten intolerance. *Interdisc Toxicol.* 2013;6(4):159–184.

25. Mao Q, Manservisi F, Panzacchi S, et al. The Ramazzini Institute 13-week pilot study on glyphosate and Roundup administered at human-equivalent dose to Sprague Dawley rats: effects on the microbiome. *Environ Health.* 2018; 17:50.

26. Argou-Cardozo I, Zeidán-Chuliá F. *Clostridium bacteria* and autism spectrum conditions: a systematic review and hypothetical contribution of environmental glyphosate levels. *Med Sci* (Basel). 2018;6(2):29.

27. Liang Y, Zhan J, Liu D, et al. Organophosphorus pesticide chlorpyrifos intake promotes obesity and insulin resistance through impacting gut and gut microbiota. *Microbiome.* 2019;7(1):19.

28. Lehmann GM, LaKind JS, Davis MH, et al. Environmental chemicals in breast milk and formula: exposure and risk assessment implications. *Environ Health Perspect.* 2018;126(9):096001.

29. Adler CJ, Dobney K, Weyrich LS, et al. Sequencing ancient calcified dental plaque shows changes in oral microbiota with dietary shifts of the Neolithic and Industrial revolutions. *Nat Genet.* 2013;45:450–455.

30. Roberts C, Manchester K. Dental disease. In *The archaeology of disease.* New York: Cornell University Press; 2005:63–83.

31. Cohen MN, Crane-Kramer GMM. Editors' summation. In *Ancient health: skeletal indicators of agricultural and economic intensification*. Gainesville: University Press of Florida; 2007:320–343.

32. Petersen PE, Bourgeois D, Ogawa H, et al. The global burden of oral diseases and risks to oral health. *Bull World Health Organ*. 2005;83:661–669.

CHAPTER 5

1. Johansson MEV, Hansson GC. Immunological aspects of intestinal mucus and mucins. *Nat Rev Immunol*. 2016;16(10):639–649.

2. Desai MS, Seekatz AM, Koropatkin NM, et al. A dietary fiber–deprived gut microbiota degrades the colonic mucus barrier and enhances pathogen susceptibility. *Cell*. 2016;167(5):1339–1353.

3. Sicard JF, Le Bihan G, Vogeleer P, et al. Interactions of intestinal bacteria with components of the intestinal mucus. *Front Cell Infect Microbiol*. 2017;7:387.

4. Payahoo L, Khajebishak Y, Alivand MR, et al. Investigation of the effect of oleoylethanolamide supplementation on the abundance of *Akkermansia muciniphila* bacterium and the dietary intakes in people with obesity: a randomized clinical trial. *Appetite*. 2019;141:104301.

5. Everard A, Belzer C, Geurts L. Cross-talk between *Akkermansia muciniphila* and intestinal epithelium controls diet-induced obesity. *Proc Natl Acad Sci*. 2013;110(22):9066–9071.

6. De Vos W. Microbe profile: *Akkermansia muciniphila*: a conserved intestinal symbiont that acts as the gatekeeper of our mucosa. *Microbiology* (Reading). 2017;163(5):646–648.

7. Wlodarska M, Willing BP, Bravo DM, Finlay BB. Phytonutrient diet supplementation promotes beneficial *Clostridia* species and intestinal mucus secretion resulting in protection against enteric infection. *Sci Rep*. 2015;5:9253.

8. Georgiades P, Pudney PDA, Rogers S, et al. Tea derived galloylated polyphenols cross-link purified gastrointestinal mucins. *PLoS ONE*. 2014;9(8):e105302.

9. Chassaing B, Koren O, Goodrich JK, et al. Dietary emulsifiers impact the mouse gut microbiota promoting colitis and metabolic syndrome. *Nature*. 2015;519(7541):92–96.

10. Laudisi F, Stolfi C, Monteleone G, et al. Impact of food additives on gut homeostasis. *Nutrients*. 2019;11(10):2334.

11. Laudisi F, Di Fusco D, Dinallo V, et al. The food additive maltodextrin promotes endoplasmic reticulum stress-driven mucus depletion and exacerbates intestinal inflammation. *Cell Mol Gastroenterol Hepatol*. 2019;7:457–473.

12. Sasada T, Hinoi T, Saito Y, et al. Chlorinated water modulates the development of colorectal tumors with chromosomal instability and gut microbiota oil Apc-deficient mice. *PLoS One*. 2015;10(7):e0132435.

13. Kim MW, Kang JH, Shin E, et al. Processed aloe vera gel attenuates non-steroidal anti-inflammatory drug (NSAID)-induced small intestinal injury by enhancing mucin expression. *Food Funct.* 2019;10(9):6088–6097.

14. Lamprecht M, Frauwallner A. Exercise, intestinal barrier dysfunction and probiotic supplementation. *Med Sport Sci.* 2012;59:47–56.

15. He J, Guo H, Zheng W, Yao W. Effects of stress on the mucus-microbial interactions in the gut. *Curr Protein Pept Sci.* 2019;20(2):155–163.

CHAPTER 6

1. Cani PD, Amar J, Iglesias MA, et al. Metabolic endotoxemia initiates obesity and insulin resistance. *Diabetes.* 2007;56(7):1761–1772.

2. Magge S, Lembo A. Low-FODMAP diet for treatment of irritable bowel syndrome. *Gastroenterol Hepatol* (NY). 2012;8(11):739–745.

3. Borghini R, Donato G, Alvaro D, Picarrelli A. New insights in IBS-like disorders: Pandora's box has been opened; a review. *Gastroenterol Hepatol Bed Bench Spring.* 2017;10(2):79–89.

4. Rezaie A, Buresi M, Lembo A, et al. Hydrogen and methane-based breath testing in gastrointestinal disorders: the North American consensus. *Am J Gastroenterol.* 2017;112(5):775–784.

5. Schink M, Konturek PC, Tietz E, et al. Microbial patterns in patients with histamine intolerance. *J Physiol Pharmacol.* 2018;69(4).

6. Parodi A, Paolino S, Greco A, et al. Small intestinal bacterial overgrowth in rosacea: clinical effectiveness of its eradication. *Clin Gastroenterol Hepatol.* 2008;6(7):759–764.

7. Romani J, Caixa A, Escote X, et al. Lipopolysaccharide-binding protein is increased in patients with psoriasis with metabolic syndrome, and correlates with C-reactive protein. *Clin Exp Dermatol.* 2013;38(1):81–84. doi:10.1111/ced.12007.

8. Lee SY, Lee E, Park YM, Hong SJ. Microbiome in the gut-skin axis in atopic dermatitis. *Allergy Asthma Immunol Res.* 2018;10(4):354–362.

9. Augustyn M, Grys I, Kukla M. Small intestinal bacterial overgrowth and nonalcoholic fatty liver disease. *Clin Exp Hepatol.* 2019;5(1):1–10.

10. Fasano A, Bove F, Gabrielli M, et al. The role of small intestinal bacterial overgrowth in Parkinson's disease. *Mov Disord.* 2013;28(9):1241–1249.

11. Roland BC, Lee D, Miller LS, et al. Obesity increases the risk of small intestinal bacterial overgrowth (SIBO). *Neurogastroenterol Motil.* 2018;30(3). https://doi.org/10.1111/nmo.13199.

12. Ghoshal UC, Shukla R, Ghoshal U. Small intestinal bacterial overgrowth and irritable bowel syndrome: a bridge between functional organic dichotomy. *Gut Liver.* 2017;11(2):196–208.

13.Weinstock LB, Walters AS. Restless legs syndrome is associated with irritable bowel syndrome and small intestinal bacterial overgrowth. *Sleep Med.* 2011;12(6):610–613.

14. Chatterjee S, Park S, Low K, et al. The degree of breath methane production in IBS correlates with the severity of constipation. *Am J Gastroenterol.* 2007;102(4):837–841.

15. Pimentel M, Wallace D, Hallegua D, et al. A link between irritable bowel syndrome and fibromyalgia may be related to findings on lactulose breath testing. *Ann Rheum Dis.* 2004;63(4):450–452.

16. Su T, Lai S, Lee A, et al. Meta-analysis: proton pump inhibitors moderately increase the risk of small intestinal bacterial overgrowth. *J Gastroenterol.* 2018;53(1):27–36.

17. Muraki M, Fujiwara Y, Machida H, et al. Role of small intestinal bacterial overgrowth in severe small intestinal damage in chronic non-steroidal anti-inflammatory drug users. *Scand J Gastroenterol.* 2014;49(3):267–273.

18. Husebye E, Skar V, Hoverstad T, et al. Fasting hypochlorhydria with gram positive gastric flora is highly prevalent in healthy old people. *Gut.* 1992;33:1331–1337.

19. Lee AA, Baker JR, Wamsteker EJ, et al. Small intestinal bacterial overgrowth is common in chronic pancreatitis and associates with diabetes, chronic pancreatitis severity, low zinc levels, and opiate use. *Am J Gastroenterol.* 2019;114(7):1163–1171.

20. Lauritano EC, Bilotta AL, Gabrielli M, et al. Association between hypothyroidism and small intestinal bacterial overgrowth. *J Clin Endocrinol Metab.* 2007;92:4180–4184.

21. Brechmann T, Sperlbaum A, Schmiegel W. Levothyroxine therapy and impaired clearance are the strongest contributors to small intestinal bacterial overgrowth: results of a retrospective cohort study. *World J Gastroenterol.* 2017;23(5):842–852.

22. Dukowicz AC, Lacy BE, Levine GM. Small intestinal bacterial overgrowth: a comprehensive review. *Gastroenterol Hepatol* (NY). 2007;3(2):112–122.

23. Cox SR, Lindsay JO, Fromentin S, et al. Effects of low FODMAP diet on symptoms, fecal microbiome, and markers of inflammation in patients with quiescent inflammatory bowel disease in a randomized trial. *Gastroenterology.* 2020;158(1):176–188.

24. Roland BC, Lee D, Miller LS, et al. Obesity increases the risk of small intestinal bacterial overgrowth (SIBO). *Neurogastroenterol Motil.* 2018;30(3). https://doi.org/10.1111/nmo.13199.

25. Chakaroun RM, Massier L, Kovacs P. Gut microbiome, intestinal permeability, and tissue bacteria in metabolic disease: perpetrators or bystanders? *Nutrients.* 2020;12(4):1082.

26. Shah A, Talley NJ, Jones M, et al. Small intestinal bacterial overgrowth in irritable bowel syndrome: a systematic review and meta-analysis of case-control studies. *Am J Gastroenterol.* 2020;115:190–201.

27. Shah A, Morrison M, Burger D, et al. Systematic review with meta-analysis: the prevalence of small intestinal bacterial overgrowth in inflammatory bowel disease. *Aliment Pharmacol Ther.* 2019;49:624–635.

28. Losurdo G, D'Abramo FS, Indellicati G, et al. The influence of small intestinal bacterial overgrowth in digestive and extra-intestinal disorders. *Int J Mol Sci.* 2020;21(10):3531.

29. Weinstock LB, Steinhoff M. Rosacea and small intestinal bacterial overgrowth: prevalence and response to rifaximin. *J Am Acad Dermatol.* 2013;68:875–876.

30. Parodi A, Paolino S, Greco A, et al. Small intestinal bacterial overgrowth in rosacea: clinical effectiveness of its eradication. *Clin Gastroenterol Hepatol.* 2008;6(7):759–764.

31. Fu P, Gao M, Yung KKL. Association of intestinal disorders with Parkinson's disease and Alzheimer's disease: a systematic review and meta-analysis. *ACS Chem Neurosci.* 2020;11(3):395–405.

32. Blum DJ, During E, Barwick F, et al. Restless leg syndrome: does it start with a gut feeling? *Sleep.* 2019;42(1):A4.

33. Stevens BR, Goel R, Seungbum K, et al. Increased human intestinal barrier permeability plasma biomarkers zonulin and FABP2 correlated with plasma LPS and altered gut microbiome in anxiety or depression. *Gut.* 2018;67(8):1555–1557.

34. Rana SV, Sharma S, Kaur J, et al. Comparison of lactulose and glucose breath test for diagnosis of small intestinal bacterial overgrowth in patients with irritable bowel syndrome. *Digestion.* 2012;85(3):243–247.

35. Birg A, Hu S, Lin HC. Reevaluating our understanding of lactulose breath tests by incorporating hydrogen sulfide measurements. *JGH Open.* 2019;3(3):228–233.

36. Fasano A. Leaky gut and autoimmune diseases. *Clin Rev Allergy Immunol.* 2012;42(1):71–78.

37. Wang W, Uzzau S, Goldblum SE, Fasano A. Human zonulin, a potential modulator of intestinal tight junctions. *J Cell Sci.* 2000;113 Pt 24:4435–4440.

38. Olsen GJ. Microbial ecology. Archaea, Archaea, everywhere. *Nature.* 1994;371(6499):657–658.

39. Brugère JF, Borrel G, Gaci N, et al. Archaebiotics: proposed therapeutic use of Archaea to prevent trimethylaminuria and cardiovascular disease. *Gut Microbes.* 2014;5:5–10.

40. Lurie-Weinberger MN, Gophna U. Archaea in and on the human body: health implications and future directions. *PLoS Pathog.* 2015;11:e1004833.

41. Takakura W, Pimentel M. Small intestinal bacterial overgrowth and irritable bowel syndrome—an update. *Front Psychiatry.* 2020;11:664.

42. Zhang J, Wang X, Chen Y, Yao W. Exhaled hydrogen sulfide predicts airway inflammation phenotype in COPD. *Resp Care.* 2015;60(2):251–258.

43. Chedid V, Dhalla S, Clark JO, et al. Herbal therapy is equivalent to rifaximin for the treatment of small intestinal bacterial overgrowth. *Glob Adv Health Med.* 2014;3(3):16–24.

CHAPTER 7

1. Sam QH, Chang MW, Chai LYA. The fungal mycobiome and its interaction with gut bacteria in the host. *Int J Mol Sci.* 2017;18:330.

2. Downward JRE, Falkowski NR, Mason KL, et al. Modulation of post-antibiotic bacterial community reassembly and host response by *Candida albicans.* *Sci Rep.* 2013;3:2191.

3. Morales DK, Hogan DA. *Candida albicans* interactions with bacteria in the context of human health and disease. *PLoS Pathog.* 2010;6:e1000886.

4. Krüger W, Vielreicher S, Kapitan M, et al. Fungal-bacterial interactions in health and disease. *Pathogens.* 2019;8(2):70.

5. Sam QH, Chang MW, Chai LYA. The fungal mycobiome and its interaction with gut bacteria in the host. *Int J Mol Sci.* 2017;18:330.

6. Erdogan A, Rao SSC. Small intestinal fungal overgrowth. *Curr Gastroenterol Rep.* 2015;17(4):16.

7. Rao SSC, Tan G, Abdull H, et al. Does colectomy predispose to small intestinal bacterial (SIBO) and fungal overgrowth (SIFO)? *Clin Transl Gastroenterol.* 2018;9(4):146.

8. Mar Rodríguez M, Pérez D, Chaves FJ, et al. Obesity changes the human gut mycobiome. *Sci Rep.* 1015;5:14600.

9. Man A, Ciurea CN, Pasaroiu D, et al. New perspectives on the nutritional factors influencing growth rate of *Candida albicans* in diabetics. An *in vitro* study. *Mem Inst Oswaldo Cruz.* 2017;112(9):587–592.

10. Jacobs C, Adame EC, Attaluri A, et al. Dysmotility and ppi use are independent risk factors for small intestinal bacterial and/or fungal overgrowth. *Aliment Pharmacol Ther.* 2013;37(11):1103–1111.

11. Graf K, Last A, Gratz R, et al. Keeping *Candida* commensal: how lactobacilli antagonize pathogenicity of *Candida albicans* in an *in vitro* gut model. *Dis Model Mech.* 2019;12(9):dmm039719.

12. Leelahavanichkul A, Worasilchai N, Wannalerdsakun S, et al. Gastrointestinal leakage detected by serum (1→3)-β-D-glucan in mouse models and a pilot study in patients with sepsis. *Shock.* 2016;46(5):506–518.

13. Panpetch W, Hiengrach P, Nilgate S, et al. Additional *Candida albicans* administration enhances the severity of dextran sulfate solution induced colitis mouse model through leaky gut–enhanced systemic inflammation and gut-dysbiosis but attenuated by *Lactobacillus rhamnosus* L34. *Microbes*. 2019;1–16.

14. Iliev ID, Funari VA, Taylor KD, et al. Interactions between commensal fungi and the C-type lectin receptor Dectin–1 influence colitis. *Science*. 2012;336:1314–1317.

15. Alassane-Kpembi I, Pinton P, Oswald IP. Effects of mycotoxins on the intestine. *Toxins* (Basel). 2019;11(3):159.

16. Alonso R, Pisa D, Marina AI, et al. Fungal infection in patients with Alzheimer's disease. *J Alzheimers Dis*. 2014;41:301–311.

17. Alonso R, Pisa D, Rábano A, Carrasco L. Alzheimer's disease and disseminated mycoses. *J Clin Microbiol Infect Dis*. 2014;33(7):1125–1132.

18. Pisa D, Alonso R, Rábano A, Rodal I, Carrasco L. Different brain regions are infected with fungi in Alzheimer's disease. *Sci Rep*. 2015;5:15015.

19. Alonso R, Pisa D, Aguado R, Carrasco L. Identification of fungal species in brain tissue from Alzheimer's disease by next-generation sequencing. *J Alzheimers Dis*. 2017;58(1):55–67.

20. Soscia SJ, Kirby JE, Washicosky KJ, et al. The Alzheimer's disease–associated amyloid beta-protein is an antimicrobial peptide. *PLoS One*. 2010;5: e9505.

21. Vendrik KEW, Ooijevaar RE, de Jong PRC, et al. Fecal microbiota transplantation in neurological disorders. *Front Cell Infect Microbiol*. 2020;10:98.

22. Hu H, Merenstein DJ, Wang C, et al. Impact of eating probiotic yogurt on colonization by *Candida* species of the oral and vaginal mucosa in HIV-infected and HIV-uninfected women. *Mycopathologia*. 2013;176:175–181.

23. Lang A, Salomon N, Wu JCY, et al. Curcumin in combination with mesalamine induces remission in patients with mild-to-moderate ulcerative colitis in a randomized controlled trial. *Clin Gastroenterol Hepatol*. 2015;13(8):1444–1449.

24. Portincasa P, Bonfrate L, Scribano MLL. Curcumin and fennel essential oil improve symptoms and quality of life in patients with irritable bowel syndrome. *J Gastrointestin Liver Dis*. 2016;25(2):151–157.

25. Praditya D, Kirchhoff L, Bruning J, et al. Anti-infective properties of the golden spice curcumin. *Front Microbiol*. 2019;10:912.

26. Ghosh SS, He H, Wang J, et al. Curcumin-mediated regulation of intestinal barrier function: the mechanism underlying its beneficial effects. *Tissue Barriers*. 2018;6(1):e1425085.

27. Zhang X, Zhao Y, Zhang M, et al. Structural changes of gut microbiota during berberine-mediated prevention of obesity and insulin resistance in high-fat diet–fed rats. *PLoS One*. 2012;7(8):e42529.

28. Zhu L, Zhang D, Zhu H, et al. Berberine treatment increases *Akkermansia* in the gut and improves high-fat diet–induced atherosclerosis in Apoe -/- mice. *Atherosclerosis.* 2018;268:117–126.

29. D'agostino M, Tesse N, Frippiat JP, et al. Essential oils and their natural active compounds presenting anti fungal properties. *Molecules.* 2019;24(20):3713.

30. Limon JJ, Skalski JH, Underhill DM. Commensal fungi in health and disease. *Cell Host Microbe.* 2017;22(2):156–165.

31. Arena MP, Capozzi V, Russo P, et al. Immunobiosis and probiosis: antimicrobial activity of lactic acid bacteria with a focus on their antiviral and antifungal properties. *Appl Microbiol Biotechnol.* 2018;102(23):9949–9958.

32. Mailander-Sanchez D, Braunsdorf C, Grumaz C, et al. Antifungal defense of probiotic *Lactobacillus rhamnosus* GG is mediated by blocking adhesion and nutrient depletion. *PLoS One.* 2017;12(10):e0184438.

CHAPTER 8

1. Chedid V, Dhalla S, Clarke JO, et al. Herbal therapy is equivalent to rifaximin for the treatment of small intestinal bacterial overgrowth. *Glob Adv Health Med.* 2014;3(3):16–24.

2. Mu Q, Tavella VJ, Luo XM. Role of *Lactobacillus reuteri* in human health and disease. *Front Microbiol.* 2018;9:757.

3. Ojetti V, Petruzziello C, Migneco A, et al. Effect of *Lactobacillus reuteri* (DSM 17938) on methane production in patients affected by functional constipation: a retrospective study. *Eur Rev Med Pharmacol Sci.* 2017;21(7):1702–1708.

4. Selle K, Klaenhammner TR. Genomic and phenotypic evidence for probiotic influences of *Lactobacillus gasseri* on human health. *FEMS Microbiol Rev.* 2013;37(6):915–935.

5. Dolin BJ. Effects of a proprietary *Bacillus coagulans* preparation on symptoms of diarrhea-predominant irritable bowel syndrome. *Methods Find Exp Clin Pharmacol.* 2009;31(10):655–659.

6. Moghadamtousi SZ, Kadir HA, Hassandarvish P, et al. A review on antibacterial, antiviral, and antifungal activity of curcumin. *Biomed Res Int.* 2014;2014:186864.

7. Zhang X, Zhao Y, Zhang M, et al. Structural changes of gut microbiota during berberine-mediated prevention of obesity and insulin resistance in high-fat diet–fed rats. *PLoS One.* 2012;7(8):e42529.

8. D'agostino M, Tesse N, Frippiat JP, et al. Essential oils and their natural active compounds presenting antifungal properties. *Molecules.* 2019;24(20):3713.

9. Pais P, Almeida V, Yilmaz M, Teixeira MC. *Saccharomyces boulardii*: What makes it tick as successful probiotic? *J Fungi* (Basel). 2020;6(2):78.

10. Kabak B, Dobson ADW. Mycotoxins in spices and herbs—an update. *Crit Rev Food Sci Nutr.* 2017;57(1):18–34.

11. Enko D, Kriegshauser G. Functional ^{13}C-urea and glucose hydrogen/methane breath tests reveal significant association of small intestinal bacterial overgrowth in individuals with active *Helicobacter pylori* infection. *Clin Biochem.* 2017;50(1–2):46–49.

12. Lauritano EC, Bilotta AL, Gabriella M, et al. Association between hypothyroidism and small intestinal bacterial overgrowth. *J Clin Endocrinol Metab.* 2007;92(11):4180–4184.

CHAPTER 9

1. Burger-van Paassen N, Vincent A, Puiman PJ, et al. The regulation of intestinal mucin MUC2 expression by short-chain fatty acids: implications for epithelial protection. *Biochem J.* 2001;420(2):211–219.

2. Rowland I, Gibson G, Heineken A, et al. Gut microbiota functions: metabolism of nutrients and other food components. *Eur J Nutr.* 2018;57(1):1–24.

3. Magnusdottir S, Ravcheev D, Crecy-Lagard V, Thiele I. Systematic genome assessment of B-vitamin biosynthesis suggests co-operation among gut microbes. *Front Genet.* 2015;6:148.

4. Frese SA, Hutton AA, Contreras LN, et al. Persistence of supplemented *Bifidobacterium longum* subsp. infantis EVC001 in breastfed infants. *mSphere.* 2017;2(6):e00501–e00517.

5. Underwood MA, German JB, Lebrilla CB, Mills DA. *Bifidobacterium longum* subspecies infantis: champion colonizer of the infant gut. *Pediatr Res.* 2015;77(1–2):229–235.

6. Nilsson AG, Sundh D, Backhed F, Lorentzon M. *Lactobacillus reuteri* reduces bone loss in older women with low bone mineral density: a randomized, placebo-controlled, double-blind, clinical trial. *J Intern Med.* 2018;284(3):307–317.

7. Levkovich T, Poutahidis T, Smillie C, et al. Probiotic bacteria induce a "glow of health." *PLoS One.* 2013;8(1):e53867.

8. Kim J, Yun JM, Kim MK, et al. *Lactobacillus gasseri* BNR17 supplementation reduces the visceral fat accumulation and waist circumference in obese adults: a randomized, double-blind, placebo-controlled trial. *J Med Food.* 2018;21(5):454–461.

9. Mailander-Sanchez D, Braunsdorf C, Grumaz C, et al. Antifungal defense of probiotic *Lactobacillus rhamnosus* GG is mediated by blocking adhesion and nutrient depletion. *PLoS One.* 2017;12(10):e0184438.

10. Ducrotté P, Sawant P, Venkataraman J. Clinical trial: *Lactobacillus plantarum* 299v (DSM 9843) improves symptoms of irritable bowel syndrome. *J World J Gastroenterol.* 2012;18(30):4012–4018.

11. Miquel S, Martín R, Rossi O, et al. *Faecalibacterium prausnitzii* and human intestinal health. *Curr Opin Microbiol.* 2013;16(3):255–261.

12. Toscano M, De Grandi R, Stronati L, et al. Effect of *Lactobacillus rhamnosus* HN001 and *Bifidobacterium longum* BB536 on the healthy gut microbiota composition at phyla and species level: a preliminary study. *World J Gastroenterol.* 2017;23(15):2696–2704.

13. Everard A, Belzer C, Geurts L. Cross-talk between *Akkermansia muciniphila* and intestinal epithelium controls diet-induced obesity. *Proc Natl Acad Sci.* 2013;110(22):9066–9071.

14. Nyangale EP, Farmer S, Cash HA, et al. *Bacillus coagulans* GBI-30, 6086 modulates *Faecalibacterium prausnitzii* in older men and women. *J Nutr.* 2015;145(7):1446–1452.

15. Imidi E, Cox SR, Rossi M, Whelan K. Fermented foods: definitions and characteristics, impact on the gut microbiota and effects on gastrointestinal health and disease. *Nutrients.* 2019;11(8):1806.

16. Gille D, Schmid A, Walther B, Verkehres G. Fermented food and non-communicable chronic diseases: a review. *Nutrients.* 2018;10(4):448.

17. Jeong D, Kim DH, Kang IB. Modulation of gut microbiota and increase in fecal water content in mice induced by administration of *Lactobacillus kefiranofaciens* DN1. *Food Funct.* 2017;8(2):680–686.

18. David LA, Maurice CF, Carmody RN, et al. Diet rapidly and reproducibly alters the human gut microbiome. *Nature.* 2013;505:559–563.

19. Sonnenburg ED, Smits SA, Tikhonov M, et al. Diet-induced extinctions in the gut microbiota compound over generations. *Nature.* 2016;529(7585):212–215.

20. Krumbeck J, Maldonado-Gomez MX, Ramer-Tait AE, Hutkins RW. Prebiotics and synbiotics: dietary strategies for improving gut health. *Curr Opin Gastroenterol.* 2016;32:110–119.

21. De Filippo C, Cavalieri D, Di Paola M, et al. Impact of diet in shaping gut microbiota revealed by a comparative study in children from Europe and rural Africa. *Proc Natl Acad Sci U S A.* 2010;107(33):14691–14696.

22. Olson CA, Vuong HE, Yano JM, et al. The gut microbiota mediates the anti-seizure effects of the ketogenic diet. *Cell.* 2018;173(7):1728–1741.

23. Zhang Y, Zhou S, Zhou Y, et al. Altered gut microbiome composition in children with refractory epilepsy after ketogenic diet. *Epilepsy Res.* 2018;145:163–168.

24. Lindefeldt M, Eng A, Darban H, et al. The ketogenic diet influences taxonomic and function composition of the gut microbiota in children with severe epilepsy. *NPJ Biofilms Microbiomes.* 2019;5:5.

25. Ulamek-Koziol M, Czuczwar SJ, Januszewski S, Pluta R. Ketogenic diet and epilepsy. *Nutrients.* 2019;11(10):2510.

26. Murtaza N, Burke LM, Vlahovich N, et al. The effects of dietary pattern during intensified training on stool microbiota of elite race walkers. *Nutrients.* 2019;11(2):261.

27. Ang QY, Alexander M, Newman JC, et al. Ketogenic diets alter the gut microbiome resulting in decreased intestinal Th17 cells. *Cell.* 2020;181(6):1263–1275.

28. Lindefeldt M, Eng A, Darban H, et al. The ketogenic diet influences taxonomic and function composition of the gut microbiota in children with severe epilepsy. *NPJ Biofilms Microbiomes.* 2019;5:5.

29. Kossoff EH, Zupec-Kania BA, Auvin S, et al. Optimal clinical management of children receiving dietary therapies for epilepsy: updated recommendations of the International Ketogenic Diet Study Group. *Epilepsia Open.* 2018;3(2):175–192.

CHAPTER 10

1. Yamamoto EA, Jorgensen TN. Relationships between vitamin D, gut microbiome, and systemic autoimmunity. *Front Immunol.* 2019;10:3141.

2. Assa A, Vong L, Pinnell LJ, et al. Vitamin D deficiency predisposes to adherent-invasive *Escherichia coli*–induced barrier dysfunction and experimental colonic injury. *Inflamm Bowel Dis.* 2015;21(2):297–306.

3. Assa A, Vong L, Pinnell LJ, et al. Vitamin D deficiency promotes epithelial barrier dysfunction and intestinal inflammation. *J Infect Dis.* 2014;210(8):1296–1305.

4. Ooi JH, Li Y, Rogers CJ, Cantoma MT. Vitamin D regulates the gut microbiome and protects mice from dextran sodium sulfate–induced colitis. *J Nutr.* 2013;143(10):1679–1686.

5. Su D, Nie Y, Zhu A, et al. Vitamin D signaling through induction of paneth cell defensins maintains gut microbiota and improves metabolic disorders and hepatic steatosis in animal models. *Front Physiol.* 2016;7:498.

6. Payahoo L, Khajebishak Y, Alivand MR, et al. Investigation of the effect of oleoylethanolamide supplementation on the abundance of *Akkermansia muciniphila* bacterium and the dietary intakes in people with obesity: a randomized clinical trial. *Appetite.* 2019;141:104301.

7. Millman J, Okamoto S, Kimura A, et al. Metabolically and immunologically beneficial impact of extra virgin olive and flaxseed oils on composition of gut microbiota in mice. *Eur J Nutr.* 2020;59(6):2411–2425.

8. Nazzaro F, Fratianni F, Cozzolino R, et al. Antibacterial activity of three extra virgin olive oils of the Campania region, Southern Italy, related to their polyphenol content and composition. *Microorganisms.* 2019;7(9):321.

9. Farras M, Martinez-Gili L, Portune K, et al. Modulation of the gut microbiota by olive oil phenolic compounds: implications for lipid metabolism, immune system, and obesity. *Nutrients.* 2020;12(8):2200.

10. Kaliannan K, Wang B, Li X-Y, et al. A host-microbiome interaction mediates the opposing effects of omega-6 and omega-3 fatty acids on metabolic endotoxemia. *Sci Rep.* 2015;5:11276.

11. Kaliannan K, Wang B, Li X-Y, et al. Omega-3 fatty acids prevent early-life antibiotic exposure–induced gut microbiota dysbiosis and later-life obesity. *Int J Obes* (London). 2016;40(6):1039–1042.

12. Lauritano EC, Bilotta AL, Gabrielli M, et al. Association between hypothyroidism and small intestinal bacterial overgrowth. *J Clin Endocrinol Metab.* 2007;92:4180–4184.

13. Roopchand DE, Carmody RN, Kuhn P, et al. Dietary polyphenols promote growth of the gut bacterium *Akkermansia muciniphila* and attenuate high-fat diet–induced metabolic syndrome. *Diabetes.* 2015;64(8):2847–2858.

14. Yuan X, Long Y, Ji Z, et al. Green tea liquid consumption alters the human intestinal and oral microbiome. *Mol Nutr Food Res.* 2018;62(12):e1800178.

15. Georgiades P, Pudney PDA, Rogers S, et al. Tea derived galloylated polyphenols cross-link purified gastrointestinal mucins. *PLoS One.* 2014;9(8):e105302.

16. Lu QY, Summanen PH, Lee RP, et al. Prebiotic potential and chemical composition of seven culinary spice extracts. *J Food Sci.* 2017;82(8):1807–1813.

17. Liu Q, Meng X, Li Y, et al. Antibacterial and antifungal activities of spices. *Int J Mol Sci.* 2017;18(6):1283.

18. Wlodarska M, Willing BP, Bravo DM, Finlay BB. Phytonutrient diet supplementation promotes beneficial Clostridia species and intestinal mucus secretion resulting in protection against enteric infection. *Sci Rep.* 2015;5:9253.

19. Kang C, Zhang Y, Zhu X, et al. Healthy subjects differentially respond to dietary capsaicin correlating with specific gut enterotypes. *J Clin Endocrin Metab.* 2016;101(12):4681–4689.

20. Valim TC, da Cunha DA, Francisco CS, et al. Quantification of capsaicinoids from chili peppers using 1H NMR without deuterated solvent. *Analytical Meth.* 2019;11(14):1939–1950.

21. Ghosh SS, Bie J, Wang J, Ghosh S. Oral supplementation with nonabsorbable antibiotics or curcumin attenuates Western diet–induced atherosclerosis and glucose intolerance in LDLR-/- mice—role of intestinal permeability and macrophages activation. *PLoS One.* 2014;9(9):e108577.

22. Zhang X, Zhao Y, Zhang M, et al. Structural changes of gut microbiota during berberine-mediated prevention of obesity and insulin resistance in high-fat diet–fed rats. *PLoS One.* 2012;7(8):e42529.

23. Zhu L, Zhang D, Zhu H, et al. Berberine treatment increases *Akkermansia* in the gut and improves high-fat diet–induced atherosclerosis in Apoe -/- mice. *Atherosclerosis.* 2018;268:117–126.

PART IV

1. Thaiss CA, Levy M, Grosheva I, et al. Hyperglycemia drives intestinal barrier dysfunction and risk for enteric infection. *Science.* 2018;359(6382):1376–1383.

2. Wang W, Uzzau S, Goldblum SE, Fasano A. Human zonulin, a potential modulator of intestinal tight junctions. *J Cell Sci.* 2000;113 Pt 24:4435–4440.

3. Zioudrou C, Streaty RA, Klee WA. Opioid peptides derived from food proteins: the exorphins. *J Biol Chem.* 1979;254(7):2446–2449.

4. Pusztai A, Ewen SW, Grant G, et al. Antinutritive effects of wheat-germ agglutinin and other N-acetylglucosamine-specific lectins. *Br J Nutr.* 1993;70(1):313–321.

5. Junker Y, Zeissig S, Kim SJ, et al. Wheat amylase trypsin inhibitors drive intestinal inflammation via activation of toll-like receptor 4. *J Exp Med.* 2012;209(13):2395–2408.

6. Bonder MJ, Tigchelaar EF, Xianghang C, et al. The influence of a short-term gluten-free diet on the human gut microbiome. *Genome Med.* 2016;8:45.

7. Wlodarska M, Willing BP, Bravo DM, Finlay BB. Phytonutrient diet supplementation promotes beneficial Clostridia species and intestinal mucus secretion resulting in protection against enteric infection. *Sci Rep.* 2015;5:9253.

8. Georgiades P, Pudney PDA, Rogers S, et al. Tea derived galloyl-ated polyphenols cross-link purified gastrointestinal mucins. *PLoS ONE.* 2014;9(8):e105302.

9. De Vos W. Microbe profile: *Akkermansia muciniphila*: a conserved intestinal symbiont that acts as the gatekeeper of our mucosa. *Microbiology* (Reading). 2017;163(5):646–648.

10. Stacy A, Andrade-Oliveira V, McCulloch JA, et al. Infection trains the host for microbiota-enhanced resistance to pathogens. *Cell.* 2021;184(3):615–627.

11. Stinton LM, Shaffer EA. Epidemiology of gallbladder disease: cholelithiasis and cancer. *Gut Liver.* 2012;6(2):172–187.

12. Festi D, Colecchia A, Orsini M, et al. Gallbladder motility and gallstone formation in obese patients following very low calorie diets. Use it (fat) to lose it (well). *Int J Obes Relat Metab Disord.* 1998;22(6):592–600.

13. Gebhard RL, Prigge WF, Ansel HJ, et al. The role of gallbladder emptying in gallstone formation during diet-induced rapid weight loss. *Hepatology.* 1996;24(3):544–548.

14. Festi D, Colecchia A, Larocca A, et al. Review: low caloric intake and gall-bladder motor function. *Aliment Pharmacol Ther.* 2000;14(suppl 2):51–53.

15. Damm I, Mikkat U, Kirchhoff F, et al. Inhibitory effect of the lectin wheat germ agglutinin on the binding of 125I-CCK-8s to the CCK-A and -B receptors of AR42J cells. *Pancreas.* 2004;28(1):31–37.

16. Wong JM, Jenkins DJ. Carbohydrate digestibility and metabolic effects. *J Nutr.* 2007;137 (suppl 11):2539S–2546S.

17. Slavin J. Fiber and probiotics: mechanisms and health benefits. *Nutrients.* 2013;5(4):1417–1435.

18. Murphy MM, Douglass JS, Birkett A. Resistant starch intakes in the United States. *J Am Diet Assn.* 2008;108(1):67–78.

19. Dreher ML. Whole fruits and fruit fiber emerging health effects. *Nutrients.* 2018;10(12):1833.

20. Lamuel-Raventos RM, St. Onge M-P. Prebiotic nut compounds and human microbiota. *Crit Rev Food Sci Nutr.* 2017;57(14):3154–3163.

21. De Bruyne T, Steenput B, Roth L, et al. Dietary polyphenols targeting arterial stiffness: interplay of contributing mechanisms and gut microbiome-related metabolism. *Nutrients.* 2019;11(3):578.

22. Van Hul M, Cani PD. Targeting carbohydrates and polyphenols for a healthy microbiome and healthy weight. *Curr Nutr Rep.* 2019;8(4):307–316.

23. Wang S, Yao J, Zhou B. Bacteriostatic effect of quercetin as an antibiotic alternative *in vivo* and its antibacterial mechanism *in vitro. J Food Prot.* 2018;81(1):68–78.

24. Wlodarska M, Willing BP, Bravo DM, Finlay BB. Phytonutrient diet supplementation promotes beneficial Clostridia species and intestinal mucus secretion resulting in protection against enteric infection. *Sci Rep.* 2015;5:9253.

25. Payahoo L, Khajebishak Y, Alivand MR, et al. Investigation of the effect of oleoylethanolamide supplementation on the abundance of *Akkermansia muciniphila* bacterium and the dietary intakes in people with obesity: a randomized clinical trial. *Appetite.* 2019;141:104301.

26. Varian BJ, Poutahidis T, DiBenedictis BT, et al. Microbial lysate upregulates host oxytocin. *Brain Behav Immun.* 2017;61:36–49.

27. Takada M, Nishida K, Kataoka-Kato A, et al. Probiotic *Lactobacillus casei* strain Shirota relieves stress-associated symptoms by modulating the gut-brain interaction in human and animal models. *Neurogastroenterol Motil.* 2016;28(7):1027–1036.

28. Messaoudi M, Lalonde R, Violle N, et al. Assessment of psychotropic-like properties of a probiotic formulation (*Lactobacillus helveticus* R0052 and *Bifidobacterium longum* R0175) in rats and human subjects. *Br J Nutr.* 2011;105(5):755–764.

SUPER GUT RECIPES

1. Poutahidis T, Kearney SM, Levkovich T, et al. Microbial symbionts accelerate wound healing via the neuropeptide hormone oxytocin. *PLoS One.* 2013;8(10):e78898.

2. Varian BJ, Poutahidis T, DiBenedictis BT, et al. Microbial lysate upregulates host oxytocin. *Brain Behav Immun.* 2017;61:36–49.

3. Jäger R, Shields KA, Lowery RP, et al. Probiotic *Bacillus coagulans* GBI-30,6086 reduces exercise-induced muscle damage and increases recovery. *Peer J.* 2016;4:e2276.

4. Mandel DR, Eichas K, Holmes J. *Bacillus coagulans*: a viable adjunct therapy for relieving symptoms of rheumatoid arthritis according to a randomized, controlled trial. *BMC Complement Altern Med.* 2010;10:1.

5. Kim J, Yun JM, Kim MK, et al. *Lactobacillus gasseri* BNR17 supplementation reduces the visceral fat accumulation and waist circumference in obese adults: a randomized, double-blind, placebo-controlled trial. *J Med Food.* 2018;21(5):454–461.

6. Shida K, Sato T, Iizuka R, et al. Daily intake of fermented milk with *Lactobacillus casei* strain Shirota reduces the incidence and duration of upper respiratory tract infections in healthy middle-aged office workers. *Eur J Nutr.* 2017;56(1):45–53.

7. Underwood MA, German JB, Lebrilla CB, Mills DA. *Bifidobacterium longum* subspecies infantis: champion colonizer of the infant gut. *Pediatr Res.* 2015;77(1–2):229–235.

8. Messaoudi M, Lalonde R, Violle N, et al. Assessment of psychotropic-like properties of a probiotic formulation (*Lactobacillus helveticus* R0052 and *Bifidobacterium longum* R0175) in rats and human subjects. *Br J Nutr.* 2011;105(5):755–764.

INDEX

acetaminophen, 178
agave nectar, 177
age reversal, 286
AIRE device, 78, 112–116
Akkermansia, 15, 51, 52, 54, 104, 157, 158, 162, 163, 170, 211, 213, 247
Akkermansia muciniphila, 32, 41, 50, 146, 158, 211
alcohol, 39, 140
alkaline phosphatase, 41
Alonso, Ruth, 99
Alzheimer's dementia, 74, 99, 106
Alzheimer's disease, 120
anthocyanins, 212
antibiotics, 178
    children receiving, 18
    exposure to, 140
    herbal, 116–119, 123
    mucus-disruptive effects of, 57
anxiety, 74, 120, 211
Asparagus, Leek, and White Bean Quiche, 267–269
autoimmune diseases, 10, 17, 30, 57, 73, 120, 154, 155

Bacillus coagulans, 89, 90, 122, 143, 146, 221, 230, 233–234, 256

bacteriocins, 29
Beef Shawarma with Super Gut Tzatziki, 265–266
benefits of Super Gut program, 219–225
    for athletes, 224
    deeper sleep, 220
    enhanced immunity, 224–225
    enhanced mental clarity, 221
    increased muscle and strength, 223
    for pregnant mothers, 224
    reduced inflammation, 221
    reduced stress, 221
    smoother skin, 220
    weight loss, 223
berberine, 103–104, 124, 160, 169–170
beverages and smoothies (recipes), 244–250
    Clove Green Tea, 246–247
    Ginger Snap Smoothie, 245–246
    Gingerbread Coffee, 249
    Matcha, Mint, and Blueberry Frozen Smoothie, 247–248
    Matcha Strawberry Key Lime Smoothie, 244–245
    Mocha Mint Kefir, 248–249

beverages and smoothies (recipes),
  [*continued*]
  Raspberry Lime Yogurt Smoothie
    for Smoother Skin, 249–250
  Strawberry, Carrot, and Dandelion
    Greens Prebiotic Smoothie, 244
Bifidobacterium, 15, 17, 23, 43, 51, 142,
    147, 148, 157, 163, 167, 202, 284
Bifidobacterium breve, 201
Bifidobacterium lactis, 201
Bifidobacterium longum, 41, 71, 145,
    166, 201, 221, 230
Bifidobacterium infantis, 17, 24, 25, 145,
    141, 216, 224, 224, 236–237, 243
bile production, 129
biliary tract cancer, 30
BioK⁺, 38
biome, rebuilding of, 135–158
  alcohol, 140
  bacterial hunger strike, 155–158
  bowel flora, 136–137
  drinking water, 139
  factors you can change, 137–140
  fermentation, 147, 151–152
  fiber, 154–155
  important species, 145–146
  management practices, 141–148
  mathematical phenomenon, 149–151
  noncaloric sweeteners, 138
  NSAIDs, 140
  organic foods, 139
  prebiotics, probiotics versus,
    147–148
  probiotics, 141
  processed foods, 138
  refrigeration, 152
  strain specificity, 143
  success story, 152–153
  sugars, 138
  wheat, 139
bisphenol A (BPA), 43
Blaser, Martin, 31
blood pressure, 165, 180
blood sugar
  normal, 179–181

reduced, 165
regulation of, 211
bowel power, 159–171
  berberine, 169–170
  capsaicin, 168
  challenge, 170
  conditions reversed, 171
  curcumin, 169
  flavonoids, 164–165
  fructooligosaccharide, 165
  goals, 159
  herbs and spices, 167–168
  iodine, 163–164
  oleic acid, 162
  olive oil, 161–162
  omega-3 fatty acids, 160, 162–163
  polyphenols, 164–165
  restoration, 171
  unsymbolized thinking, 165–166
  vitamin D, 160–161
BPA. *See* bisphenol A
brown sugar, 177
butyrate, 211

Campylobacter, 75
CandiBactin-AR/CandiBactin-BR
  regimen, 85, 105, 116
Candida, 106, 125, 199
Candida albicans, 11, 86, 94, 104, 170,
    227
Candida glabrata, 11, 94
Cani, Patrice, 65
cannabidiol (CBD), 162
Cano, Raul, 143
capsaicin, 168, 213–214
carbohydrates, 56, 155, 178, 208
carboxymethylcellulose, 55, 56, 88,
    177
carrageenan, 177
casein beta A1, 228
catechins, 212
CBD. *See* cannabidiol
CCK. *See* cholecystokinin
CDC. *See* Centers for Disease
  Control and Prevention

celiac disease, 54, 120
Centers for Disease Control and
    Prevention (CDC), 5
cervical cancer, 96
Cesarean sections (C-section), 13
CFUs. *See* colony-forming units
Chassaing, Benoit, 55
chlorpyrifos, 43
Chocolate Chip Frozen Yogurt, 270
cholecystokinin (CCK), 183
cholesterol, 5, 39, 64, 179
ciprofloxacin, 282
Citrobacter, 15
Clostridium difficile, 37, 123, 167
Clove Green Tea, 246–247
coconut milk (recipe), 241–242
coconut sugar, 177
colon cancer, 63, 96 165
colony-forming units (CFUs), 95,
    141, 105
colorectal cancer, 120
colorful compounds (vegetables and
    fruit), 211–212
Cooper, Bradley, 285
coronary artery disease, 62
COVID-19, 64
C-reactive protein, 9
Cream of Mushroom Soup, 255
Crohn's disease, 14, 36, 54, 56, 71, 95,
    120
curcumin, 101–103, 104, 124, 160,
    169, 192–193, 212
Curried Cauliflower with Peas, 254

dairy products, issues with, 228
Dandelion Greens and Raw Potato
    Salad with Avocado Lime
    Dressing, 258
dementia, 63
Dengue fever, 135
dental decay, 44–45
depression, 9, 19, 74, 120, 221
desserts (recipes), 270–274
    Chocolate Chip Frozen Yogurt,
    270

One-Minute Strawberry Ice Cream,
    271
Orange Clove Scones, 271–272
Raspberry Cream Pie, 273–274
Desulfovibrio, 84, 156
dextrose, 177
DHA, 188
diabetes
    type 1, 73, 79
    type 2, 10, 11, 30, 36, 39, 40, 43, 56,
    61, 73, 90, 119, 171, 284
diclofenac, 56
die-off reaction, 86, 117
dietary fat, 39–41
disaccharides, 71
disappearing microbiome, 4
diseases of civilization, 4
diverticular disease, 19, 63, 120
DNA markers, 22
drinking water, 139, 178
dysbiosis, 12, 31, 40, 42, 54, 56, 84, 95,
    183, 196

emulsifiers, 55–56, 138
emulsifying agents, 177
endocannabinoid, 162
endotoxemia, 19, 57
    bacterial overpopulation and, 10
    LPS and, 8, 10, 81
    main driver of, 8
Enterococcus 11, 121
EPA, 188
epigallocatechin, 165, 212
Escherichia coli, 8, 23, 32, 45, 65, 75, 86,
    94, 156, 161, 184
essential oils, 104–105, 124–125
eugenol, 53, 104, 167, 213
Evivo, 224
extremophiles, 82

Faecalibacterium prausnitzii, 71, 145,
    157, 168, 211, 213
fatty liver, 19, 40, 62, 73, 75, 186
FC-Cidal/Dysbiocide regimen, 85,
    105, 116, 123

fecalization, 35–45, 54, 121
    antibiotics and, 36–37
    causes of, 35
    Clostridium difficile, 37–38
    coprolites, 44
    dental decay and, 44–45
    description of, 35
    dietary fat, 39–41
    disruptive chemicals and, 43
    Enterobacteriaceae species,
        overproliferation of, 45
    factors disrupting bowel flora, 39
    fecal transplants, 38
    herbicides and pesticides and, 42
    trimethylamine oxide, 42
fermentation, 241
    -friendly food, 243
    prebiotic fiber and, 217
    projects, 230
    vegetable, 202–204
fermented foods, 147, 197
Fermented Roasted Peppers, 256–257
fiber, 154–155
fibromyalgia, 10, 49, 62, 65, 75, 90,
    119, 136
fish oil, 188
flavonoids, 164–165
flours and meals (alternative),
    190–191
flow cytometry, 228
FODMAPs, 71, 78, 115
food intolerances, 69, 284
foods, frequently used, 277–278
Ford, Henry, 283
FOS. *See* fructooligosaccharide
fructooligosaccharide (FOS), 165,
    187, 207, 213, 246
fruits, pureed (recipe), 243

gallstones, 10, 178, 183–184
garam masala, 265
gastrointestinal (GI) tract, 3–12
    antibiotics and, 36–37
    bacterial colonization of, 18

bacterial species feeding on mucus
    lining of, 32
bacterial species occupying
    unexpected locations, 11
CT scan of, 35
depression and, 9
disappearing microbiome, 4
diseases of civilization, 4
effect of fats on, 41
health epidemic, 5
inflammation and, 9
metabolic endotoxemia, 8
microorganisms, evolution of, 4
natural antibiotics in, 29
rosacea and, 19
small intestine, 5–9
species of bowel flora in, 15
violent coup in, 45
gastrointestinal (GI) tract, mucus
    lining of, 47–57
    Akkermansia, 51, 52–53
    antibiotics, 57
    bacterial digestion, 48
    colon, 49
    dietary factors, mucus production
        and, 53
    emulsifying agents, 55–56
    eugenol, 53
    fiber in diet, 49–51
    green tea catechins, 54
    importance of mucus, 47–48
    motile bacteria, 54
    mucus-disrupting factors, 56
    prebiotic fiber, 48
    production of mucus, 51
GI tract. *See* gastrointestinal tract
Ginger Chicken, 261–262
Ginger Snap Smoothie, 245–246
Gingerbread Coffee, 249
gliadin, 70, 80, 182, 223
glucomannan powder, 210
glucose, 76
glyphosate, 14, 15, 19, 32, 42, 43, 63,
    286

goiters, 164
grand mal seizures, 157
green tea, 160
    catechins, 54, 165, 211, 212
    polyphenols, 165

Hadza (Tanzanian), 23, 136, 285
Hashimoto's thyroiditis, 49, 61, 65
heart disease, 8, 42, 179
Helicobacter pylori, 30–31, 70, 87, 128, 129
hemoglobin A1c (HbA1c) test, 170
herbal antibiotics, 116–119, 123
Herbed Focaccia Bread, 252–253
herbicides
    glyphosate, 14, 15, 19, 32, 42, 43
    Roundup, 32
herbs and spices, 167–168
Herxheimer, Karl, 86
high-fructose corn syrup, 177
High-Potency Probiotic Yogurt, 239
Homo sapiens, 30, 48
Hot Chili Fries, 253–254
Hulberg, Russell, 165
hummus (recipe), 243
hunter-gatherers, 23, 44, 190, 207
hydroxytyrosols, 212
hypertension, 96
hypothyroidism, 70, 164, 189

IBS. *See* irritable bowel syndrome
IBS-D. *See* irritable bowel syndrome with diarrhea
ibuprofen, 56, 178
indomethacin, 56
infant's microbiome. *See* microbiome (maternal)
inflammation, 103
    endotoxemia and, 19
    GI tract and, 9
    rise of, 57
inflammatory bowel disease, 56, 73
inner extinction event. *See* lost microbes

inner primate. *See* biome, rebuilding
insomnia, 176–177
insulin resistance, 43, 56, 178, 185
intelligence quotient (IQ), 17
intestinal alkaline phosphatase, 163
iodine, 163–164, 185, 189
irritable bowel syndrome (IBS), 10, 15, 54, 71, 73, 75, 95, 120, 136
irritable bowel syndrome with diarrhea (IBS-D), 81
Italian Sausage Soup, 262–263

Jarisch, Adolf, 86
Jarisch-Herxheimer reaction, 86, 116

kefir, 200–202
ketogenic diets, 157
ketones, 156
Klebsiella, 8, 15, 45, 67, 85, 86, 104, 170, 184, 196
Kluyveromyces, 199

lactic acid, 147, 151, 217
Lactobacillus, 15, 17, 23, 32, 43, 51, 67, 100, 147, 148, 167, 284
Lactobacillus acidophilus, 200, 201
Lactobacillus brevis, 202
Lactobacillus bulgaricus, 200, 228
Lactobacillus casei, 200, 201, 215, 235
Lactobacillus cremoris, 201
Lactobacillus delbrueckii, 201
Lactobacillus gasseri, 87, 89, 121, 145, 196, 216, 220, 230, 234–235
Lactobacillus helveticus, 166, 215, 221, 237, 247
Lactobacillus lactis, 201
Lactobacillus paracasei, 201
Lactobacillus plantarum, 24, 145, 201, 202
Lactobacillus reuteri, 25, 83, 89, 110, 121, 145, 166, 196, 201, 215, 216, 232–233
Lactobacillus rhamnosus, 105, 125, 144, 145, 201

lactose, 148, 217, 228, 241
lactulose, 76
lecithin, 177
Leuconostoc, 147
Leuconostoc mesenteroides, 201 202
levothyroxine, 70
life quality, goal of improving, 285
lipopolysaccharide (LPS), 8
    artificial increase in, 9
    chlorpyrifos and, 43
    curcumin and, 169
    disabling of, 163
    endotoxemia and, 8, 10, 81, 169
    endotoxin, 9, 86, 166
    intestinal permeability to, 80
    psychological issues and, 74
    SIBO and, 65
lost microbes, 21–33
    ancient microbiomes, 22
    Bifidobacterium infantis, 24–25
    DNA identification methods, 22
    Helicobacter pylori, 30–31
    hunter-gatherers, 23
    inner extinction event, 21
    Lactobacillus reuteri, 25–29
    Oxalobacter species, 24
    oxytocin, 26–28
    replacement of lost species, 24
    success story, 29
    vanished species, 23
Lou Gehrig's disease, 100
LPS. *See* lipopolysaccharide

magnesium supplementation, 192
magnesium, 192
main dishes (recipes), 260–270
    Asparagus, Leek, and White Bean
        Quiche, 267–269
    Beef Shawarma with Super Gut
        Tzatziki, 265–266
    Ginger Chicken, 261–262
    Italian Sausage Soup, 262–263
    Salmon with Avocado Lime Sauce,
        265
    Sicilian Pizza, 263–264

Spiralized Zucchini Pasta with
    Oregano Pesto, 260–261
Turmeric Flaxseed Wrap, 267
Yakisoba Noodles, 269–270
malaria, 135
Malassezia, 11
maltitol, 177
maltodextrin, 177
maltose, 177
management of SIBO and SIFO,
    109–131
    AIRE device, 112–116
    bacterial probiotics, 125–126
    berberine, 124
    choices, 110
    curcumin use, 169
    curcumin, 124
    decision-making, 111
    die-off management, 116–117
    essential oils, 124–125, 167
    FODMAPs, 115
    ground rules, 110–111
    herbal antibiotics, 116–119
    ignoring SIBO, 119–120
    manifestation of, 7
    power over health conditions,
        130–131
    probiotics, 120–121
    reducing fungal overgrowth,
        122–126
    Saccharomyces boulardii, 125
    SIBO recurrences, prevention of,
        126–130
    telltale signs, 66, 67, 111
    yogurt, 121–122
Massachusetts Institute of Technology
    (MIT), 25
Matcha, Mint, and Blueberry Frozen
    Smoothie, 247–248
Matcha Strawberry Key Lime
    Smoothie, 244–245
maternal microbiome, 13–20
    altered microbiome, 14
    antibiotics, 18
    bowel flora (child), 15

Cesarean sections, 13
commercialization of motherhood, 13
disrupted microbiomes, 16
herbicides and, 14, 15, 19
infant formula, 16–17
modern lifestyle habits and, 19
premature infants, 14
Matsés (Peru), 23
MCTs. *See* medium-chain triglycerides
medium-chain triglycerides (MCTs), 157
menu plan and shopping lists, 275–280
metabolic endotoxemia, 8
Methanobrevibacter smithii, 24, 82
microbes, lost. *See* lost microbes
microbiome (maternal), 13–20
altered microbiome, 14
antibiotics, 18
bowel flora (child), 15
Cesarean sections, 13
commercialization of motherhood, 13
disrupted microbiomes, 16
herbicides and, 14, 15, 19
infant formula, 16–17
modern lifestyle habits and, 19
premature infants, 14
MIT. *See* Massachusetts Institute of Technology
Mixed-Culture *Lactobacillus reuteri* Yogurt, 238–239
Mocha Mint Kefir, 248–249
monosaccharides, 71
Moroccan Roasted Vegetables, 251
morphine, 182
mucus gatekeepers, 213
mucus-building tea, 187–188
mucus lining (GI tract), 47–57
Akkermansia, 51, 52–53
antibiotics, 57
bacterial digestion, 48
colon, 49

dietary factors, mucus production and, 53
emulsifying agents, 55–56
eugenol, 53
fiber in diet, 49–51
green tea catechins, 54
importance of mucus, 47–48
motile bacteria, 54
mucus-disrupting factors, 56
prebiotic fiber, 48
production of mucus, 51
multiple sclerosis, 100, 120

NAC. *See* N-acetyl cysteine
N-acetyl cysteine (NAC), 87
naproxen, 56
necrotizing enterocolitis, 25
neurodegenerative disorders, 10, 120, 136
nonsteroidal anti-inflammatory drugs (NSAIDs), 18, 19, 56, 140, 178
NSAIDs. *See* nonsteroidal anti-inflammatory drugs

obesity, 10, 39, 40, 43, 56, 72, 73, 90, 119
obstipation, 182
OEA. *See* oleoylethanolamide
oleic acid, 41, 52, 162, 213
oleoylethanolamide (OEA), 162
oleuropeins, 212
oligosaccharides, 18, 71
olive oil, 42, 51, 52, 114, 161–162
Olsen, Gary, 81
omega-3 fatty acids, 41, 160, 162–163, 175, 188
omega-6-rich oils, 41
omeprazole, 69, 104
One-Minute Strawberry Ice Cream, 271
opioids, 70, 129, 182
Orange Clove Scones, 271–272
organic foods, 139, 178
Osfortis, 232
oxalate kidney stones, 24

Oxalobacter species, 24
oxycodone, 182
oxytocin, 26–28, 223, 232

pancreatic cancer, 30
pancreatic enzyme production, 129
panic attacks, 281
pantoprazole, 69
Parkinson's disease, 30, 73, 120, 284
past microbes, 21–33
    ancient microbiomes, 22
    Bifidobacterium infantis, 24–25
    DNA identification methods, 22
    Helicobacter pylori, 30–31
    hunter-gatherers, 23
    inner extinction event, 21
    Lactobacillus reuteri, 25–29
    Oxalobacter species, 24
    oxytocin, 26–28
    replacement of lost species, 24
    success story, 29
    vanished species, 23
PCBs. *See* polychlorinated biphenyls
Pediococcus, 147
pesticides, chlorpyrifos, 43
Pimentel, Mark, 7, 83
polychlorinated biphenyls (PCBs), 43
polyols, 71
polyphenols, 164–165, 211
polysorbate 80, 55, 56, 88, 177
prebiotic fibers, 48, 156, 158, 206. *See
    also* week 3 (program)
prebiotics, 148
    FOS, 187
    probiotics versus, 147–148
prediabetes, 56
Prevotella, 157
Prilosec (omeprazole), 104
proanthocyanidins, 165
probiotics, 120–121, 148
    bacterial, 125–126
    commercial, 141, 196, 197, 224
    creation, 197, 198–200
    intolerance to, 198

prebiotics versus, 147–148
second-generation, 283
third-generation, 284
program benefits, 219–225
    for athletes, 224
    deeper sleep, 220
    enhanced immunity, 224–225
    enhanced mental clarity, 221
    increased muscle and strength, 223
    for pregnant mothers, 224
    reduced inflammation, 221
    reduced stress, 221
    smoother skin, 220
    weight loss, 223
Protonix (pantoprazole), 140
Pseudomonas, 11, 23, 65, 68, 104, 170
psoriatic arthritis, 57
pureed fruits, sweet potatoes (recipe),
    243

quercetin, 212

Raspberry Cream Pie, 273–274
Raspberry Lime Yogurt Smoothie for
    Smoother Skin, 249–250
Reagan, Ronald, 21
recipes, 227–274
    beverages and smoothies, 244–250
    coconut milk, 241–242
    desserts, 270–274
    hummus, 243
    main dishes, 260–270
    pureed fruits, 243
    pureed sweet potatoes, 243
    salsa, 243
    small dishes, side dishes, and
        condiments, 250–259
    yogurt, 230–241
restless leg syndrome, 10, 74, 75
resveratrol, 212
rheumatoid arthritis, 284(fa)
rice syrup, 177
rifaximin, 85
rosacea, 19, 65, 281

Rosemary Turnips, 257
Roundup herbicide, 32
rutin, 212

Saccharomyces, 199
Saccharomyces boulardii, 105, 125, 141
Saccharomyces cerevisiae, 105, 125
Salmon with Avocado Lime Sauce,
    265
Salmonella, 15, 65, 67, 68, 75, 104, 148,
    156, 162, 170, 184, 196, 213
salsa (recipe), 243
sexually transmitted disease. *See*
    syphilis
Shigella, 23, 32
shopping lists, 277–280
Shortt, Aonghus, 78
SIBO. *See* small intestinal bacterial
    overgrowth
SIBO and SIFO, management of,
    109–131
  AIRE device, 112–116
  bacterial probiotics, 125–126
  berberine, 124
  choices, 110
  curcumin use, 169
  curcumin, 124
  decision-making, 111
  die-off management, 116–117
  essential oils, 124–125, 167
  FODMAPs, 115
  ground rules, 110–111
  herbal antibiotics, 116–119
  ignoring SIBO, 119–120
  manifestation of, 7
  power over health conditions,
      130–131
  probiotics, 120–121
  reducing fungal overgrowth, 122–126
  Saccharomyces boulardii, 125
  SIBO recurrences, prevention of,
      126–130
  telltale signs, 66, 67, 111
  yogurt, 121–122

Sicilian Pizza, 263–264
SIFO. *See* small intestinal fungal
    overgrowth
small bowel feces sign, 35
small dishes, side dishes, and
    condiments (recipes), 250–259
  Cream of Mushroom Soup, 255
  Curried Cauliflower with Peas, 254
  Dandelion Greens and Raw
      Potato Salad with Avocado Lime
      Dressing, 258
  Fermented Roasted Peppers,
      256–257
  Herbed Focaccia Bread, 252–253
  Hot Chili Fries, 253–254
  Moroccan Roasted Vegetables, 251
  Rosemary Turnips, 257
  Spicy Garlic Pickles, 259
  Super Gut Tzatziki, 250–251
small intestinal bacterial overgrowth
    (SIBO), 61–91. *See also* SIBO and
    SIFO, management of
  AIRE device, 78, 79
  antibiotic regimens used to manage,
      105
  biofilm disrupter, 87
  capsaicin and, 168
  conditions associated with, 72–74
  curcumin and, 103, 193
  description of, 64–65
  endotoxemia in, 67, 139
  epidemic of, 72
  FODMAPs, 71–72
  H. pylori and, 30, 31
  hydrogen production, 75–78
  hydrogen sulfide, 83–84
  identification of, 6, 97
  infestation of, 12
  iodine intake and, 189
  killing off microbes, 86
  lethal combinations, 80–81
  LPS levels and, 65
  manifestation of, 7
  as man-made condition, 64

small intestinal bacterial overgrowth
    (SIBO) [*continued*]
methanogenic, 81–83
modern phenomena, 64
monster of, 84–85
mucus production and, 57
peristalsis and, 182
population statistics on, 10
probiotics eradicating, 284
protection against recurrence of,
    232, 234
rebuilding of bowel health after
    reversing, 54
red flag conditions, 75
scourges, 63–64
SIFO and, 90–91
species most responsible for, 38,
    42, 45
telltale signs, 66, 67–70
therapeutic test for, 210
ubiquity of, 7, 96, 148
uncorrected, consequences of, 62
unhealthy species, 63
vitamin D deficiency and, 161
yogurt, 88–90 225, 240
small intestinal fungal overgrowth
    (SIFO), 6, 93–107. *See also* SIBO
    and SIFO, management of
bacterial probiotics, 105–106
berberine and, 103–104
brain and, 99–101
challenge, 95
curcumin and, 101–103
endotoxemia of, 139
essential oils, 104–105
eugenol and, 213
fungal overgrowth, identification
    of, 101
fungal proliferation, 94, 95
infections, 94
iodine intake and, 189
manifestation of, 97–98
occurrence of, 96–97
probiotics eradicating, 284

protection against recurrence of,
    232, 234
rebuilding of bowel health after
    reversing, 54
Saccharomyces boulardii, 105
SIBO and, 90–91
sugar and, 96, 98
ubiquity of fungi, 93
smallpox, 64
smoothies and beverages (recipes),
    244–250
Clove Green Tea, 246–247
Ginger Snap Smoothie, 245–246
Gingerbread Coffee, 249
Matcha, Mint, and Blueberry
    Frozen Smoothie, 247–248
Matcha Strawberry Key Lime
    Smoothie, 244–245
Mocha Mint Kefir, 248–249
Raspberry Lime Yogurt Smoothie
    for Smoother Skin, 249–250
Strawberry, Carrot, and Dandelion
    Greens Prebiotic Smoothie,
    244
sodium stearoyl lactylate, 177
Spicy Garlic Pickles, 259
Spiralized Zucchini Pasta with
    Oregano Pesto, 260–261
Staphylococcus, 104, 170
Staphylococcus aureus, 15, 85, 227
statin drugs, 5, 39, 64, 175, 178, 286
stomach cancer, 30
strain specificity, 88, 143–144
Strawberry, Carrot, and Dandelion
    Greens Prebiotic Smoothie,
    244
Streptococcus, 104, 121, 170
Streptococcus diacetylactis, 201
Streptococcus florentinus, 201
Streptococcus thermophilus, 228
Streptococcus thermophilus, 200
sucrose, 177
sugar, 71, 138, 191. *See also specific
    forms*

super fertilizers, 212–214
Super Gut program, 173–280
  menu plan and shopping lists,
    275–280
  recipes, 227–274
Super Gut program (week 1), 175–193
  blood sugar, 179–181
  bowel flora disruption, 176, 177
  curcumin, 192–193
  flours and meals (alternative),
    190–191
  gallstones, 183–184
  insulin resistance, 185
  iodine deficiency, 185
  iodine, 189–190
  magnesium, 192
  mucus-building tea, 187–188
  week 1 (program), nutrients,
    186–193
  omega-3 fatty acids, 188
  overview, 176
  single-ingredient foods, 178
  steps, 177–178
  success story, 188–189
  summary, 175–176
  sweeteners (alternative), 191
  weight loss, 184–186
  wheat and grains, 181–183, 185
Super Gut program (week 2),
    195–204
  fermented foods, 197
  kefir, 200–202
  overgrowth conditions, 198
  probiotic choice, 196
  probiotic creation, 197, 198–200
  summary, 195
  vegetable fermentation, 202–204
Super Gut program (week 3),
    205–214
  colorful compounds (vegetables and
    fruit), 211–212
  foods rich in prebiotic fibers,
    207–209
  mucus gatekeepers, 213

prebiotic fiber intake (goal), 206–207
  strategies, 205–206
  summary, 205
  super fertilizers, 212–214
  third-generation probiotics, 212
  variety, 212
Super Gut program (week 4),
    215–226
  beneficial microbes, 215
  benefits, 216, 219–225
  factors behind the magic,
    216–217
  fermentation, 216–217
  liberated bowel, 225–226
  psychobiotics, 221–223
  SIBO yogurt, 225
  success story, 218–219
  summary, 215
  yogurt, 217–218
Super Gut SIBO Yogurt, 240–241
Super Gut Tzatziki, 250–251
sweet potatoes, pureed (recipe), 243
sweetener alternatives, 177, 191
sweeteners (alternative), 191
syphilis, 63, 64, 86, 116

tetrahydrocannabinol (THC), 162
THC. See tetrahydrocannabinol
third-generation probiotics, 284
thyroid status, 189
TMAO. See trimethylamine oxide
triglycerides, 186
trimethylamine oxide (TMAO), 42
turbinado sugar, 177
Turmeric Flaxseed Wrap, 267

ulcerative colitis, 14, 36, 49, 54, 56, 63,
    71, 95, 120, 281
unsymbolized thinking, 165–166

vegetable fermentation, 202–204
vitamin D, 160–161, 186–187
vitamin supplements, reduced need
    for, 284

week 1 (program), 175–193
    blood sugar, 179–181
    bowel flora disruption, 176, 177
    curcumin, 192–193
    flours and meals (alternative),
        190–191
    gallstones, 183–184
    insulin resistance, 185
    iodine deficiency, 185
    iodine, 189–190
    magnesium, 192
    mucus-building tea, 187–188
    week 1 (program), nutrients,
        186–193
    omega-3 fatty acids, 188
    overview, 176
    single-ingredient foods, 178
    steps, 177–178
    success story, 188–189
    summary, 175–176
    sweeteners (alternative), 191
    weight loss, 184–186
    wheat and grains, 181–183, 185
week 2 (program), 195–204
    fermented foods, 197
    kefir, 200–202
    overgrowth conditions, 198
    probiotic choice, 196
    probiotic creation, 197, 198–200
    summary, 195
    vegetable fermentation, 202–204
week 3 (program), 205–214
    colorful compounds (vegetables and
        fruit), 211–212
    foods rich in prebiotic fibers,
        207–209
    mucus gatekeepers, 213
    prebiotic fiber intake (goal),
        206–207
    strategies, 205–206
    summary, 205

super fertilizers, 212–214
third-generation probiotics, 212
variety, 212
week 4 (program), 215–226
    beneficial microbes, 215
    benefits, 216, 219–225
    factors behind the magic, 216–217
    fermentation, 216–217
    liberated bowel, 225–226
    psychobiotics, 221–223
    SIBO yogurt, 225
    success story, 218–219
    summary, 215
    yogurt, 217–218
weight loss, 184–186, 223
Western diet, 56(fa)
WGA. See Wheat germ agglutinin
wheat, 178, 179, 181–183
Wheat germ agglutinin (WGA), 182
whey protein, 228
World Health Organization, 15, 45

Yakisoba Noodles, 269–270
Yakult, 235
Yanomami (Amazonian), 23, 136, 285
yogurt (recipes), 230–241
    Bacillus coagulans Yogurt, 233–234
    Bifidobacterium infantis Yogurt,
        236–237
    High-Potency Probiotic Yogurt,
        239
    Lactobacillus casei Shirota Yogurt,
        235
    Lactobacillus gasseri Yogurt, 234–235
    Lactobacillus helveticus and
        Bifidobacterium longum Yogurt,
        237
    Lactobacillus reuteri Yogurt, 232–233
    Mixed-Culture *Lactobacillus reuteri*
        Yogurt, 238–239
    Super Gut SIBO Yogurt, 240–241